Milady Illustrated Cosmetology Dictionary

By

Bobbi Ray Madry

MILADY PUBLISHING CORPORATION

3839 WHITE PLAINS ROAD BRONX, NEW YORK 10467

Author: Bobbi Ray Madry
Coordinator: Deborah J. Perry
Associate Editor: Mary Healy
Associate Editor: Miriam Helbok
Art Director: John P. Fornieri
Illustrator: Shiz Horii
Anatomy Tables: Diane Sarnataro

MILADY PUBLISHING CORP.

Bronx, N.Y.

Printed in the United States of America.

ISBN 087350-402-X

Table of Contents

PREFACE	v
KEY TO PRONUNCIATION	vii
PREFIXES	ix
SUFFIXES	x
THE MILADY ILLUSTRATED COSMETOLOGY DICTIONARY: A-Z	1

CHARTS AND TABLES

ANATOMY TABLE I:	THE SKELETAL SYSTEM ANTERIOR VIEW	264
ANATOMY TABLE II:	THE SKELETAL SYSTEM POSTERIOR VIEW	265
ANATOMY TABLE III:	CRANIUM, FACE AND NECK BONES	266
ANATOMY TABLE IV:	THE MUSCULAR SYSTEM—ANTERIOR VIEW	267
ANATOMY TABLE V:	THE MUSCULAR SYSTEM—POSTERIOR VIEW	268
ANATOMY TABLE VI:	MUSCLES OF THE HEAD, FACE AND NECK	269
ANATOMY TABLE VII:	THE NERVOUS SYSTEM	270
ANATOMY TABLE VIII:	NERVES OF THE HEAD, FACE AND NECK	271
ANATOMY TABLE IX:	NERVES OF THE ARM AND HAND	272
ANATOMY TABLE X:	MOTOR NERVE POINTS OF THE FACE AND NECK	273
ANATOMY TABLE XI:	THE CIRCULATORY SYSTEM	274
ANATOMY TABLE XII:	ARTERIES OF THE HEAD, FACE AND NECK	275
ANATOMY TABLE XIII:	VEINS OF THE HEAD, FACE AND NECK	276
ANATOMY CHART XIV:	BLOOD SUPPLY FOR THE ARM AND HAND	277
ANATOMY CHART XV:	ANATOMY OF THE HEART	278
ANATOMY TABLE XVI:	THE DIGESTIVE SYSTEM	279
ANATOMY TABLE XVII:	THE ENDOCRINE SYSTEM	280
ANATOMY TABLE XVIII:	THE RESPIRATORY SYSTEM	281
ANATOMY TABLE XIX:	THE LYMPHATIC SYSTEM	282
ANATOMY TABLE XX:	THE INTEGUMENTARY SYSTEM (SKIN) AND THE HAIR AND SCALP	283

TABLE OF ELEMENTS 284
THE pH SCALE 285
CHART OF DISINFECTANTS COMMONLY USED IN COSMETOLOGY 286
CHART OF ANTISEPTICS COMMONLY USED IN COSMETOLOGY 286
WEIGHTS AND MEASURES WITH METRIC EQUIVALENTS 287
METRIC CONVERSION FACTORS 288
EVERYDAY METRIC AID 289
VITAMIN AND MINERAL INFORMATION CHART 290

Preface

As new techniques and methods are developed in the cosmetology arts and sciences, new words are created that become a part of cosmetology terminology. Although many words used in relation to the practice of cosmetology and its related fields can be found in a standard or conventional dictionary, words with more than one meaning can be confusing. For this reason, the "Milady Illustrated Cosmetology Dictionary" is comprised of words and phrases which are used in connection with cosmetology and are defined in their sense of relationship to anatomy, cosmetic chemistry, electricity, dermatology, esthetics, hair structure and chemistry, nutrition, color, massage therapy and professional skills.

This dictionary has been prepared to keep abreast of the times in cosmetology language usage and to provide clear definitions as they relate to cosmetology and associated fields. It has been designed to provide cosmetologists with a practical reference that is comprehensive and professionally correct, yet not so technical that it fails to serve the needs of today's students, teachers, managers, salon owners and practitioners. It can also serve as an ideal instrument for classroom instruction for use in preparing for state licensing examinations.

For the convenience of teachers and students, many of the main ingredients used in cosmetic preparations have been listed in this dictionary.

The terminology used in cosmetology reflects the mind and spirit of an industry. When a profession or vocation is developing new techniques, its language will be expanding and moving forward. Every new thought and every new fact becomes fixed in words and language which reflect the spirit and progress of the industry itself. This dictionary is intended to capture that reflection of spirit and progress and make it available to the entire industry.

We wish to express our sincere appreciation to the many cosmetology educators who have contributed their much valued advice during the preparation of this dictionary. We wish to also thank Pivot Point International, Inc. for their courtesy in granting permission to include a number of widely used Pivot Point terms in the "Milady Illustrated Cosmetology Dictionary."

MILADY PUBLISHING CORPORATION

Key to Pronunciation

Dictionaries often differ in the use of diacritical marks (a mark added to a letter to indicate its pronunciation or to distinguish it from another letter). The editors of the "Milady Illustrated Cosmetology Dictionary" have selected the most widely used and easy-to-understand diacritical marks to indicate pronunciation and accents. The schwa (shwa) represented by the symbol (ə) for unstressed vowel sounds has been omitted. The pronunciation of a word is shown after the word: hairbrush (har′-brush). The hyphen symbol (-), marks syllable division. The symbol (′) accent mark, indicates the syllable given the strongest emphasis or accent; e.g., later, lā′-tẽr. A symbol (′) indicates that a syllable is given a softer pronunciation than one having no stress symbol; e.g., hairstylist, hâr′ stīl-ĭst; antibody, ăn′ tĭ-bŏd′ ē.

SYMBOL

A
ă at, am
ā fate, way
â senate, carbonate
â final, alcohol
ä arm, car
ă sofa, camera
â care, hair
au̇ now, proud
E
ĕ end, bent
ē heat, receive
ê event, degrade
ê recent, hen
ẽr ever, roller
I
ĭ ill, big
ī ice, find
O
ŏ odd, cot
ō bold, lobe
ô obey, biology
ô connect, bronchus
ô orb, bought
o͞o food, too
o͝o foot, cook
oi choice, ointment
ou̇ house, spout
oy boy, oil
yo͞o use, utensil
U
ŭ up, cut
ū use, duty
û unite, university
û us, circus
û urn, turn
ü shoe, blue

Full Pronunciation Key

A
b bee, robe
ch child, which
d do, did
E
f if, fifth
g big, go
h how, ahead
hw when, wheat
I
j enjoy, edge
k kind, cook
l lip, cool
m am, meet
n in, not
ng long, singing

O	**U**
p purpose, lamp	v vital, live
q (kw) quick, quarter	w we, wash
r rain, wrong	x x-ray
s see, yes (sh) she, tension	y yet, you
t too, it (th) then, the	z zero, please (zh) leisure, pleasure

Prefixes

A careful study of the following prefixes will enable you to grasp the meaning of many anatomical, medical and electrical terms or words.

Ad: to; toward; addition; intensification.
Anti: opposite; contrary.
Auto: self; acting upon one's self; of or by itself.
Bi: two; twice; double.
Cliedo: relation to the clavicle.
Contra: against; opposite; contrary.
De: from; down; away.
Di: two-fold; double; twice; separation or reversal.
Dia: through; apart; asunder between.
Dis: apart; away; asunder; between.
Ecto: without; outside; external.
Endo: inner; within.
Epi: upon; beside; over; among.
Ex: out of; from; away from.
Hydro: water; hydrogen.
Hyper: excessive; above normal; over; above; beyond.
Hypo: under; beneath; lower state of oxidation.
In: not; negation; within; inside.
Infra: below; lower.
Inter: between; among; amid.
Leuco: white; colorless.
Mal: ill; evil; bad.
Mega: great; extended; powerful; a million.
Meso: in the middle; intermediate.
Micro: very small; trivial; slight; millionth part of, as in the metric system.
Mid: the middle part.
Mono: uni; singly.
Non: not.
Onycho: relating to nail.
Para: alongside of; beyond; beside; against; near.
Per: through; throughout; by; for.
Peri: around; about; near.
Post: back; after.
Pyro: fire; prepared by fire.
Re: back to original or former state or position.
Sterno: denoting connection with the sternum (breast-bone).
Sub: under; below.
Super: over; above; beyond.
Supra: over; above; on top of; beyond; besides; more than.
Syn: along with; together; at the same time.
Trans: over; across; through; beyond.
Ultra: beyond on the other side; excessively; exceedingly; extraordinarily; abnormally.
Un: not; contrary.
Uni: one; once.

Suffixes

Many medical and anatomical words are of Latin origin. The following endings will enable you to tell at a glance whether they are singular, plural or possessive.

ENDINGS OF REGULAR LATIN NOUNS

Singular:	**Plural:**	**Possessive Singular:**
. . . **us** —Nasus	. . . **i** —Nasi	. . . **i** —Nasi
. . . **a** —Ala	. . . **ae**—Alae	. . . **ae**—Alae
. . . **um**—Labium	. . . **a** —Labia	. . . **i** —Labii

. . . **tis, sis:** a termination denoting inflammation of a part to the name of which it is attached; such as pityria**sis,** dermati**tis.**

. . . **al:** termination denoting belonging to, of, or pertaining to; such as nas**al.**

. . . **oma:** termination properly added to words derived from Greek roots, denoting a tumor; such as cyst**oma.**

. . . **ize:** termination forming transitive verbs; such as steril**ize.**

. . . **ive:** termination signifying relating or belonging to; such as act**ive.**

. . . **ide:** termination forming names of compounds, such as bacteric**ide,** germic**ide.**

Contents

1 A-B

33 C-D

77 E-F

103 G-H

125 I-J

137 K-L

149 M-N

167 O-P

193 Q-R

205 S-T

243 U-V

253 W-X

263 Y-Z

A

abampere (ăb-ăm′pēr): the cgs electromagnetic unit of electric current equivalent to 10 amperes.

abbreviate (ă-brē′vē-āt): to make shorter; to reduce; make briefer.

abdomen (ăb′dă-měn): the belly; the cavity in the body between the thorax and the pelvis.

abducent (ăb-dū′sênt): drawing away from, as muscles draw away.

abducent nerve (ăb-dū′sênt nûrv): the sixth cranial nerve; a small motor nerve supplying the external rectus muscle of the eye.

abductor (ăb-dŭk′tēr): a muscle that draws a part away from the median line (opp., adductor).

ability (ă-bĭl′ĭ-tē): the quality or state of being able to perform.

abiogenesis (ab-ē-ō-jěn′ē-sĭs): the generating or springing up of living from nonliving matter; spontaneous generation.

abiosis (ăb-ē-ō′sĭs): absence of life.

abirritant (ăb-ĭr′ě-tănt): a soothing agent that relieves irritation.

abnormal (âb-nôr′mâl): irregular; contrary to the natural law or customary order.

abnormality (ăb-nôr-măl′ě-tē): the state or condition of being abnormal or unusual.

abohm (ăb-ōm′): the cgs electromagnetic unit of resistance equal to one millionth of an ohm.

aboral (ă-bōr′âl): located or situated opposite to or away from the mouth.

abrade (ă-brād′): to remove or roughen by friction or rubbing.

abrasion (ă-brā′zhûn): scraping of the skin; rubbing or wearing off the surface; an irritation; a scraped or scratched area of the skin.

abrasive (ă-brā′sĭv): a substance used for smoothing, as in dermabrasion, the sanding or brushing of the skin.

abreast (ă-brěst): in line with; side by side with; up to the mark.

abruption (ă-brŭp′shûn): a sudden breaking off.

abscess (ă′sěs): a collection or pocket of pus in any part of the body, characterized by dead tissue and inflammation.

absolute (ăb-sŭ-lūt′): pure, as a liquid; perfect, beyond a doubt.

absorb (ăb-sôrb′): to take in and make part of an existing whole; to suck up or take up; as a towel absorbs water.

absorbefacient (ăb-sôr-bă-fā′shěnt): substance causing or promoting absorption.

absorbent (ăb-sôr′běnt): able to absorb.

absorption (ăb-sôrp′shûn): assimilation of one body by another; act of absorbing.

abstract design (ăb′străkt dĭ-zīn′): cosmetology; a hairstyle with broken lines, planned to give a casual, relaxed effect; informal hairstyle.

absurd (ăb-sûrd′): inconsistent with reason.

abundance (ă-bûn′dăns): ample, plentiful quantity.

abuse (ă-by-ōōz′): to misuse; to use improperly.

academic (ăk-ă-děm′ĭk): pertaining to an academy, school, college or university; scholarly.

acanthosis (ă-căn-thō′sĭs): altered skin

metabolism that can produce thickening of the stratum corneum.

acariasis (ăk-ă-rī′ŭh-sĭs): any condition, usually dermatitis, caused by an acarid (tick or mite).

acarid (ăk′ă-rĭd): any of an order of arachnids, including mites and ticks.

accelerate (ăk-sĕl-ă-rāt): increase speed; hasten action.

acceleration (ăk-sĕl-ă-rā-shûn): an increase in speed; the process of moving or developing faster.

accelerator (ăk-sĕl′ĕr-rāt-ĕr): any agent which hastens or quickens action.

accent (ăk′sĕnt): to give special force or emphasis; to highlight or give added color tone.

accentuate (ăk-sĕn′chōō-āt): to emphasize; to heighten effect; in makeup, to emphasize the features of the face.

accessory (ăk-sĕs′ô-rē): a person or item which aids subordinately or assists; something added.

accessory nerve (ăk-sĕs′ô-rē nûrv): spinal accessory nerve; eleventh cranial nerve; affects the sterno-cleido-mastoid and trapezius muscles of the neck.

accidental (ăk-sĭ-dĕn′tâl): happening by chance; not planned.

acclimate (ă-klī′măt): to adapt or become adapted to environment, climate or situation.

accord (ă-kôrd′): to bring into agreement or harmony.

accreditation (ă-krĕd-ă-tā′shûn): the granting of approval and status to an institution by an accrediting body after its credentials are approved.

accretion (ă-krē′shûn): growth or increase by external additions; something added; pathology: an accumulation of foreign matter in a body cavity.

acellular (ā-sĕl′ū-lâr): containing no cells, as a noncellular substance.

acentric (ā-sĕn′trīk): off center; not centered; not arising centrally, as from a nerve center.

acetic (ă-set′ĭk): pertaining to vinegar; sour.

acetic acid (ă-sēt′ĭk ăs′ĭd): a colorless, pungent, liquid acid that is the chief acid of vinegar.

acetone (ăs′ĕ-tōn): a colorless, inflammable liquid, miscible with water, alcohol, and ether, and having a sweetish odor and burning taste; used as a solvent.

acetyl (ă-sēt′′l): pertaining to that which is derived from acetic acid and found in compounds.

acetylated (ă-sēt′′l-āt′ĕd): any organic compound that has been heated with acetic anhydride or acetyl chloride to remove water.

acetylated lanolin (ă-sēt′′l-āt′ĕd lăn′′l-ĭn): lanolin treated to be water resistant; used in cosmetics to reduce water loss from the skin; an emollient.

acetylcholine (ăs-ē-tĭl-kō′lēn): the acetic acid ester of choline, a constituent of many body tissues; used in treatment of some diseases and for lowering of blood pressure.

ache (āk): a dull, distressing and often persistent pain.

Achilles heel (ă-kĭl′ēz hēl): calcaneal tendon; a tender or vulnerable spot associated with the Achilles tendon, which joins the muscles of the calf of the leg to the bone of the heel; named for the Greek hero, Achilles.

achromasia (ă-krō-mā′zhŭh): a condition such as albanism or vitiligo where there is loss of normal color or lack of melanin in the skin.

acid (ăs′ĭd): having a sour taste; a substance containing hydrogen replaceable by metals to form salts and capable of dissociating in aqueous solution to form hydrogen ions; having a pH number below 7.0.

acid balanced (ăs′ĭd băl′ânst): describes a product whose pH level is stabilized; commonly used to refer to products such as shampoos and conditioners that are balanced to the pH of skin and hair which is 4.5–5.5.

acidic (ă-sĭd′ĭk): containing a high percentage of acid; having properties of an acid.

acidify (ă-sĭd′ĕ-fī): to change into an acid; to lower the degree of alkalinity.

acid mantle (ăs′ĭd măn′t'l): the natural acidity of the skin or hair which helps to retard irritation or bacterial growth.

acidosis (ăs-ĭ-dō′sĭs): a condition in which there is an excess of acid products in the blood or excreted in the urine.

acid peel (ăs′ĭd pēl): a skin peeling treatment or process using a diluted acidic substance.

acid rinse (ăs′ĭd rĭns): a solution or emulsion that has acidic properties; commonly used to close the cuticle of the hair after shampooing or chemical services.

acidulate (ă-sĭj′o͞o-lāt): to make acid or sour.

acidum boricum (ăs′ĭ-dûm bôr′ĭ-kŭm): boric acid; a white crystalline compound used as a preservative and as an antiseptic.

acid wave (ăs′ĭd wāv): permanent wave with lotion that has a pH of 7.0 or below and requiring heat or other form of activator to speed processing.

acne (ăk′nē): a skin disorder characterized by inflammation of the sebaceous glands from retained secretions.

acne albida (ăk′nē ăl′bī-dă): milium; whitehead.

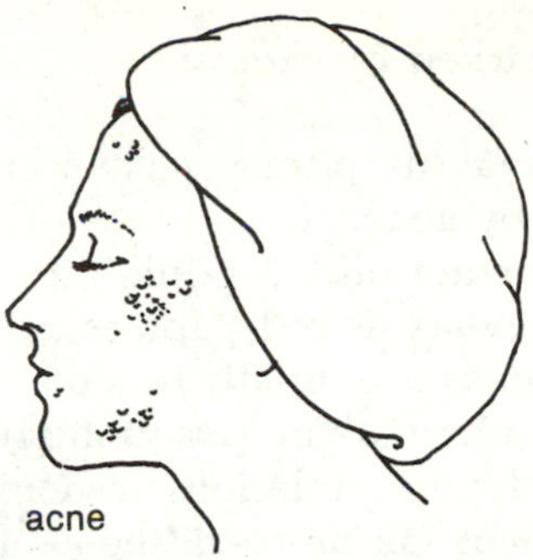

acne

acne artificialis (ăk′nē är-tĭ-fĭsh-ē-ăl′ĭs): pimples due to external irritants.

acne atrophica (ăk′nē ă-trŏf′ĭ-kă): acne in which the lesions leave a slight amount of scarring.

acne cachecticorum (ăk′nē kă-kĕk-tĭ-kōr′ûm): pimples which sometimes occur when anemia or some debilitating constitutional disease is present.

acne conglobata (ăk′nē kŏn-glō-bā′tŭh): a severe and stubborn form of acne that usually affects the back, buttocks, the face and sometimes the thighs; often causes scarring.

acne cream (ăk′nē krēm): a facial cream, containing medicinal substances or agents, used in the treatment of acne.

acne cystica (ăk′nē sĭs′tĭ-kŭh): a form of acne with lesions that are primarily cysts.

acne hypertrophica (ăk′nē hī-pĕr-trŏf′ĭ-kă): pimples in which the lesions on healing leave conspicuous pits and scars.

acne indurata (ăk′nē ĭn-dū-rä′tă): deeply seated pimples with hard tubercular lesions or papules occurring chiefly on the back.

acne keratosa (ăk′nē kĕr-aă-tō′să): an eruption of papules consisting of horny plugs projecting from the hair follicles, accompanied by inflammation.

acne miliaris (ăk′nē mĭl-ē-âr′rĭs): a condition marked by excessive whiteheads (milia).

acne pits (ăk′nē pĭts): pit-like scars produced by acne.

acne punctata (ăk′nē pŭnk-tä′tă): acne that appears as red papules in which blackheads are usually found.

acne pustulosa (ăk′nē pŭs-tû-lō′să): acne in which pustular lesions predominate.

acne rosacea (ăk′nē rō-zā′shē-ă): a form of acne usually occurring around the nose and cheeks, in which the capillaries become dilated and sometimes broken.

acne simplex (ăk′nē sĭm′plĕks): acne vulgaris; simple uncomplicated pimples.

acne vulgaris (ăk′nē vŭl-găr′ĭs): acne simplex; simple uncomplicated pimples.

acoustic (ă-kōōs′tĭk): pertaining to the science of sound or the sense or organs of hearing.

acoustic nerve (ă-kōō′tĭk nûrv): eighth cranial nerve, controlling the sense of hearing.

acquire (ă-kwīr′): to receive; to attain; to master.

acrolein (ă-krō′lê-ĭn): a light, volatile, oily liquid that gives off an irritating vapor.

acromion process (ă-krō′mē-ŏn prŏs′ĕs): the outward extension of the spine of the scapula, forming the point of the shoulder.

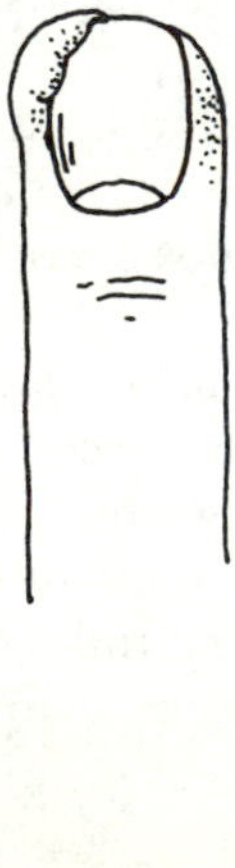

acronyx (ăk′rō-nĭks): an ingrowing nail.

acrylic acid (ă-krĭl′ĭk ăs′ĭd): unsaturated aliphatic acids used in the making of plastics, which are used in the manufacture of items useful to cosmetology. (combs, brushes, capes, etc.).

actinic (ăk-tĭn′ĭk): relating to the chemically active rays of the spectrum.

actinic carcinoma (ăk-tĭn′ĭk kär-sĭn-ō′mă): a basal cell carcinoma of the face or body due to prolonged exposure to the sun.

actinic dermatosis (ăk-tĭn′ĭk dûr-mă-tō′sĭs): an inflammatory condition of the skin caused by strong sunlight; it may be uticarial, papular or eczematous.

actinic ray (ăk-tĭn′ĭk rā): an invisible ray which produces chemical action; a ray of light beyond the violet spectrum that is capable of bringing about chemical changes.

actinodermatitis (ăk′tĭn-ō-dûr-mă tī′tĭs): dermatitis caused by overexposure to sunlight, actinic rays or X rays.

actinomycosis (ăk′tĭ-nō-mī-kō′sĭs): a chronic, infectious disease that affects animals and people, caused by bacteria and characterized by the forming of lesions and tumors around the jaws.

actinotherapy (ăk′tĭn-nō-thĕr′â-pē): the treatment of disease by use of sunlight, X rays and ultraviolet rays.

activate (ăk′tĭ-vāt): to make active; to start the action of hair coloring products.

activator (ăk′tĭ-vā-tẽr): a chemical agent employed to start the action of chemical products on hair.

activator machine (ăk′tĭ-vā-tẽr mă-shēn′): a device employed in facial therapy which helps to cleanse, stimulate and firm the skin.

active immunity (ăk′tĭv ĭ-myōō′nĭ-tē): acquired immunity.
activity (ăk-tĭv′ĭ-tē): natural or normal function or operation; physical motion or exercise of force.
aculeate (ă-kyōō′lē-ăt): causing a sting as from a pin prick.
acuminate (ă-kyōō′mă-nāt): to sharpen to a point or taper.
acupuncture (ăk′yōō-pŭnk-chĕr): puncturing the skin with needles at specific points for therapeutic purposes.
acute (ă-kūt′): coming to a crisis quickly, as opposed to chronic: said of a disease having a rapid onset, severe symptoms and short course.
ad (ăd): a prefix denoting to, toward; addition, intensification.
adapt (ă-dăpt′): to make suitable; to alter so as to fit a new use.
adaptable (ă-dăpt′ă-b'l): capable of or given to adapting one's self to new conditions and uses.
additive (ăd′ĭ-tĭv): a substance which is to be added to another product.
adductor (ă-dŭk′tĕr): a muscle that draws a part toward the median line of the body or toward the axis of an extremity.
adenitis (ăd-ĕ-nī′tĭs): inflammation of the lymph nodes.
adenoid (ăd′ĕ-noyd): an enlarged lymphoid growth located behind the pharynx.
adenology (ăd ê-nŏl′ē-jē): the branch of anatomy concerned with glands.
adenoma (ă-dĕn-ō′mă): a tumor of glandular origin.
adenoma sebaceum (ă-dĕn-ō-mă sĕ-bā′sē-ûm): a small tumor of translucent appearance, originating in the sebaceous glands.
adermogenesis (ā-dŭr-mō-jen′ĕ-sĭs): imperfect development or healing of the skin.
adhere (ăd-hēr′): to remain in contact; to unite.
adhesive (ăd-hē′sĭv): a sticky substance used for holding something fast.
adhesive patch (ăd-hē′sĭv păch): a small area of the underside of a man's hairpiece which is covered with oiled silk.
adiaphoretic (ā-dī-ă-fō-rĕt′ĭk): any agent, drug or cosmetic preparation that reduces, checks or prevents perspiration.
adipic acid (ā-dĭp′ĭk ăs′ĭd): hexanedioic acid; an agent derived from beets; used in hair coloring products for its buffering and neutralizing qualities.
adipose (ăd′ĭ-pōs): relating to fat.
adipose tissue (ăd′ĭ-pōs tĭsh′ū): areolar connective tissue containing fat cells: subcutaneous tissue.
adjacent (ă-jā′sĕnt): lying near or adjoining.
adjust (ă-jŭst′): to make exact; to fit; to bring into proper relationship.
adjustable block holder (ă-jŭst′ă-b'l blŏk hōld′ĕr): a metal bracket, which can be screwed to a work bench, used to hold the wooden or malleable head block in position while working on a hairpiece or mannequin head.

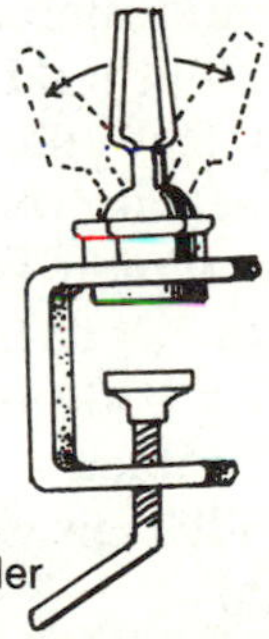

adjustable block holder

adjustable wig (ă-jŭst′ă-b'l wĭg): a wig designed for ready-to-wear use, constructed with an elastic insert at the back to make it easily adjustable for various head sizes.

admix (ăd-mĭks′): to mix with something else.

adnata alopecia (ăd-nā′tă ăl-ô-pē′shē-ă): baldness at birth.

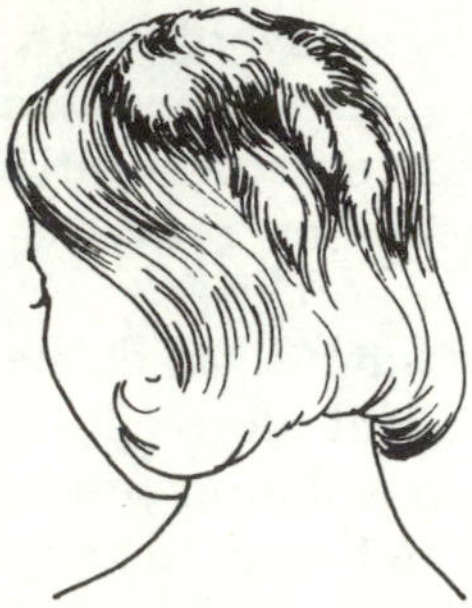

adnata alopecia

adolescence (ăd-ô-lĕs′êns): state or process of growing from childhood to adulthood: the period of time encompassing that process.

adorn (ă-dôrn′): to decorate a person or object.

adrenal (ăd-rē′nâl): an endocrine gland situated on top of the kidneys.

adrenaline (ă-drĕn′â-lĕn): a hormone secreted by the adrenal glands; it stimulates the nervous system, raises metabolism, increases cardiac pressure and output and increases blood pressure.

adroit (ă-drôyt′): skillful, dexterous; having physical and mental capabilities.

adsorption (ăd-sôrp′shûn): the adhesion of an extremely thin layer of one substance (a gas or liquid) to the surface of a solid body or liquid with which it is in contact.

adult (ă-dŭlt′): grown to full age, size or strength.

adulterate (ă-dŭl′tĕr-āt): to falsify; to alter; to make impure by the addition of other substances.

advanced (ăd-vănst′): progressive; ahead of the times; beyond the elementary or introductory.

advisable (ăd-vīz′ă-b'l): proper to be done or practiced; expedient.

adynamia (ăd-ĭ-nā′mē-ă): loss of physical strength; weakness.

aerate (âr′āt): to supply or charge with air or gas; to oxygenate.

aeration (ăr-ā′shûn): exposure to air; saturating a fluid with air or gas; conversion of venous to arterial blood.

aerification (âr-ĭ-fĭ-kā′shûn): the process of converting into gas, air or vapor.

aerobe (âr′ōb): a microorganism that can live only in the presence of oxygen.

aerobic (âr-ō′bĭk): living or occurring only in the presence of oxygen: a term applied to modern dance exercises.

aerosol (âr′ă-sōl): colloidal suspension of liquid or solid particles in a gas; container filled with liquefied gas and dissolved or suspended in ingredients which can be dispersed as a spray; used for cosmetic and food preparations.

aerotherapeutics (âr-ō-thêr-ă-pyōō′tĭks): a system by which disease is treated by varying the pressure or the composition of the air breathed.

aesthetician (esthetician) (ĕs-thĕ-tĭsh′ên): a specialist in esthetics; one who works in a profession dedicated to the cleansing and maintenance of the health and beauty of the skin.

aesthetics (esthetics) (ĕs-thĕt′ĭks): a branch of philosophy pertaining to or dealing with the forms and nature of beauty and judgments concerning beauty; the branch of cosmetology dealing with skin care.

afferent (ăf′ĕr-ênt): bearing or carrying toward the center; inward.

afferent nerves (ăf′ĕr-ĕnt nûrvz): nerves that convey stimuli from the external organs to the brain.

affinity (ă-fĭn′ĭ-tē): attraction; in chemistry: the characteristic which impels certain atoms to unite with certain others to form compounds.

affix (ă-fĭks′): to attach, fix or fasten.

affixative (ă-fĭks′ă-tĭv): a product, hair spray or setting lotion used in holding the finished style in place.

Afro-comb (ăf′rō-kōm): a comb designed especially for thick curly hair; hair lifter.

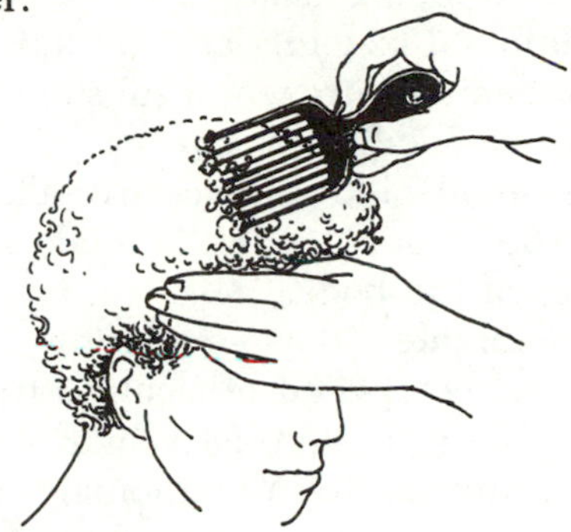

Afro lifter or comb

Afro-lifter (ăf′rō-lĭft′ĕr): a fork-like comb for styling and lifting curly hair.

Afro-pick (ăf′rō-pĭk): a styling tool with long fork-like prongs used to pick the hair into place.

Afro-styling (ăf′rō-stīl′ĭng): styling and shaping excessively curly or kinky hair in accordance with its natural tendencies and the facial features of the client.

after-image (ăf′tĕr-ĭm′ĭj): an image or sensation that stays or comes back after the external stimulus has been withdrawn; e.g., as seeing spots after looking at the sun.

after rinse (ăf′tĕr rĭns): a prepared cosmetic product used to rinse hair following a hair treatment, to accomplish some special purpose; a color, cream or finishing rinse.

agenesis (ā-jĕn′ĕ-sĭs): the imperfect development of any part of the body.

agent (ā′jênt): an active power which can produce a physical, chemical or medicinal effect.

aggravate (ăg′ră-vāt): to make worse; intensify, as an illness or skin condition.

aging skin (ā′jĭng skĭn): skin that has lost its elasticity and has developed lines or wrinkles.

agitate (ăj′ă-tāt): to stir up; shake; disturb.

agonist (ăg′ŭ-nĭst): a contracting muscle that executes movements of a part and is opposed by an antagonistic muscle.

air purifier (âr pyōōr′ă-fī-ĕr): an apparatus which removes impure substances from the air.

air waving (âr wāv′ĭng): a technique of rolling the hair over the fingers while air drying the hair; drying, combing and styling of the hair with a hand hair dryer.

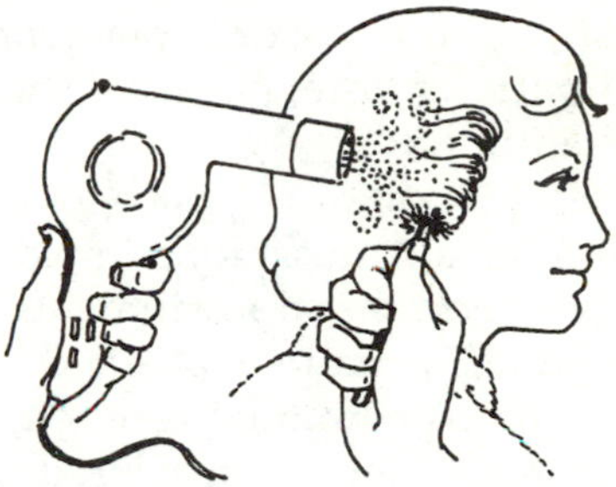

air waving

al (âl): a word termination denoting belonging to, of, or pertaining to.

ala (ā′lă); pl., **alae** (ā′lē): a wing-like structure, as the wing of the nose.

alae nasi (ā′lē nā′zī): the wing cartilage of the nose.

albida, acne (ăl′bĭ-dă ăk′nē): whitehead; milium.

albinism (ăl′bĭ-nĭz′m): congenital leucoderma or absence of pigment in the skin and its appendages; it may be partial or complete.

albino (ăl-bī′nō): an individual affected with albinism; having little or no coloring pigment in the skin, hair or iris of the eyes.

albumen (ăl-byōō′mĕn): the white of an egg; the nutritive protein substance in germinating animal or plant cells; sometimes used in facial masks for its tightening effect.

albumin (ăl-byōō′mĭn): any of a class of proteins naturally occurring, soluble in water, coagulated by heat and found in eggs, milk, muscle tissue, blood and in many vegetable tissues.

albuminous (ăl-byōō′mĭ-nûs): relating to albumen.

albumose (ăl-byōō′mōs): a substance formed from protein during digestion; chemical compounds derived from albumins by the action of certain enzymes.

alcohol (ăl′kô-hôl): a readily evaporating, colorless liquid with a pungent odor and burning taste; powerful stimulant and antiseptic.

alcohol 70% (ăl′kô-hôl): alcohol used as a disinfectant to sanitize implements, surfaces and metal instruments.

algae (ăl′jē): primitive plants found in fresh or salt water (seaweed, kelp, stoneworts, etc.); considered a nutrient.

algin (ăl′jin): the dried gelatinous form of various seaweeds, especially kelp, used as an emulsifier, thickening and ripening agent.

align (ă-līn): to bring into place or line.

aliment (ăl′ĭ-mênt): nourishment; food or anything which feeds or adds to a substance in natural growth.

alimentary (ăl-ĭ-mĕn′tă-rē): relating to food or nutrition; the canal which extends from the mouth to the anus.

alkali (ăl′kă-lī): a class of compounds which react with acids to form salts, turn red litmus blue, saponify fats and form soluble carbonates; having a pH number above 7.0.

alkalimeter (ăl-kă-lĭm′ă-tẽr): an apparatus for measuring the amount of alkali in a mixture or solution and quantity of carbon dioxide in solids.

alkaline (ăl′kă-līn): having the qualities of or pertaining to, an alkali.

alkalinity (ăl′kă-lĭn′ĭ-tē): the quality or state of being alkaline.

alkaloid (ăl′kă-loid): any organic base containing nitrogen; a substance containing alkaline properties.

alkalosis (ăl′kă-lō′sĭs): excessive alkalinity of the blood, other body fluids and tissues of the body.

alkanolamine (ăl-kăn-ô-lă′mīn): a substance comprised of alcohols from alkene (a saturated, fatty hydrocarbon) and amines (from ammonia); used in cosmetic creams as a solvent.

alkylation (ăl-kă-lā′shûn): the introduction of an alkyl group into an organic compound.

allantoin (ăl-ăn′tō-ŭn): a uric acid derivative originally found in foetal allantoic fluid and in some roots, bark and grain; used in healing and cleansing preparations.

allergic (ăl-ẽr′jĭk): pertaining to having an allergy, aversion or disagreeable sensitivity.

allergy (ăl′ẽr-jē): a disorder due to extreme sensitivity to certain foods, chemicals or other substances.

allergy test (ăl′ẽr-jē tĕst): a test to determine the existence or nonexistence of extreme sensitivity to certain substances, foods or chemicals which do not adversely affect most individuals; a test used before applying hair color or facial cosmetics; a test done on a small section of skin or scalp.

almond (ä′mûnd, äl′mûnd): the kernal

or seed of the fruit of the almond tree; used in facial and other cosmetic preparations.

almond meal (äl′mûnd mēl): pulverized, blanched almonds; a powder used in the manufacture of cosmetics and some fragrances.

almond oil (äl′mûnd oyl): emolient; natural vegetable oil pressed from almonds and having penetrating and softening powers; used in some cosmetic preparations.

aloe (ăl′ō): any member of a genus of plants of the lily family; used in some cosmetic preparations and as a cathartic.

aloe vera (ăl′ō vē′ră): a juice extracted from the South African aloe plant leaf; contains water, amino acids and carbohydrates; used in some cosmetic and medicinal preparations.

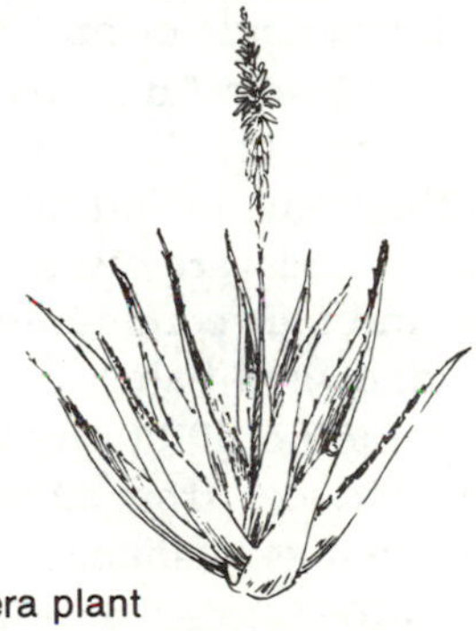

aloe vera plant

alopecia (ăl-ô-pē′shē-ă): deficiency of hair; baldness.

alopecia adnata (ăl-ô-pē′shē-a ăd-nă′tă): baldness at birth.

alopecia areata (ăl-ô-pē′shē-ă ā-rê-ă′tă): baldness in spots or patches.

alopecia cicatrisata (ăl-ô-pē′shē-ă sĭ-kă-trĭ-sä′tă): baldness in uneven patches caused by atrophy of the skin.

alopecia dynamica (ăl-ô-pē′shē-ă dī-năm′ĭ-kă): loss of hair due to destruction of the hair follicle by ulceration or some disease process.

alopecia follicularis (ăl-ô-pē′shē-ă fŏl-ĭk-ū-lăr′ĭs): loss of hair due to inflamed hair follicles.

alopecia localis (ăl-ô-pē′shē-ă lō-kā′lĭs): loss of hair occurring in patches on the course of a nerve at the site of an injury.

alopecia maligna (ăl-ô-pē′shē-ă mă-lĭg′nă): a term applied to the form of alopecia that is severe and persistent.

alopecia prematura (ăl-ô-pē′shē-ă prē-mă-tū′ră): baldness beginning before middle age.

alopecia seborrheica (ăl-ô-pē′shē-ă sĕb-ôr-ē′ĭ-kă): baldness caused by diseased sebaceous glands.

alopecia senilis (ăl-ô-pē′shē-ă sĕ-nĭl′ĭs): baldness occurring in old age.

alopecia syphilitica (ăl-ô-pē′shē-ă sĭf-ĭl-ĭt′ĭ-kă): loss of hair resulting from syphilis, occurring in the second stage of the disease.

alopecia traction (ăl-ô-pē′shē-ă trăk′-shûn): hair loss caused by holding the hair tight and under tension for long periods of time.

alopecia universalis (ăl-ô-pē′shē-ă ūn-ĭ-vĕr-să′lĭs): a condition manifested by general falling out of the hair of the body.

alpha (ăl′fă): beginning or first of anything; alpha and omega, the first and last or beginning and the end.

alpha helix (ăl′fă hē′lĭks): term indicating the spiral of the polypeptide chains within the hair cortex in the first or unstretched position.

alphosis (ăl-fō′sĭs): pertaining to lack of skin pigmentation, as in albinism.

alternate (ôl′tĕr-năt): to do by turns; being one of two or more choices.

alternating (ôl′tĕr-nāt-ĭng): occurring in reciprocal succession.

alternating current, A.C. (ôl′tĕr-nāt-ĭng kŭr′ênt): a current which rises and falls in strength of flow, alternating in opposite directions at regular intervals.

alternating rod (ôl′tĕr-nāt′ĭng rŏd): a permanent waving technique recommended for fine or weak hair; this method alternates rods having two different circumferences.

alternator (ôl′tĕr-nāt′ĕr): a generator giving an alternating current of electricity.

alum, alumen (ăl′ŭm ă-lū′mên): an aluminum salt; sulphate of potassium and aluminum; an astringent; used as a styptic and in mouthwashes, shave lotions, etc.

aluminum (ă-lū′mĭ-nŭm): silver-white metal with low specific gravity, noted for its lightness and resistance to oxidation; often used in the manufacture of combs, rollers, etc.

aluminum acetate solution (ă-lū′mĭ-nŭm ăs′ê-tāt sō-lū′shûn): a solution diluted with water and used as an antiseptic and astringent.

aluminum chloride (ă-lū′mĭ-nŭm klôr′-īd): a crystalline powder, soluble in water; used as an astringent, antiseptic or deodorant.

aluminum sulfate (ă-lū′mĭ-nŭm sŭl′fāt): cake alum; used in antiseptics, astringents and in some deodorant preparations.

alveola (ăl-vē′ô-lă); pl., **alveolae** (-lē): a small hollow alveolae border; the portion of the jaws bearing the teeth; branch of the internal maxillary artery.

alveolar ducts (ăl-vē′ô-lär dŭkts): air passages in the lungs branching from the respiratory bronchioles leading to the alveolar sacs.

alveolar nerve (ăl-vē′ô-lär nûrv): a nerve servicing the teeth.

alveolar process (ăl-vē′ô-lär prŏ′sĕs): the ridge of bone in the maxilla and in the mandible, containing the alveolar of the teeth.

alymphia (ā-lĭm′fē-ŭh): absence or deficiency of lymph.

amber (ăm′bĕr): a fossil resin of pine trees found in northern Europe; it becomes negatively electrified in friction: the oil is sometimes used as a stimulant.

amber color (ăm′bĕr kŭl′ĕr): a yellow-brown color resembling amber.

ambergris (ăm′bĕr-grĭs): an opaque, grayish secretion from the sperm whale; used in perfumery.

ambidextrous (ăm-bĭ-dĕk′strĕs): able to use both hands equally well.

amines (ă′mēnz): compounds that are the basic ingredients of proteins.

amino acid (ă-mē′nō ăs′ĭd): the chemical building blocks of all proteins that make up the body, including skin and hair; amino acids are used in some shampoos and hair conditioners to recondition damaged hair.

amino dye (ă-mē′nō dī): a synthetic, organic tint produced from a coal tar derivative known as analine.

amitosis (ăm-ĭ-tō′sĭs): cell multiplication by direct division of the nucleus in the cell.

ammonia (ă-mō′nē-ă): a colorless gas with a pungent odor; very soluble in water.

ammonium bisulfide (ă-mō′nē-ŭm bī-sŭl′fīd): a chemical used in cosmetology products, such as hair relaxers in permanent waving.

ammonium hydroxide (ă-mō′nē-ŭm hī-drŏks′īd): an alkaline base formed from ammonia and water; used in products such as hair tints and cleansing solutions.

ammonium persulfate (ă-mō′nē-ŭm pĕr-sŭl′fāt): ammonium salt; soluble in water; used as an oxidizer and bleach in some hair and skin cosmetics; an ingredient used in some disinfectants and deodorants.

ammonium stearate (ă-mō′nē-ŭm stĕr′-āt): stearic acid; ammonium salt; powder used as a texturizer in some cosmetic creams such as vanishing creams.

ammonium sulfide (ă-mō′nē-ŭm sŭl′fīd): a combination of ammonia and sulfur.

ammonium sulfite (ă-mōn′nē-ŭm sŭl′fīt): a combination of ammonia and salt of sulfuric acid.

ammonium thiocyanate (ă-mō′nē-ŭm thī-ō-sī′ă nāt): a combination of ammonia and thiocyanic acid.

ammonium thioglycolate (ă-mō′nē-ŭm thī-ō-glī′kō-lāt): a combination of ammonia and thioglycolic acid; reducing agent used primarily in permanent waving and hair relaxing solutions and creams.

amotile (ā-mō′tĭl): incapable of movement, as a muscle; opposite of motile, to move.

amp (ămp): amperage; the strength of an electric current.

ampere (ăm′pēr): the unit of measurement of strength of an electric current.

amphetamine (ăm-fĕt′ă-mēn): an acrid, colorless liquid compound used as an inhalant or stimulant for relief of colds.

amphoteric (ăm-fĕ-tĕr′ĭk): having the characteristics of both an acid and an alkali; a substance used in cleaning agents.

ampule (ăm′pūl): a small glass container used for one application of a product; a glass attachment used for vacuuming.

amyl acetate (ăm′ĭl ăs′ê-tāt): banana oil; a colorless, aromatic and inflammable liquid employed as a solvent in making nail polishes.

amyl alcohol (ăm′ĭl ăl′kô-hŏl): a colorless, strong smelling alcohol, obtained by the fermentation of starchy substances; found naturally in oranges; used as a solvent in nail polish.

amylase (ăm′ĭl-āz): an enzyme that helps to change starch into sugar; found in pancreatic secretions; used as a texturizer in cosmetics; also used in some medications to reduce inflammation.

amylopectin (ăm′il-ō-pĕk′tĭn): amioca; a substance derived from starch, almost insoluble; used as a texturizer in cosmetics.

anabolism (ăn-ăb′ō-lĭz′m): constructive metabolism; the process of assimilation of nutritive matter and its conversion into living substance.

anagen phase (ăn′ă-jĕn fāz): the phase during which new hair is synthesized; the early productive phase of the hair cycle in a follicle.

analgesic (ăn′âl-jē′zĭk): a drug for the alleviation of pain.

analine derivative tint (ăn′ĭ-lĭn dê-rĭv′ă-tĭv tĭnt): a synthetic, organic hair tint produced from a coal tar product (see: amino dye).

analogous (ăn-ăl′ă-găs): similar or comparable in certain respects.

analysis (ă-năl′ĭ-sĭs): the process by which the nature of a substance is recognized and its chemical or physical composition determined.

analysis, hair (ă-năl′ĭ-sĭs hâr): examination to determine the condition of the hair prior to a hair treatment.

analyze (ăn′ă-līz): to make an analysis.

anaphoresis (ăn-ă-fôr-ē′sĭs): the process of forcing liquids into the tissues from the negative toward the positive pole.

anaplastic (ăn-ŭ-plăs′tĭk): pertaining to the restoration of lost or absent parts, as in reconstructive surgery.

anaplasty (ăn′ŭ-plăs-tē): an operation for the restoration of lost parts; plastic surgery.

anaplerosis (ăn-ă-plê-rō′sĭs): plastic surgery; replacement of defective parts of the body, caused by injury or disease.

anatomy (â-năt′ô-mē): the study of the gross structure of the body which can be seen with the naked eye; the science of the structure of organisms, or of their parts.

androgen (ăn′drō-gĕn): any of various hormones that control the development of masculine characteristics.

androsterone (ăn-drŏs′tĕr-ōn): a male sex hormone.

anemia, anaemia (ă-nē′mē-ă): a condition in which the blood is deficient in red corpuscles or in hemoglobin, or both.

anesthesia, anaesthesia (ăn-ēs-thē′sē-ă): a state of insensibility, local or general, with or without loss of consciousness.

anesthetic, anaesthetic (ăn-ĕs-thĕt′ĭk): substance producing anesthesia.

anesthetize (ă-nĕs′thê-tīz): to render insensible by use of an anesthetic; to make unable to feel sensation, such as pain, cold, or extreme heat.

anethole (ăn′ĕ-thōl): a colorless crystalline compound from anise and fennel oils, used in perfumery.

angelica (ăn-jĕl′ĭ-kă): an herb of the parsley family used in fragrances, mouth wash, toothpastes and medicinal preparations.

angiectid (ăn-jē-ĕc′tĭd): abnormal dilation of the blood vessels causing tension and tenderness in the skin.

angiodermatitis (ăn′jē-ō-dûr-mă-tī′tĭs): inflammation of the blood vessels of the skin.

angiology (ăn-jē-ŏl′ô-jē): the science of the blood vessels and lymphatic system.

angioma (ăn-jē-ō′mă): a tumor formed of blood vessels or lymphatic vessels.

angiorhexis (ăn-jē-ō-rĕk′sĭs): rupture of a blood vessel.

angle (ān′g'l): the space between two lines or surfaces that intersect at a given point; in haircutting, the hair is held away from the head to create elevation; degree of elevation used to determine base relationship in setting the hair.

angora (ăng-gôr′ă): long, silky hair from the angora goat; used in some mannequin heads for its superior white, glossy finish.

angstrom (ăng′strôm): a unit of measurement for the wave length of light.

angular artery (ăng′û-lär är′tĭr-ē): the terminal part of the facial artery which supplies the lacrimal sac and the eye muscles.

angular chelitis (ăng′û-lär kī′lī-tĭs): an acute or chronic inflammation of the skin around the corners of the mouth.

anhidrosis (ăn-hī-drō′sĭs): partial or complete lack of perspiration.

anhydration (ăn-hī-drā′shûn): dehydration; removal of water; lacking moisture.

anhydrous (ăn-hī′drŏs): without water; not hydrated.

anidrosis (ăn-ĭ-drō′sĭs): a deficiency in producing perspiration.

aniline (ăn′ĭ-lĭn, an′ĭ-lēn): a colorless liquid with a faint characteristic odor, obtained from coal tar and other nitrogenous substances; combined with other substances, it forms the aniline colors or dyes derived from coal tar.

aniline dye (ăn′ĭ-lĭn dī): any dye produced synthetically from coal tar; used in the manufacture of hair coloring products and fragrances.

animal-human hair (ăn′ĭ-mâl hū′mân hâr): a blend of animal and human hair which is used in the manufacture of wigs.

anion (ăn′ī-ôn): the ion which carries a charge of negative electricity; the element which, during electrolysis of a chemical compound, appears at the positive pole or anode.

anise (ăn′ĭs): the fragrant seed of the anise plant, used in medicine, cookery and in some cosmetic preparations.

ankle (ăng′kĕl): the joint connecting the foot and the leg.

ankle bone (ăng′kĕl bōn): the talus; the proximal bone of the foot.

annular (ăn′û-lăr): ring-like.

annular finger (ăn′û-lăr fĭn′gĕr): the ring finger or third finger of the left hand.

anode (ăn′ōd): the positive terminal of an electric source.

anodermous (ăn-ō-dûr′mûs): lacking skin.

anomalous (ă-nŏm′ă-lûs): abnormal; unusual; irregular.

anoxia (ăn-ŏk′sē-ă): condition of inefficient oxygen supply to body tissues.

antacid (ănt-ăs′ĭd): a substance that relieves or neutralizes acidity.

antagonist (ăn-tăg′ă-nĭst): in anatomy, a muscle that acts counter to another muscle.

antalkali (ănt-ăl′kă-lī): any substance able to neutralize alkalis.

anterior (ăn-tĭr′ē-ĕr): situated before or in front of; the ventral side of the body.

anterior auricular artery (ăn-tĭr′ē-eĕr ô-rĭk′yo͞o-lär är′tĭr-ē): artery which supplies blood to the anterior part of the ear.

anterior auricular muscle (ăn-tĭr′e-ĕr ô-rĭk′yo͞o-lär mŭs′′l): the muscle in front of the ear.

anterior auricular nerve (ăn-tĭr′ē-ĕr ô-rĭk′yo͞o-lär nûrv): nerve found in the skin anterior to the external ear.

anterior cardiac vein (ăn-tĭr′ē-ĕr kär′dē-ăk vān): vein located anterior (in front of) the right ventricle; vein affecting the heart.

anterior facial veins (ăn-tĭr′ē-ĕr fā′shăl vānz): veins located on the anterior sides of the face; draws into the internal jugular vein located on the sides of the neck.

anterior interosseous artery (ăn-tĭr′ē-ĕr ĭn′tĕr-ŏs′ē-ês är′tĭr-ē): supplies blood to the anterior part of the forearm.

anterior jugular vein (ăn-tĭr′ē-ĕr jŭg′ū-lär vān): vein located near the midline of the neck that drains into the external jugular or subclavian veins.

anthrax (ăn′thrăks): a disease found in man and some animals; has characteristic carbuncle-like lesions.

anti (ăn′tī): prefix meaning against or opposed to.

antibacterial (ăn′tī-băk-tē′rē-âl): destructive to or preventing the growth of bacteria.

antibiotic (ăn′tĭ-bī-ŏ′tĭk): a drug, such as penicillin, made from substances derived from mold or bacterium which inhibits the growth of bacteria.

antibody (ăn′tĭ-bŏd-ē): a substance in the blood which builds resistance to disease.

anticatalyst (ăn′tĭ-kăt′ă-lĭst): a substance that stops or inhibits a chemical reaction.

anticathode (ăn′tĭ-kăth′ōd): the electrode in an electron or X-ray tube that receives and reflects rays emitted from a cathode.

antidote (ăn′tĭ′dōt): an agent preventing or counteracting the action of poison.

antifungal (ăn′tĭ-fŭn′gâl): pertaining to a substance that stops or inhibits the growth of fungi.

antigen (ăn′tĭ-jĕn): any of several substances such as toxins, enzymes, or foreign proteins, that stimulates the development of antibodies.

antioxidant (ăn′tĭ-ŏk′sĭ-dănt): preservative that prevents fats from spoiling; that which prevents oxidation.

antiperspirant (ăn′tĭ-pĕr′spĭ-rênt): a strong astringent liquid or cream used to stop the flow of perspiration in the region of the armpits, hands or feet.

antiphlogistic (ăn′tē-flō-jĭs′tĭk): reducing or preventing fever or inflammation.

antisepsis (ăn′tĭ-sĕp′sĭs): a method by which a substance, item or organism is kept sterile, by preventing the growth of pathogenic bacteria.

antiseptic (ăn′tĭ-sĕp′tĭk): a chemical agent that prevents the growth of bacteria.

antisepticize (ăn′tĭ-sĕp′tĭ-sīz): to make antiseptic by treating with antiseptic preparations.

antitoxin (ăn′tĭ-tŏk′sĭn): a substance in serum which binds and neutralizes toxin (poison).

antixerotic (ăn′tē-ză-rŏt′ĭk): preventing dryness of the skin.

anus (ā′nûs): the lower opening of the digestive tract, through which fecal matter is extruded.

aorta (ā-ôr′tă): the main arterial trunk leaving the heart and carrying blood to the various arteries throughout the body.

apex (ā′pĕks): the summit or extremity; the upper end of a lung or the heart; the high part of the arch of the eyebrow.

apocrine glands (ăp′ō-krĭn glănz): sweat glands that produce a characteristic odor; found in the underarms and pubic areas of the body.

aponeurosis (ăp-ô-nū-rō′sĭs): a broad, flat tendon that serves to connect muscle to the part that it moves.

apparatus (ăp′ă-rā′tûs): a collection of instruments or devices adapted for a specific purpose.

appendage (ă-pĕn′dêg): an outgrowth attached to an organ or part of the body and dependent upon it for growth; a limb or limb-like structure.

appendix (ă-pĕn′dĭks): the vermiform appendix, a small appendage of the intestine.

apple blossom (ăp′′l blŏs′ŏm): essence of flowers from the apple tree; used in fragrances.

appliance (ă-plī′ăns): a device or implement used for a certain purpose.

applicator (ăp′lĭ-kā-tẽr): an instrument or item used to apply products; as brushes, combs, spatulas, containers, etc.

apposition (ăp-ô-zĭsh′ŭn): the act of fitting together or being fitted together.

apprentice (ă-prĕn′tĭs): one who learns a trade by working and studying under the direction of others who are already skilled in that trade.

appropriate (ă-prō′prē-ât): suitable; fitting.

approximately (ă-prŏk′sĭ-mât-lē): about; nearly.

apricot (ā′prĭ-kŏt): a yellow, juicy fruit similar to a peach whose kernel produces an oil used in some cosmetic preparations; a pinkish-orange color.

aptitude (ăp′tĭ-to͞od): natural or acquired ability that makes one suited to pursue a specific activity or career.

aptitude test (ăp′tĭ-to͞od tĕst): a test designed to determine the ability of an individual to engage in certain activities or to pursue specific career goals.

aqueous (ā′kwē-ûs): watery; pertaining to water.

arc (ärk): part of the circumference of a circle; an incomplete circle; in hairstyling, the first half of a shaping is referred to as base direction and the last half of the shaping is called the arc.

arch (ärch): a curved or arch-like part of the body such as the arch of the foot; dental arch.

area (â′rê-ă): an open space; a limited extent of surface.

areata, alopecia (ā-rê-ă′tă ăl-ô-pē′shē-ă): baldness appearing in spots or patches.

areola (ă-rē′ô-lă): any small ring-like discoloration; the pigmented ring surrounding the nipple of the breast.

areolar tissue (ă-rē′ô-lăr tĭsh′ū): loose connective tissue with many interspaces.

arm (ärm): the part of the human anatomy from the shoulder joint to the wrist.

arnica (är′nĭ-kă): an aromic plant containing astringent and healing qualities; used in cosmetic and medicinal preparations.

aroma (ă-rō′mă): a distinctive flavor, fragrance or odor.

aromatherapy (ă-rō′mă-thĕr′ă-pē): the use of aromatic fragrances to induce relaxation; used in the practice of esthetics; facial and body treatments using aromatic oils.

aromatic (ăr-ô-măt′ĭk): pertaining to or containing aroma; fragrant.

aromatic bitters (ăr-ô-măt′ĭk bĭt′ẽrz): obtained from bitter herbs such as ginger and cinnamon; used in the manufacture of fragrances.

arrectores pilorum (ă-rĕk-tŏ′rēz pī-lôr′-ûm): the minute involuntary muscle fiber in the skin attached to the base of the hair follicles.

arrector pili (ă-rĕk′tôr pī′lī): (plural of arrectores pilorum) involuntary muscle fibers in the skin attached to the base of the hair follicles.

arrowroot (âr′ō-ro͞ot): named for its use in healing wounds caused by arrows; the root of a starchy plant; used in the manufacture of dusting powders and hair coloring products.

arsenical compound (är-sĕn′ĭ-kôl kŏm′-pound):a compound used in some hair products and skin medications; it can have a highly caustic action on the skin.

art (ärt): skill; dexterity facility in performing any operation, intellectual or physical, acquired by experience or study, as the art of hairdressing or hairstyling.

arterial (är-tĭr′ē-âl): pertaining to an artery.

arteriole (är-tĭr′ē-ôl): a minute artery; a terminal artery continuous with the capillary network.

arteriosclerosis (är-tĭr′ē-ô-sklê-rō′sĭs): an abnormal condition of the arteries marked by loss of elasticity; hardening and thickening of the arterial walls.

artery (är′tĭr-ē): a vessel that conveys blood from the heart to other parts of the body.

arthritic (är-thrĭt′ĭk): pertaining to or affected with arthritis; inflammation of a joint.

articular (är-tĭk′û-lär): pertaining to the junction of two or more skeletal parts, or to the muscle or ligament associated with a joint.

articulate (är-tĭk′ū-lāt): divided into individual points; made up of distinctive parts.

articulation (är-tĭk-û-lā′shûn): in anatomy, the junction of two or more skeletal parts.

artificial (är-tĭ-fĭsh′âl): not natural; imitation.

artificial eyelashes (är-tĭ-fĭsh′âl ī′lăsh-ĕz): eyelashes made from synthetic or human hair to be glued to or in place of one's own lashes.

artificial hair (är-tĭ-fĭsh′âl hâr): manufactured hair-like fiber made of dynel, nylon, etc., which is employed in the construction of lower-priced wigs and hairpieces.

artificialis, acne (är-tĭ-fĭsh-ē-âl′ĭs ăk′nē): a papular eruption caused by external irritants such as tar.

artificial nails (är-tĭ-fĭsh′âl nālz): plastic nails formed and hardened on the fingers, or pre-manufactured and then glued to the natural nails.

artist (är′tĭst): one who is skilled in fine arts; in cosmetology, one skilled in the artistry of hairstyling and/or makeup application.

ascertain (ăs-ĕr-tān′): to acquire an accurate knowledge of.

ascorbic acid (ăs-skôr′bĭk ă′sĭd): chemical component of vitamin C; scurvy preventing vitamin found in fruits and vegetables.

asepsis (ā-sĕp′sĭs): a condition in which pathogenic bacteria are absent.

aseptic (ā-sĕp′tĭk): free from pathogenic bacteria.

ash (ăsh): a drab shade containing no red or gold tones; green or blue-based.

ash blond (ăsh blŏnd): whitish-grey light hair color with no red or gold tones.

Asiatic hair (ā-zhĭ-ăt′ĭk hâr): human hair from eastern nations; dark, straight, coarse hair generally used in inexpensive wigs and hairpieces.

asperation (ăs′pĕr-ā′shûn): a mechanical method used to remove dead surface cells from the skin.

asphyxia (ăs-fĭk′sē-ă): a lack of oxygen or excess of carbon dioxide in the body causing unconsciousness.

asphyxic skin (ăs-fĭk′ĭk skĭn): skin lacking oxygen.

aspirator (ăs′pĭ-ra-tĕr): an appliance for drawing fluids from the body by suction.

assimilate (ă-sĭm′ĭ-lāt): to absorb; to incorporate into the body; to digest.

assimilation (ă-sĭm-ĭ-lā′shûn): the incorporation of materials prepared by digestion of food, into the tissues of the body.

asteatosis (ăs-tē-ă-tō′sĭs): dry and scaly skin due to a deficiency or absence of the sebaceous secretion, called sebum.

asthma (ăz′mă): a condition characterized by coughing and difficulty in breathing.

astrictive (ă-strĭk′tĭv): astringent; styptic.

astringent (ă-strĭn′jĕnt): a substance in cosmetics and medicines that causes contraction of the tissues and checks secretions.

asymmetric (ā-sĭ-mĕt′rĭk): lacking symmetrical balance; off center.

asymmetrical (ā-sĭ-mĕt′rĭ-kâl): off center; unbalanced; unequal in proportion; a

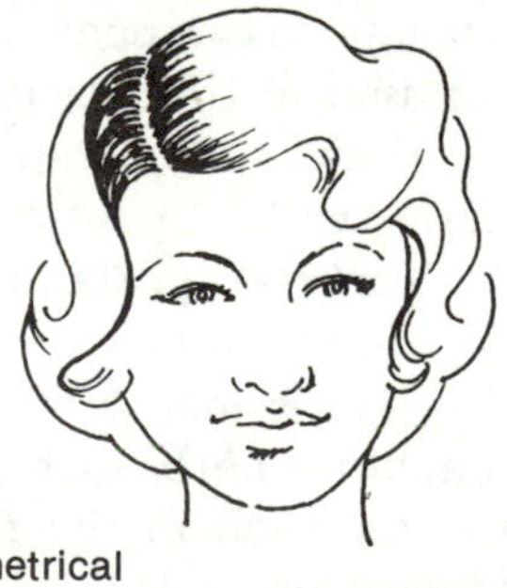

asymmetrical

hairstyle that has unequal proportions designed to balance facial features.

ataxia (ă-tăk′sē-ă): a term used in physical therapy pertaining to irregularity in bodily functions or muscular movements; inability to coordinate voluntary movements.

athlete's foot (ăth′lēts fo͞ot): a fungal foot infection; medical name, epidermophytosis.

atlas (ăt′lăs): in anatomy, the first cervical vertebra in the spinal column.

atmosphere (ăt′mûs-fēr): the whole mass of air surrounding the earth; the effect produced by decor, furnishings or the environment.

atom (ăt′ûm): the smallest quantity of an element that can exist and still retain the chemical properties of the element.

atomize (ăt′ă-mīz): to reduce to minute particles or to a fine spray.

atomizer (ăt′ă-mīz-ēr): a container used to spray a fine liquid mist of perfume, hairspray or other product.

atrichia (ă-trĭk′ē-ă): absence of hair; congenital or acquired.

atrium (ā′trē-ûm): the auricle or upper chamber of the heart.

atrophy (ăt′rô-fē): a wasting away of the tissues of the body or of a part of the body from lack of nutrition or because of injury or disease.

attachment (ă-tăch′mĕnt): the physical connection by which one thing is fastened to another.

attenuate (ă-tĕn′û-āt): to make thin; to increase the fluidity or thinness of the blood or other secretions; to lessen the effect of an agent.

attolens aurem (ăt′ô-lĕnz ô′rêm): auricularis superior; muscle that elevates the ear slightly.

attrahens (ăt′ră-hĕnz): a muscle that draws or pulls forward.

attrahens aurem (ăt′ră-hĕnz ô′rĕm): a muscle which pulls the ear forward.

attune (ă-tūn′): to bring into harmony with.

auburn (ô′bûrn): a reddish brown color.

auditory nerve (ô′dĭ-tō-rė nûrv): eighth cranial nerve, controlling the sense of hearing.

aurantiosis cutis (ô-răn-tī′ă-sĭs kū′tĭs): a condition of the skin that renders it a golden yellow; sometimes caused by excessive intake of carotene.

auricle (ô′rĭ-k'l): the external ear; one of the upper cavities of the heart.

auricular (ô-rĭk′û-lâr): pertaining to the ear or cardiac auricle.

auricular anterior artery (ô-rĭk′û-lâr ăn-tĭr′ē-ēr är′tĭr-ē): artery that supplies blood to the anterior part of the ear.

auricularis, anterior (ô-rĭk-û-lâr′ĭs ăn-tĭr′ē-ēr): the anterior auricularis; the muscle that draws the ear forward.

auricularis, posterior (ô-rĭk-û-lâr′ĭs pŏs-tĭr′ē-ēr): the muscle that draws the ear backward.

auricularis superior (ô-rĭk-û-lâr′ĭs sū-pĭr′ē-ēr): muscle that draws the ear upward.

auricular nerve (ô-rĭk′û-lâr nûrv): nerve that receives stimuli from the skin around the ear.

auricular posterior artery (ô-rĭk′û-lâr pŏs-tĭr′ē-ēr är′tĭr-ē): posterior artery that supplies blood to the scalp and paratid gland.

auriculotemporal nerve (ô-rĭk′û-lō-tĕm′-pôr-âl nûrv): sensory nerve affecting the temple and external ear; distrib-d in the skin of the scalp and at the temples.

auto (ô′tô): denoting self; acting upon one's self, or by itself.

autoclave (ô′tō-klāv): a vessel or chamber producing steam for the sterilization of instruments.

auto condensation (ô′tō kŏn-dĕn-sā′-shûn): a method of applying high frequency current for therapeutic purposes by making the patient part of the condenser.

autolysis (ô-tŏl′lĭ-sĭs): the disintegration of cells and tissues by the action of enzymes already present; self digestion of tissues within a living body.

automatic (ô-tō-măt′ĭk): acting from forces within; self-acting; largely or entirely involuntary.

autonomic; autonomous (ô-tŭ-nŏm′ĭk; ô-tŏn′ă-mûs): independent in origin, action or function; self governing.

autonomic nervous system (ô-tŭ-nŏm′ĭk nûrv′ûs sĭs′tĕm): the part of the nervous system that controls the involuntary muscles.

avitaminosis (ā-vī′tă-mĭn-ō′sĭs): a disease that results from lack of vitamins in the diet, such as scurvy (vitamin C) or rickets (vitamin D).

avocado (ă-vă-kä′dō): a pear-shaped, green pulpy fruit whose oils are used in some cosmetics and in facial masks to cleanse and moisturize the skin.

axilla (ăk-sĭl′ă): armpit; the region between the arm and the thoracic wall bounded by the pectoralis major muscle and the latissimus dorsi muscle.

axillary (ăk′sĭ-lĕr′ē): pertaining to the axilla or armpit.

axillary artery (ăk′sĭ-lĕr′ē är′tĭr-ē): artery associated with the region of the muscles of the upper arm, chest, shoulder and the skin of the pectoral region.

axillary glands (ăk′sĭ-lĕr′ē glăndz): the axillary lymph nodes.

axillary nerves (ăk′sĭ-lĕr′ē nûrvz): nerves located in the shoulder and armpit regions which stimulate deltoid muscles.

axillary veins (ăk′sĭ-lĕr′-ē vānz): veins located within the regions of the armpits.

axiom (ăk′sē-ŭm): an established principle or rule.

axis (ăk′sĭs): the line around which a body turns or rotates, or around which parts are arranged.

axon (ăk′sŏn): a long nerve fiber extending from the nerve cell body.

azo dye (ā′zō dī): a group of synthetic dyes derivable from azobenzene; used in some hair coloring products.

azuline (azk′ū-lēn): an intensely blue liquid hydrocarbon found in the oil of chamomile flowers; used as a coloring agent and in some shampoos.

azure (āzh′ĕr): pertaining to the color of a clear, blue sky; sky blue.

B

babassu (bä′bä-so͞o′): the oil from nuts produced by the Brazilian palm tree; widely used in making soap and similar products.

baby fine hair (bā′bē fīn hâr): a hair fiber that is extremely fine due to its very small cortex diameter and delicate construction.

baby oil (bā′bē oyl): a product made of mild, soothing oils such as lanolin, vegetable or mineral oils.

bacillus (bă-sĭl′ûs); pl., **bacilli** (-ī): rod-shaped bacterium.

back (băk): the rear or posterior part of the body or head; the part of the body nearest the spine.

backbone (băk′bōn): the spinal or vertebral column.

back brushing (băk brŭsh′ĭng): a method used in styling hair; while holding the ends of hair strands up and outward, the strands are brushed back toward the scalp to create a look of softness and bulk in some hair designs.

back combing (băk kōm′ĭng): combing small sections of hair from the ends toward the scalp, causing shorter hair to mat at the scalp, forming a cushion or base; also called teasing.

back design (băk dĭ-zīn′): design of the hairstyle at the back of the head.

backhand (băk-hănd): a movement made with the back of the hand turned in the direction of the movement; used in barbering techniques.

back of head (băk ŏf hĕad): the area of the head behind the ears.

backsweep (băk′swēp): sweeping the hair backward with comb or brush; also upsweep: hair is swept upward into the desired style.

backward curls (băk′wûrd kûrlz): curls wound in a counterclockwise direction on the left side of the head; curls wound in a clockwise direction on the right side of the head; curls whose stems are directed toward the back of the head.

backward direction (băk′wûrd dī-rĕk′-shûn): movement used when brushing, combing, winding or wrapping the hair away from the face.

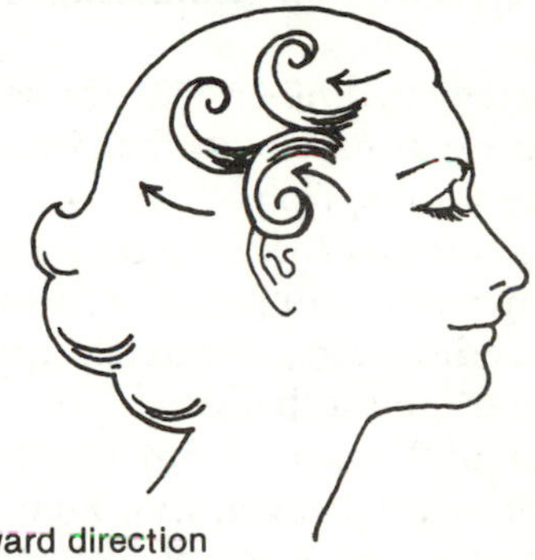

backward direction

bacteria (băk-tĭr′ē-ă); pl., **bacterium:** widely distributed unicellular microorganisms with both plant and animal characteristics; the three varieties are bacillus, coccus, and spirillum; some harmful; some are harmless; commonly known as microbes or germs.

bacterial (băk-tĕr′ē-âl): pertaining to bacteria.

bactericide (băk-tĭr′ă-sīd): an agent that destroys bacteria.

bacteriology (băk-tĭr-ē-ŏl′ô-jē): the science which deals with bacteria.

bacterium (băk-tĭr′ē-ûm); pl., **bacteria:** unicellular vegetable microorganism.

bakelite shield (bāk′līt shēld): a shield made of a substance that strongly resists chemicals; used as a scalp protector.

balance (băl′âns): harmony or proportion created in a hairstyle by the proper degree of height and width.

baldness (bôld′nês): a deficiency of hair; hair loss.

balm (bäm): an aromatic resinous substance used as a medicine or fragrance.

bal masque makeup (bâl măsk māk′ŭp): a fantasy makeup applied with exaggerated colors and designs; makeup based on a fantasy theme as an added attraction at hairdressing and cosmetology shows, or in makeup competitions.

balneology (bâl′nē-ŏl′ô-jē): the science of treating disease by baths in the waters of mineral springs.

balneotherapy (bâl′nē-ō-thĕr′ă-pē): the science of treating disease, burns, emotional disorders, or skin diseases by use of therapeutic baths.

balsam of Peru (bâl′săm of pĕ-ro͞o′): a thick, dark brown, oily fluid exuded from the cut bark of Tolurfera pereirae; used as an antiseptic and astringent.

banana oil (bă-nă′nă oyl): oil from the fruit of the banana (isoamye acetole) used in cosmetics and medicinal preparations.

band (bănd): a narrow strip of hair that is discolored; a narrow strip of material placed around the hairline when giving facials or applying makeup; elastic fastener on permanent wave rod.

bandeau hairpiece (băn-dō hâr′pēs): hairpiece sewn to a headband covering the hairline; band wig.

band wig (bănd wĭg): bandeau-style hairpiece.

bang (băng): front hair cut so as to fall over the forehead; often used in the plural, as to "wear bangs."

bang frame (băng frām): the shaping of bangs so as to frame the face.

banker's pin (băng′kẽrz pĭn): also called a "T" pin. It resembles the letter "T" and is used to secure a hairpiece to the styling block.

barba (bär′bă): the growth of beard hair of either men or women.

barber (bär′bẽr): one whose occupation includes haircutting, hairdressing, shaving and trimming beards and related services.

barber chair (bär′bẽr châr): a specially designed chair for barber clients; a hydraulic, reclining chair with adjustable footrest and headrest.

barber comb (bär′bẽr kōm): a comb of plastic or hard rubber with a ¾-inch-wide set of teeth tapering to a narrow end about ¼-inch wide with a set of fine teeth; an implement for combing and styling the hair.

barber science (bär′bẽr sī′êns): the study of the beard and hair and their treatment.

barber shop (bär′bẽr shŏp): the place of business where the barber's clients receive services.

barber's itch (bär′bẽrz ĭch): tinea sycosis; ringworm of the beard; chronic inflammation of the hair follicles.

barbiturate (bär-bĭch′ă-răt): a sedative or sleeping pill; a drug which can interfere with healthy body metabolism when taken in excess.

barium sulfide (bă′rê-ûm sŭl′fīd): a yellowish powder which decomposes in water with liberation of hydrogen sulfide gas; used in dipilatory preparations.

barrel (băr′ăl): the part of a thermal heating iron or curling iron that contains the heating element.

barrel curl (băr′ăl kûrl): a curl, wound in croquignole fashion, with large center opening and fastened to the head in a standing position; a pin curl technique used in place of rollers.

barrette (bä-rĕt′): a small bar with a clasp used to pin the hair in place.

basal (bās′âl): foundation; located at the base which is the lowest or supporting part of anything; lowest or least.

basal layer (bās′âl lā′ẽr): the layer of cells at the base of the epidermis closest to the dermis.

base (bās): a cosmetic preparation applied to the face to form a foundation upon which to apply other cosmetics such as powder and cheek color; in wiggery, the foundation upon which the hair is attached in order to form a wig; in hairstyling, the portion of a curl that is attached to the scalp; in chemistry, the chief substance of a compound; an electropositive element that unites with an acid to form a salt.

base coat (bās kōt): a clear liquid similar to nail enamel which is applied to fingernails before the application of colored polish; also used as a protective top coat.

base cream (bās crēm): an oily cream used to protect the scalp during a hair straightening process.

base direction (bās dī-rĕk′shûn): a line of motion from the starting point or foundation created in setting the hair.

base of a curl (bās of a kûrl): that portion of the hair strand nearest the scalp which is being curled.

base part (bās pärt): the working part of the hair toward which the curl is rolled.

base, protective (bās prô-tĕk′tĭv): in hairdressing: a petroleum base applied to the entire scalp in order to protect it from the active agents contained in the chemical hair relaxer.

base substance (bās sŭb′stăns): a supporting or carrying ingredient in a preparation which serves as a vehicle for active ingredients in some medicinal and cosmetic preparations.

basic (bās′ĭk): pertaining to the fundamental or foundation knowledge and skills of any craft, skill or profession.

basify (bā′sĭ-fī): to change into a base by chemical means; to make alkaline.

basil (bās′ĭl): any of certain aromatic plants of the mint family; used in cookery and in some cosmetics.

basilar plexis vein (bās′ĭ-lär plĕk′sĭs vān): vein located at the base part of the occipital bone.

basilic vein (bă-sĭl′ĭk vān): the large vein on the inside of the arm.

basin (bas′ĭn): a shallow vessel with sloping sides used to hold liquids, as a shampoo bowl or a small vessel for manicures or pedicures.

bath (bäth): to wash or dip in water or other liquid.

bath lotion (bäth lō′shûn): a fragrant emollient applied after the bath.

bath oil (bäth oyl): emulsifying oil; a fragrant oil, usually vegetable or mineral oil used after the bath or in the bath water to soften and soothe the skin.

bath powder (bäth paŭ′dẽr): dusting powder, usually of scented talcum powder to which boric, starch and zinc may have been added.

bath salts (bäth sôltz): rock salt to which fragrances and color are usually added;

used to soften water and aid in cleansing the skin.

battery (băt′ĕr-ē): an apparatus containing two or more cells for generating electricity.

bayberry plant (bā′bĕr-ē plănt): the leaves of myrcia acris which yield oil of bay used to make bay rum.

bayberry wax (bā-bĕr′ē wăx): wax from the bayberry shrub used in some hair tonics and soaps.

bay rum (bā rŭm): an after-shave lotion; a tonic and astringent.

beaker (bēk′ĕr): a vessel of glass with a lip for pouring; used in chemical analyses and in mixing preparations.

beard (bērd): the hair on a man's face, especially on the chin (the hair over the upper lip is usually called a mustache, which may be a part of a full beard).

beat (bēt): to whip or stir rapidly.

beautician (bū-tĭsh′an): a term used to describe one skilled in the art of beautifying the appearance of a person; licensed to perform cosmetology services.

beauty clinic (bū′tē klĭn′ĭk): a space set aside in a cosmetology school where students can practice their skills on clients before becoming employed in a salon.

beauty culture (bū′tē kŭl′tûr): pertaining to cosmetology; the study and practice of the improvement of personal appearance; personal grooming performed on another person.

beauty operator (bū′tē ŏp′ĕr-ā-tĕr): a term, considered outdated, used to describe one who works as a hairdresser and cosmetologist.

beauty parlor (bū′tē pär′lôr): an outdated term used to describe the place of business of a hairdresser or cosmetologist; also called a beauty shop or beauty salon.

beauty salon (bū′tē săl′ŏn; să-lŏn′): the term used to describe the place of business of a cosmetologist or hairdresser (also called hairdressing or facial salon); a full service salon supplies all cosmetology services, such as care of hair, skin, or nails; a facial salon supplies facial services, such as massage, treatments, and makeup.

beauty spot (bū′tē spŏt): a small patch or mark put on the face as an accent; a mole or other natural mark that is accented; originally, a small patch of fabric used to cover a blemish.

bed hair (bĕd hâr): hair which has separated from the papilla and lies loosely in the follicle.

beehive (bē′hīv): a hairstyle shaped like a beehive, popular in the 1960's; the hair was teased, pulled back and formed into the desired shape.

beer (bĭr): a fermented beverage made from grain and hops; used as a hair rinse to add body.

beeswax (bēz′wăks): wax given out by bees, from which they make their honeycomb; used in making of hairpieces to add strength to sewn parts; also used to dress unruly ends.

beige (bāj): a color term used to describe hair that is pale yellow-gray or pale gray-brown; a type of blond.

belly (bĕl′ē): the abdomen; the prominent part of a bulging muscle.

benign (bĭ-nīn′): mild in character; in relation to tumors, the opposite of malignant; characterizing any growth not likely to reoccur after removal.

bentonite (bĕn′tō-nīt): a porous clay from volcanic ash; used as a facial mask to absorb oil on the face; used in a variety of cosmetic products to thicken lotions, emulsify oils and suspend pigments.

benzine (bĕn′zēn): an inflammable liquid derived from petroleum and used as a cleaning fluid.

benzoic acid (bĕn′zô-ĭk ăs′ĭd): a preservative and antiseptic substance used in mouthwashes, after shave lotions, deodorants and creams.

benzoin (bĕn′zô-ĭn): a balsamic resin used as a stimulate and also as a perfume.

benzoldehyde (bĕn-zŏl′dă-hīd): a liquid with an odor similar to that of almonds; used in the dye and perfume industries.

benzoyl peroxide (bĕn′zô-ĭl pĕr-ŏks′īd): an ingredient used in cosmetic preparation and used to treat skin eruptions such as acne.

bergamot oil (bûr′gă-măt oyl): oil extracted from the rind of citrus fruits; used in some perfumes and lotions.

beriberi (bĕr′e-bĕr′ē): a deficiency disease characterized by weakness, anemia, etc.; due to lack of vitamin B1 in the diet.

berloque dermatitis (bĕr-lôk′ dûr-mă-tī′tĭs): a skin eruption characterized by red patches on the face and neck, generally caused by a reaction to a chemical (bergapten) found in some perfumes and other liquid cosmetics.

beta helix (bā′tă hē′lĭks): term indicating that the spiral of the body of the poly peptide chains within the cortex of the hair are in the second position; the spiral is stretched but can return to its alpha or first position when released.

bevel (bĕv′êl): to slope the edge of a surface; in haircutting; to taper the ends of the hair.

bevel cut (bĕv′êl kŭt): haircutting technique of rolling a strand of hair upward before cutting so that top of strand is slightly shorter, encouraging the hair to turn upward.

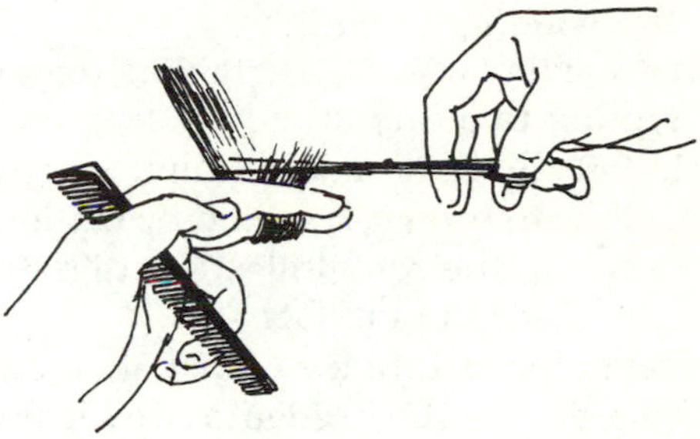

bevel cut

beveling (bĕv′êl-ĭng): a technique for creating fullness in a haircut; cutting the ends of the hair at a slight taper.

bi (bī): a prefix denoting two, twice, double.

bias (bī′ăs): a diagonal or slanted line; to cut on the bias.

bib (bĭb): an item of plastic or cloth placed across the client's chest and shoulders and around the back to protect clothing; a neutralizing bib has a pocket hem to catch solution.

bicarbonate of soda (bī-kär′bân-ât of sō′dă): baking soda; relieves burns, itching, urticarial lesions and insect bites; is often used in bath powders as an aid to cleansing oily skin; adding baking soda to the water in which instruments are to be boiled will keep them bright.

biceps (bī′sĕps): a muscle having two heads or points of attachment, as the biceps brackic which rotates and flexes the forearm, and the biceps femores, which flexes the knee and extends the hip joint.

bichloride (bī-klôr′īd): a compound having two parts or equivalents of chlorine to one of the other elements.

bicipital (bī-sĭp′ĭ-tâl): pertaining to the biceps.

bigoudi (bĭg-ū′dē): a small wooden curler employed in the formation of wigs for the winding of curls.

bilateral (bī-lăt′ĕr-âl): pertaining to or affecting two sides.

bile (bīl): a bitter alkaline fluid, greenish yellow to brown, secreted by the liver; it aids in the remulsification, digestion and absorption of fats.

bi-level haircut (bī-lĕv′l hâr′kŭt): a style that divides the head into two separate design lines.

binder (bīnd′ĕr): a substance such as gum arabic, glycerin and sorbitol with the ability to increase consistency and hold ingredients together; used in compact powders, toothpaste and like cosmetics.

binding (bīnd′ĭng): in wiggery, ribbon used at the edges of the netting to secure the edges and to connect two pieces together; also used for reinforcement; tubular binding is used to contain wire and springs.

binocular (bĭn-ŏk′ū-lâr): referring to the use of both eyes; a binocular optical instrument.

biocatalyst (bī′ō-kăt′ă-lĭst): a substance that acts to promote or modify some physiological process, especially an enzyme, vitamin or hormone.

biochemistry (bī′ō-kĕm′ĭs-trē): the chemistry of living animals and plants; the study of chemical compounds and processes occurring in living organisms.

biodegradable (bi′ō-dê grād′ăble): the ability of a substance to decay organically or naturally.

bioelectricity (bī′ō-ēlĕc-trĭs′ĭ-tē): electric phenomena occurring in living tissues; effects of electric current on living tissues.

bioesthegenics (bī′ō-ĕs′thē-jĕn-ĭks): the scientific study of the skin as an organ; relating to organic skin care.

bioflavonoid (bī′ō-flā′vă-noyd): a biologically active flavonoid; also called vitamin P; considered an aid to healthy skin and found most abundantly in fruits of the citrus variety.

biology (bī-ŏl′ô-jē): the science of life and living things.

biorhythm (bī′ō-rĭth-ûm): any regular pattern or change of cycle in an organism, such as periodic variations in body temperature, blood pressure, etc.

biostimulant (bī′ō-stĭm′ū-lânt): an agent used to stimulate activity in living tissue.

biotin (bī′ô-tĭn): a vitamin B complex, found in small amounts in plant and animal tissue.

biphosphate (bī-fŏs′fāt): a salt of phosphoric acid in which one of the three hydrogen atoms of the acid is replaced by a base.

bipolar (bī-pō′lăr): of or having two poles; characterized by opposite natures.

bipolarity (bī′pō-lăr′ĭ-tē): the use of two electrodes in the stimulation of muscles or nerves; the condition of having two processes extending from opposite poles.

birchwood stick (bûrch′wŏŏd stĭk): a thin stick used as a swab or stirring implement, similar to an orangewood stick which is used as a manicure implement.

birthmark (bûrth′märk): any mark on the face or body which is present at birth, usually lasting; a form of nevus.

bisulfate (bī-sŭl′fāt): an acid sulfate.

bisulfide (bī-sŭl′fīd): a compound containing two atoms of sulfur; a disulfide.

bisulfite (bī-sŭl′fīt): an acid sulfite.

biterminal (bī-tûr′mĭ-nâl): two terminals or poles of an electric source.

black (blăk): a neutral hue having no brightness or color; the maximum degree of darkness in hair coloring; a term used to describe dark skin and hair; the opposite of white.

blackhead (blăk′hĕd): a comedone; a plug of sebaceous matter that has darkened upon contact with air.

bladder (blăd′ẽr): a membranous sac which serves as a reservoir for holding urine.

bland (blănd): pertaining to nonirritating substances such as a bland, mild diet free of roughage or irritating spices; a smooth mild facial.

blastema (blăs-tē′mă): the hypothetical lymph or fluid from which cells and organs are formed; the formative cellular matrix from which an organ, tissue or part is derived.

bleach (blēch): a chemical preparation used to remove the color from hair; also used in some preparations to lighten skin pigmentation.

bleached hair (blēcht hâr): hair from which the color has been wholly or partially removed by means of a bleaching or lightening agent.

bleaching solution (blēch′ĭng sô-lū′-shûn): hydrogen peroxide with the addition of ammonia.

bleach pack (blēch păk): a bleach formula prepared in a thick consistency.

bleb (blēb): a blister of the skin filled with watery fluid.

blemish (blĕm′ĭsh): a mark, spot or defect on the skin.

blemish cover (blĕm′ĭsh kŭv′ẽr): a cosmetic in stick or cream form, based on alcohol, oil, wax and pigments; used to conceal minor blemishes.

blend (blĕnd): to meet or join; in hair coloring: to mix or blend colors to achieve various hair colors; in haircutting: to graduate from shorter to longer lengths; in makeup: to mix together so there is no line of demarcation.

blending (blĕnd′ĭng): the physical act of fusing the color of hair during tinting and lightening applications; mixing of makeup colors; connection between two or more shapes in hair design.

blepharoplasty (blĕf′ă-rō-plăs-tē): plastic surgery of the eyebrows and/or eyelids.

blister (blĭs′tẽr): a vesicle; a collection of serous fluid causing an elevation of the skin.

block (blŏk′): to mark off or indicate sections in an outline to be followed when subsectioning the hair.

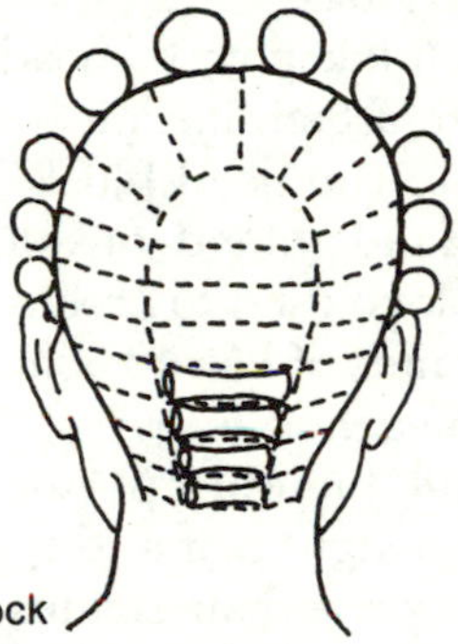
block

blockhead (blŏk′hĕd′): a head shaped form usually made of canvas covered cork, to which a wig is secured for fitting, cleaning and styling.

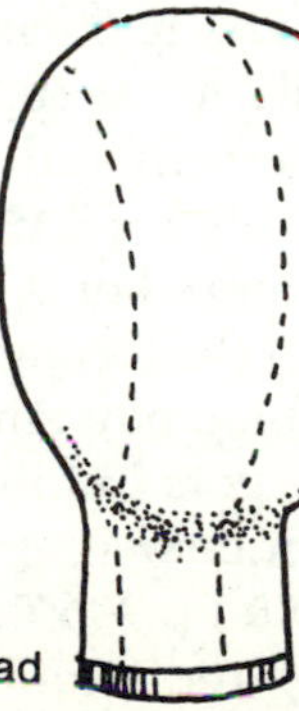
blockhead

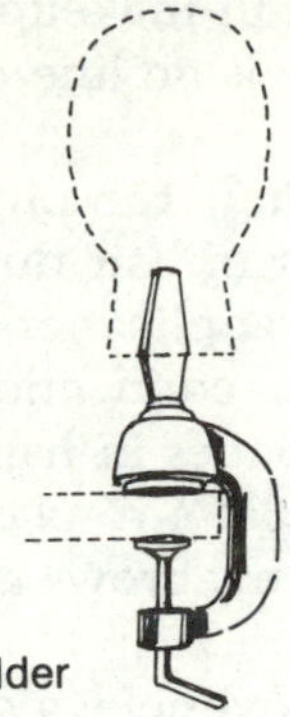

block holder (blŏk hōld′ĕr): a clamping device used to hold a blockhead form to a table.

blocking (blŏk′ĭng): the act of dividing the hair into sections in order to work on smaller parts.

block point (blŏk poynt): headless steel pin used to attach hairpieces or other materials to the head block.

blond on blond (blŏnd on blŏnd): two shades (colors) used to create light and darker strands of hair to achieve a natural sun-bleached look.

blonde; blond (blŏnd): a person with fair complexion, light hair and eyes; a term used to describe hair shades and tints that range from light yellowish brown to platinum or silver white.

blonding (blŏnd′ĭng): the process of lightening the hair in preparation for the application of a toner.

blood (blŭd): the nutritive fluid circulating through the body (heart, veins, arteries and capillaries) to supply oxygen and nutrients to cells and tissues.

blood platelets (blŭd plāt′lĕts): blood cells smaller than red or white corpuscles which aid in the formation of clots.

blood poisoning (blŭd poy′zĭn-ĭng): an infection which gets into the bloodstream (see septicemia).

blood pressure (blŭd prĕsh′ĕr): the pressure exerted by the circulatory blood on the walls of the blood vessels or heart.

blood stream (blŭd′strēm): the flow of blood in its circulation through the body.

blood vascular system (blŭd văs′kû-lăr sĭs′tĕm): the group of structures: the heart, arteries, veins and capillaries which distribute blood throughout the body.

blood vessel (blŭd vĕs′êl): an artery, vein or capillary.

blotch (blŏch): a spot or eruption on the skin.

blouse (blaůs): in hairstyling, a loose fitting at the base of a pin curl or wound perm rod; to push up to create fullness or puffiness.

blow-dry (blō′-drī′): to use a blow-drying machine to dry and style the hair in a single process, usually without presetting; a service performed after a haircut and shampoo when a soft style is desired.

blower (blō′ĕr): a small hand-held hair dryer used when styling and blow-drying the hair.

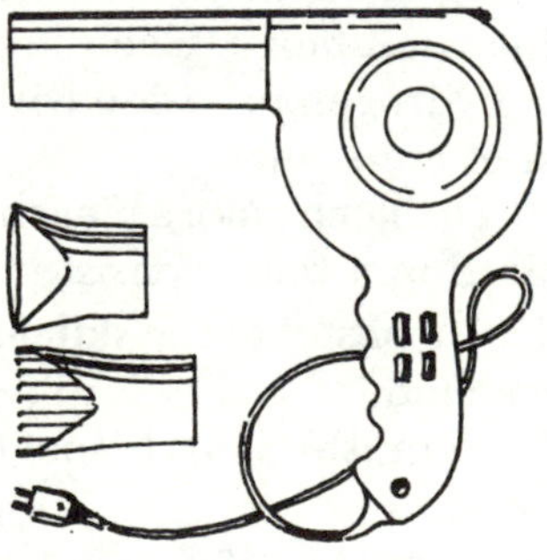

blow-out (blō′-oůt): a term used to describe styling of the hair when it is done with a blower and brush; the process in which hair is styled with a blower and brush.

blow-out perm (blō′-oůt pûrm): a permanent wave that is styled with a blow dryer, brush and comb; a permanent wave that does not require setting with rollers or pin curls.

blow-style (blō′-stīl): a hairstyle created with the blow-dryer, brush and comb.

blue (bloo͞): the color of a clear sky, between green and violet in the spectrum; a primary color; the color of venous blood that shows through the skin as in a bruise.

blue light (bloo͞ līt): a therapeutic lamp used to soothe the nerves.

blue nevus (blū nē′vûs): a nevus (birthmark) composed of spindle-shaped pigmented melanocytes usually in the middle and lower portions of the dermis.

bluing rinse (bloo͞′ĭng rĭns): a temporary coloring used to neutralize the unbecoming yellowish tinge in gray or white hair.

blunt (blŭnt): having a thick or rounded edge or end.

blunt cutting (blŭnt cŭt′ĭng): cutting straight across a strand of hair without thinning or tapering. (see: club cutting).

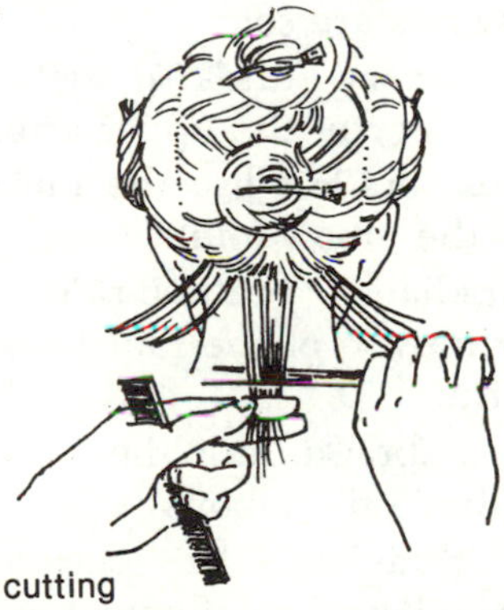

blunt cutting

blusher (blŭsh′ĕr): a powdered substance, also called "rouge" used to add color or highlights to the cheeks or to shade areas of the face.

boar bristle brush (bôr brĭs′âl brŭsh): a brush made with the short, stiff hairs from a wild boar; considered to be less damaging to hair than other types of bristle; also called "natural bristle brush."

boardwork (bôrd′wûrk): the art of making hairpieces.

boardworker (bôrd-wûr′kĕr): one who makes hairpieces.

bob (bŏb): pertaining to a short, blunt haircut for women and children; to cut long hair to shoulder length or shorter.

bobby pin (bŏb′ē pĭn): a long "U" shaped clamp or clasp-like pin with the ends pressing close together, used to hold the hair in place in a style or hair set.

body (bŏd′ē): in anatomy: the human or animal frame and its organs; in cosmetology: the consistency or solidarity of texture or quality of liveliness and springiness which the hair possesses.

body brushing (bŏd′ē brŭsh′ĭng): a treatment for the body which benefits circulation and removes dead surface cells from the epidermis.

body cream (bŏd′ē krēm): a creamy substance used for smoothing and softening the skin of the entire body.

body image (bŏd′ē ĭm′ĭj): the conscious and unconscious concept a person has of his or her body as it may be perceived by others.

body lotion (bŏd′ē lō′shûn): a smooth liquid to be used on the body following the bath or a skin treatment; a lotion applied after the removal of superfluous hair from any part of the body.

body perm (bŏd′ē pûrm): a permanent wave given to impart body rather than curl or visible wave to the hair.

body surface area (bŏd′ē sûr′fŭs â′rē-ă): the area covered by a person's skin, expressed in square meters.

body wave (bŏd′ē wāv): a large wave pattern created by a permanent wave as a foundation for a style.

body wrap (bŏd′ē răp): a wrapping treatment used to treat cellulite, the condition of fatty deposits; the substances used and the wrapping technique have a diuretic effect which sometimes aids weight reduction.

boil (boy′l): a furuncle; a subcutaneous abscess caused by bacteria which enter through the hair follicles.

boiling point (boy′l′ĭng poynt): 212° F. (fahrenheit) or 100° C. (Celsius); the temperature at which a liquid begins to boil.

bond (bŏnd): the attractive force that binds one atom to another in a molecule, resulting from the transfer or sharing of one or more electrons, often represented in formulas by a line or dot.

bond breaker (bŏnd brāk′ĕr): a substance which has the ability to disrupt or destroy the bond units of chemical compounds.

bone (bōn): the hard tissue forming the framework of the body.

bonnet (bŏn′ĕt): in hairstyling, a head covering with perforations used for frosting, highlighting or glazing strands of hair.

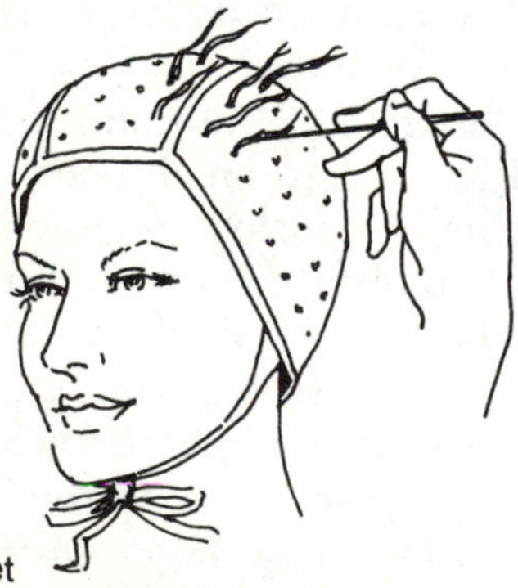

bonnet

book end wrap (bo͞ok ĕnd răp): technique of protecting hair ends with porous paper by folding single end paper over the hair strands like an envelope; conducive to the use of concave rods.

boom boom iron (bo͞om bo͞om ī′ĕrn): also called bop iron. A thermal curling iron with oversized rod and groove.

booster (bo͞ost′ĕr): oxidizer added to hydrogen peroxide to increase its chemical action.

borax (bō′răks): sodium tetraborate; a white powder used as an antiseptic and cleansing agent.

borderline (bôr′dĕr-līn): pertaining to being neither normal nor abnormal; doubtful; difficult to classify; a line of demarcation; between.

boric acid (bō′rĭk ăs′ĭd): acidum boricum; used as an antiseptic dusting powder and in liquid form as an eyewash.

bouffant (bo͞o-fănt′): the degree of fullness, height and width in a particular hairstyle; a wide, full, teased hairstyle popular in the 1960s and early 1970s.

boutique (bo͞o-tēk′): a specialty shop or department which may be situated within a salon, in which cosmetics or accessories are sold.

brachial artery (brā′kĭ-âl är′tĭr-ē): the main artery of the upper arm.

brachialis (brā′kĭ-ā′lĭs): the muscle that flexes the elbow joint.

brachioradialis (brā′kĭ-ô-rā′dĭ-ā′lĭs): a flexor muscle of the radial side of the forearm.

brachium (brā′kĭ-ŭm): the part of the arm above the elbow.

bracing (brās′ĭng): the cotton which holds a hairpiece foundation in the proper position on the wooden block during the process of manufacture.

braid (brād): three interwoven strands of hair that form a repetitive pattern; a braided or coiled hair switch which is used to create different hairstyles; a three stemmed switch joined with a loop at the top; to weave, entwine or enterlace hair strands.

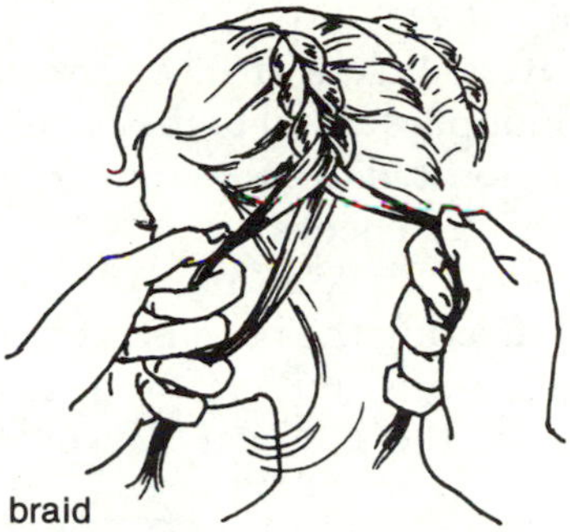

braid

brain (brān): that part of the central nervous system contained in the cranial cavity, and consisting of the cerebrum, the cerebellum, the pons, and the medulla oblongata.

brassy tone (brăs′ē tōn): in hair coloring; a harsh, brass-like color quality exhibiting excess red or yellow tones.

breakage (brāk′ĭj): a condition in which hair splits and breaks off; caused by damage to the hair.

breastbone (brĕst′bōn): the sternum; the narrow flat bone located in the middle of the chest.

brewer's yeast (broo͞′ĕrz yēst): a yellowish substance consisting of small plants or cells that grow rapidly in a liquid containing sugar; a natural source of vitamin B complex and protein.

brightening (brīt′ĕn-ĭng): adding highlights and luster to the hair by lightening or toning the natural shade.

brilliantine (brĭl′yân-tēn): an oily preparation that imparts luster to the hair.

bristle (brĭs′l): the short stiff hair of a brush; short stiff hair of an animal used in brushes.

brittle hair (brĭt′l hâr): hair that is dry and fragile and is easily broken.

broad (brôd): wide; having great breadth as distinguished from length; having much width or breadth; not narrow.

bromide (brō′mīd): a compound which is formed by the replacement of the hydrogen in hydrobromic acid by a metal or organic radical; such substances are used to allay nervous excitement and are employed as sedatives.

bromidrosis (brō-mĭ-drō′sĭs): excretion of perspiration (sweat) which has an unpleasant odor.

bromo-acid (brō-mō-ăs′ĭd): a soluble dye used to impart a red indelible color in lipsticks and similar cosmetics.

bromoderma (brō′mō-dûr′mă): a skin eruption due to the ingestion of bromides.

bronchial (brŏn′kē-âl): pertaining to or involving the bronchi and their branches.

bronchus (brŏn′kûs); pl., **bronchi** (-kē): the main branch of the windpipe.

bronze powder (bränz paů′dĕr): fine flakes of a metal such as copper alloy or aluminum; used as a pigment in cosmetics to impart a "frost" or sheen.

brow (braů): the upper anterior portion of the head; the forehead; the supraorbital ridge; the hair above the eyes called the eyebrows.

bruise (broo͞z): an injury without laceration which produces capillary hemorrhage beneath the surface of the skin causing a bluish discoloration; to injure.

bruised fingernails (broo͞z′d fĭng′ĕr-nālz): bluish spots underneath the nails caused by a blow or other injury.

brunet, brunette (broo͞-nĕt′): a person having brown or olive skin, brown or black hair and dark eyes; term used to describe dark hair color.

brush (brŭsh): a grooming tool with a handle and rows of bristles embedded in the other end.

brush blow-drying (brŭsh blō′-drī′ĭng): the use of a hand-held blow-dryer and a brush to style the hair.

brush combing (brŭsh kōm′ĭng): back combing the hair with a brush.

brush-curl (brŭsh-cûrl): to turn, bend or form the hair into ringlets by means of a hairbrush and the fingers.

brush dryer (brŭsh drī′ẽr): a hand-held hair dryer or blower with a brush attachment.

brush electrode (brŭsh ē-lĭk′trōd): an electrode resembling a brush which is used for the application of electricity.

brushing machine (brŭsh′ĭng mă-shēn′): a machine with a facial brush attachment which rotates at varied speeds and is used for facial and body treatments to increase circulation.

brushless shaving cream (brŭsh′lĕs shāv′ĭng krēm): a cream for shaving that does not have the lathering action of soap: brushless creams usually contain lanolin or mineral oil, stearic acid, gums and thickeners.

brush-out (brŭsh-oủt): the use of a brush and comb to achieve the opening and blending of the hair set (its curls and waves) into the finished coiffure.

brush roller (brŭsh rōl′ẽr): wire or plastic mesh hair roller with fine brush bristles to hold the hair to the roller while it is rolled into place.

brush waves (brŭsh wāvz): a series of alternating rows of pin curls which are then brushed into waves.

bubble bath (bŭb′l bäth): crystals or powders that form surface bubbles when used in bath water; usually contain sodium lauryl sulfate, sodium chloride, alcohol and fragrance.

bubo (bū′bō): an inflammatory condition causing enlargement of the lymph nodes.

bucca (bŭk′ă): the hollow part of the cheek.

buccal artery (bŭk′âl är′tĭr-ē): the artery which supplies blood to the buccinator muscle located in the mucus membrane of the cheeks.

buccal nerve (bŭk′âl nûrv): a motor nerve affecting the buccinator and the orbicularis-oris muscle; the sensory branch of the modular nerve of the cheek.

buccinator (bŭk′sĭ-nā-tẽr): the thin, flat muscle of the cheek, shaped like a trumpet.

buckle (bŭk′'l): distortion of a curl caused by a bend in its formation.

buffer (bŭf′ẽr): a manicuring implement used with powdered polish or buffering cream to import a sheen to the nails and to improve circulation of blood to the nail area.

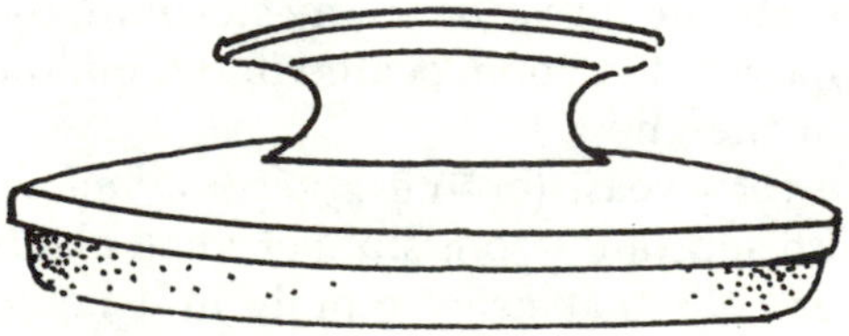

buffer

buffer activity (bŭf′ẽr ăk-tĭv′ĭ-tē): the action of a buffer solution which has a tendency to resist changes in its pH when treated with strong acids or bases.

buildup (bĭld′ŭp): in hairstyling, an accumulation of excess foreign matter deposited in the hair shaft; in manicuring, an accumulation of substance to create artificial nails.

buildup cut (bĭld′ŭp kŭt): to cut hair so that it appears fuller.

bulb (bŭlb): the lowest area or part of a hair.

bulbous (bŭl′bûs): pertaining to or like a bulb in shape and structure.

bulk (bŭlk): in haircutting and hairstyling, the density, thickness, textured, length and volume of the hair.

bulky (bŭl′kē): pertaining to hair that is thick and heavy; having great thickness and weight.

bulla (bo͞ol′ă): a large bleb or blister.

bullous pemphigoid (bo͞ol′ŭs pĕm′fĭ-goyd): a chronic skin disease characterized by large bulla which heal without leaving scars.

bump (bŭmp): an area of raised, swollen tissue.

bun (bŭn): a roll of hair shaped like a bun or small roll of bread.

bundle (bŭn′d'l): a structure composed of a group of fibers, muscular or nervous.

bunion (bŭn′yŭn): a swelling of a bursa of the foot, generally affecting the joint of the great (big) toe.

burdock root (bûr′dŏk ro͞ot): a coarse, biennial weed used as an ingredient in some hair and skin care products formulated to control excess oil secretions.

burn (bûrn): the tissue reaction or injury resulting from application of extreme heat, cold, friction, electricity, radiation or caustic substances.

burrowing hair (bûr′ō-ĭng hâr): a condition where the hair does not emerge from the skin but grows beneath the surface and may become infected.

butter (bŭt′ĕr): in cosmetology, a substance that is solid at room temperature but melts at body temperature; cocoa butter and lip lubricants are examples and are manufactured in stick or molded forms: cosmetic butters usually contain hydrogenated oils, lanolin, wax, preservative and coloring ingredients.

butterfly clamp (bŭt′ĕr-flī klămp): a clamping device designed to hold the hair in place while sectioning, subsectioning or during other procedures.

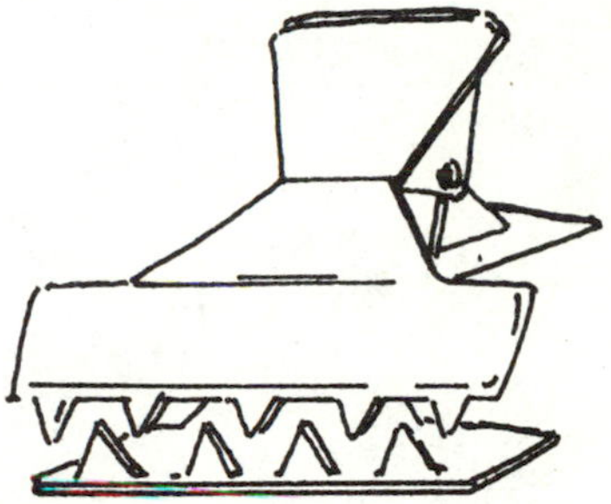

butterfly clamp

butyl alcohol (byo͞ot′l ăl′kô-hŏl): any of four isomeric alcohols obtained from petroleum products; used as a clarifying agent in shampoos.

butylene glycol (byo͞ot′-l-ēn glī′kôl): a substance made from acetylene formaldehyde and hydrogen, used in hair sprays and hair setting preparations.

butyl stearate (byo͞ot′'l stēr′āt): stearic acid; butyl ester; used in nail polish, lipstick, creams and bath oils.

C

cacao (kă-kā′ō): the seeds or beans from the theobroma cacao; used in making cocoa butter which is used to relieve dryness and tautness of the skin.

cachecticorum, acne (kă-kĕk-tĭ-kōr′ûm ăk′nē): pimples occurring in subjects of anemia or some debilitating constitutional disease.

cadmium sulfide (kăd′mē-ûm sŭl′fīd): a yellow-orange powder, insoluble in water, used in shampoo for the treatment of scalp diseases.

cake makeup (kāk māk′ŭp): a shaped, solid mass usually containing finely ground pigment, kaolin, zinc, titanium oxide, calcium carbonate, iron oxide, lanolin or other oils, sorbital and fragrance; a moistened cosmetic sponge is used to apply the makeup to the face; gives good coverage.

cake mascara (kāk mäs-kâr′ă): a makeup for the eyelashes applied with a moistened brush or applicator; comes in dry molded form or a more liquid product in a cylinder or tube: ingredients usually used in mascara are carnauba wax, paraffin, lanolin, carbon black, triethanolamine stearate and propylparaben.

caking (kāk′ĭng): the process in which small particles cling and form a thick or hardened mass such as caking of powder or lipstick when applied.

calamine (kăl′ă-mĭn): zinc carbonate; a pinkish powder of zinc oxide and ferric oxide used to treat skin ailments.

calamine lotion (kăl′ă-mīn lō′shûn): zinc carbonate in alcohol used as a mild astringent and healing lotion, especially for skin irritations.

calcaneal nerve (kăl-kān′ē-âl nûrv): nerve that receives stimuli from the skin of the heel.

calcaneus (kăl-kā′nē-ûs): the heel bone; the large tarsal bone.

calcified tumor (kăl′sĭ-fīd tū′mẽr): any cutaneous neoplasm containing calcium.

calcium (kăl′sē-ûm): a silvery-white metal; in compounds, a component of bone.

calcium carbonate (kăl′sē-ûm kär′bôn-āt): chalk; a tasteless, odorless, absorbent powder that occurs in coral, limestone and marble; used as a whitener in cosmetics and as a buffer in face powders; also used in toothpaste or powders, in deodorants and some medicinal preparations.

calcium propionate (kăl′sē-ûm prō′pē-ō-nāt′): propanoic acid; calcium salt; used as a preservative in cosmetics.

calefacient (kăl′ĕ-fā′shŭnt): a substance that produces a sensation of heat and warmth; ingredients used in a facial mask or body wrap.

calendula (kă-lĕn′jă-lâ): commonly known as the marigold plant; used in some skin care preparations as a softening agent.

caliber, calibre (kăl′ĭ-bẽr): the diameter of a tube, such as the esophagus, urethra or artery.

calibrate (kăl′ĭ-brāt): to correct, graduate or adjust the scale of a measuring instrument such as a pH meter.

caliper (kăl′ĭ-pĕr): an instrument used for measuring diameters, thickness and distance between surfaces; often used to measure facial proportions.

callosity (kă-lŏs′ĭ-tē): a portion of skin that has been thickened by persistent friction or pressure, caused by hypertrophy of the horny layer of the epidermis; dry, hard, calloused skin.

callous, callus (kăl′ûs): hardened skin usually appearing on the feet and palms of the hands.

callus remover (kăl′ûs rê-mōōv′ĕr): an implement, usually rounded or cylinder-shaped and covered with emery paper, used to smooth and remove calluses during a manicure or pedicure.

calomel (kâl′ō-mĕl): a white powder, insoluble in water; used in ointment form as an antibacterial.

calor (kăl′âr): pertaining to heat; one of four classic signs of inflammation: color, heat; dolar, pain; rubor, redness; and tumor, swelling.

calorie (kăl′ă-rē): a measurement of heat or energy; the amount of heat necessary to raise the temperature of water from zero to one degree centegrade; a unit of heat used to express the heat-energy producing content of foods; see kilogram; calorie.

calvaria (kăl-vâr′ē-ă): the upper part of the skull.

calvities (kăl-vĭsh′ĭ-ēz): baldness; baldness of the anterior and upper part of the head.

camomile, chamomile (kăm′ă-mēl): an herb whose leaves produce an oily substance that is used in lotions for the skin; used in concentrated form as a hair lightener; a soothing tea.

camphor (kăm′fĕr): oil distilled from the bark and wood of the camphor tree; used with other ingredients such as castor oil and wax to produce a product that is healing to chapped skin; it is slightly anaesthetic and cooling.

canaliculas (kăn-ă-lĭk′ū-lûs): a small canal or groove, as in a bone.

cancellous (kăn′sĕ-lûs): pertaining to bone; having a porous or spongy structure.

cancer (kăn′sĕr): a malignant tumor.

candlestick curl (kăn′d'l-stĭk kûrl): a hair setting technique in which rollers are placed vertically; elongated, spiral wound curls; also called "long" or "poker" curls.

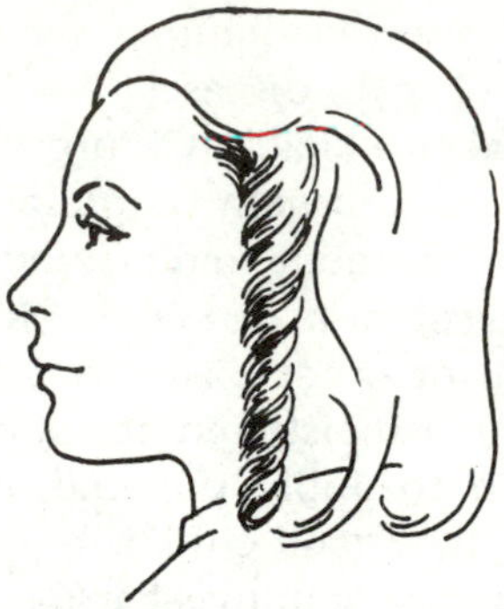

candlestick curl

caninus (kā-nīn′ûs): the levator anguli oris muscle which lifts the angle of the mouth.

canitics (kă-nĭt′ĭks): the study of canities; the graying of the hair.

canities (kă-nĭsh′ē-ēz): grayness or whiteness of the hair.

canities, accidental (ka-nĭsh′ē-ēz ăk-sĭ-dĕn′tâl): grayness of hair caused by fright.

canities, congenital (kă-nĭsh′ē-ēz kôn-jĕn′ĭ-tâl): a type of grayness or whiteness of the hair which is hereditary.

canities, premature (kă-nĭsh′ē-ēz prē′mă-tūr′): graying of the hair before the usual age for this occurrence.

canities senile (kă-nĭsh′ē-ēz sĕn′īl): grayness of hair that is associated with advanced age.

canities unguium (kă-nĭsh′ē-ēz ŭn-give′ŭm): abnormal whiteness or white spots on nails.

canker (kâng′kĕr): an ulceration usually affecting the mucous membranes of the mouth.

cantharides (kăn-thăr′ĭ-dēz): a powerful counterirritant.

canthus (kăn′thŭs): the corner of each side of the eye where the upper and lower lids meet.

cap (kăp): the netting and binding of a hairpiece which together form the base to which the hair is attached.

cap coiffure (kăp kwă-fūr′): a cap-like haircut that is short and closely trimmed at the nape line.

cape (kāp): a sleeveless garment of cloth or plastic used to protect the client's clothing during cosmetology services.

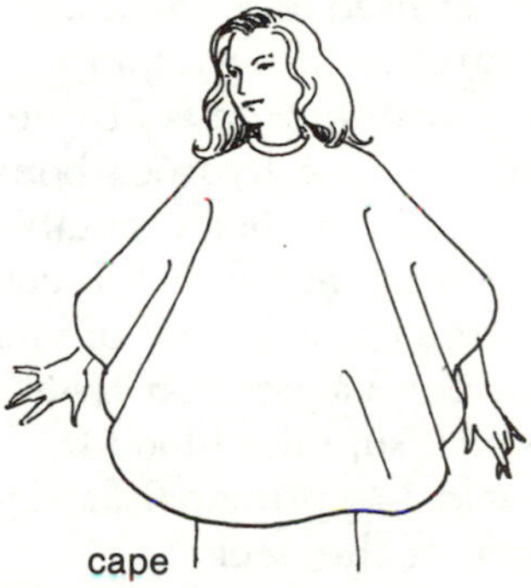

cape

capillarectasia (kăp′ĭ-lăr′ă-ĕk-tā′zē-ă): dilation of the capillaries.

capillaritis (kăp-ĭ-lăr-ī′tĭs): a progressive pigmentary disorder of the skin which has no inflammation but causes dilation of the capillaries.

capillarity (kăp-ĭ-lăr′ĭ-tē): elevation or depression of liquids in narrow tubes due to the surface tension that exists between the molecules of the liquid and those of the solid tube.

capillary (kăp′ĭ-lĕ-rē): any one of the minute blood vessels which connect the arteries and veins; hairlike blood vessels.

capillary hemangioma (kap′ĭ-lĕ-rē hē-măn-jē-ō′mă): a benign vascular tumor made up largely of capillaries.

capillurgy (kăp-ĭ-lûr′jē): the art of destroying superfluous hair.

capitate (kăp′ĭ-tāt): shaped like or forming a head as the rounded end of a bone; the large bone of the wrist; the largest carpal bone.

capsicum (kăp′sĭ-kŭm): an herb of the nightshade family, including varieties of red pepper, used in condiments for food and in medical preparations as gastric stimulants.

capsule (kăp′sūl): a membranous or saclike structure enclosing a part of an organ; a small case to enclose substances of disagreeable taste.

caput (kā′pût): a head or head-like part.

caramel (kär′ă-m′l): burnt sugar used to color and flavor foods; in cosmetology, used as a soothing agent in skin lotions.

carbohydrate (kär-bô-hī′drāt): a substance containing carbon, hydrogen, and oxygen, the two latter in proportion to form water; sugars, starches and cellulose belong to class of carbohydrates.

carbolic acid (kär-bŏl′ĭk ăs′ĭd): phenol, a caustic and corrosive poison found in coal tar used in dilute solution as an antiseptic.

carbomer (kär′bō-mûr): a polymer of acrylic acid; when cross-linked with other agents it forms a substance

C-D

which is used for preparing suspensions and emulsifiers.

carbon (kär′bôn): an element in nature which predominates in all organic compounds and occurs in three distinct forms: black lead, charcoal and lamp black (soot) the symbol for carbon is the capital letter "C."

carbona (kär-bō′nă): a trade name for a cleaning fluid containing carbon tetrachloride, which is sometimes used in giving a dry shampoo and for cleaning wigs.

carbon arc lamp (kär′bôn ärk lămp): an instrument which produces ultraviolet rays.

carbonate (kär′bôn-āt): a compound of carbonic acid and a base; to charge with carbon dioxide.

carbon dioxide (kär′bûn dī-ŏk′sīd): carbonic acid gas; product of the combustion of carbon with a free supply of air.

carbonic acid (kär-bôn′ĭk ăs′ĭd): an acid formed by the union of carbon dioxide and water.

carbon monoxide (kär′bûn mŏn-ŏk′sīd): a colorless, odorless and poisonous gas, its toxic action being due to its strong affinity for hemoglobin.

carbon tetrachloride (kär′bôn tĕ-tră-klôr′ĭd): a non-flammable, colorless liquid used as a solvent in cleaning mixtures.

carbuncle (kär′bŭn-k'l): a large circumscribed inflammation of the subcutaneous tissue, similar to a furuncle (boil) but more extensive.

carcinogen (kär-sĭn′ô-jĕn): a cancer-causing agent or substance.

carcinoma (kär-sĭ-nō′mă): a malignant tumor.

carcinomatous dermatitis (kär-sĭ-nō′mă-tûs dẽr-mă-tī′tĭs): reddening of the skin associated with carcinoma; inflammatory carcinoma.

card (kärd): a device, mounted on a workbench, consisting primarily of sharp, steel prongs; the instrument used for disentangling hair which is to be used in a hairpiece; also used to direct all the hair imbrications in one direction to prevent tangling.

cardiac (kär′dē-ăk): pertaining to the heart.

cardiac cycle (kär′dē-ăk sī′kâl): the rhythmic cycle of contraction, dilation and relaxation of all four chambers of the heart, both atris and ventricles.

cardiac glands (kär′dē-ăk glănz): the glands of the cardia of the stomach.

cardiac muscle (kär′dē-ăk mŭs′âl): the involuntary muscle that makes up the heart.

cardiac nerves (kär′dē-ăk nûrvz): nerves affecting the heart.

carnation (kär-nā′shûn): a bright pink or red flower used in some cosmetics and as a fragrance in perfumery.

carotene (kâr′ô-tēn): any of three orange colored isomeric hydrocarbons found in carrots and similar vegetables; used as a coloring material for cosmetics; used in the manufacture of vitamin A.

carotid artery (kă-rŏt′ĭd är′tĭr-ē): the artery which supplies blood to the head and neck; the principal artery on either side of the neck.

carotid nerves (kă-rŏt′ĭd nûrvz): sympathetic nerves associated with glands and smooth muscles of the head.

carpal (kär′pâl): pertaining to the wrist or carpus.

carpus (kär′pûs): the wrist; the group of eight bones between the metacarpals and the radius and ulna.

carrot (kăr′ĕt): the long, orange root used as a vegetable and source of vitamin

A; carrot oil is used in some cosmetics to treat skin blemishes.

cartilage (kär′tĭ-lĭj): gristle; a nonvascular connective tissue softer than bone.

carve (kärv): in hairsetting: to pick up or slice a strand of hair from a shaping.

carved curl (kärvd kûrl): a pin curl, sliced from a shaping and formed without lifting the hair from the head.

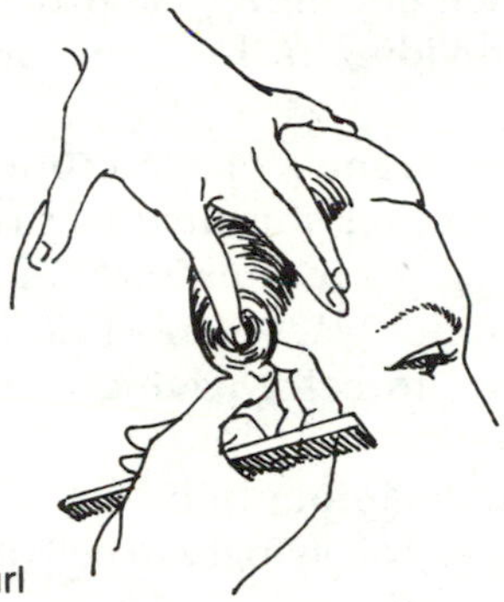

carved curl

cascade (kăs-kād′): a hairpiece with an oblong-shaped base, worn primarily at the back of the head where it falls (cascades) like a waterfall.

cascade curl (kăs-kād′ kûrl): a strand of hair held directly up from the scalp and wound with a large center opening, in croquignole fashion; the curl is fastened to the head in a standing position to allow the hair to flow upward and then downward.

casein (kā′sē-ên, kā-sēn′): a phosphoprotein found in milk and constituting the principal ingredient in cheese; used in the manufacture of plastics and resins.

cassia oil (kăsh′ă oyl): oil made from a variety of cinnamon which is used in some skin care preparations to speed surface circulation of the blood.

Castile soap (kăs-tēl sōp): a hard, white soap containing olive oil and other oils; originally from the region of Castile, Spain.

castor oil (kăs′tĕr oyl): oil obtained from the castor bean; used as a lubricant and in some laxative preparations.

casual (kăzh′o͞o-âl): in dress or hairstyling; informal, natural and relaxed.

catabolism (kă-tăb′ă-lĭz′m): the phase of metabolism which involves the breaking down of complex compounds within the cells, often resulting in the liberation of energy.

catagen faz (kăt′ă-jĭn fāz): the brief transitional period between growth and inactive stage of a hair follicle.

catalysis (kă-tăl′ĭ-sĭs): an increase in the rate of a chemical reaction, caused by the presence of a substance that is not altered by the reaction.

catalyst (kăt′ă-lĭst): any substance that increases the reaction time of physical and chemical processes and remains unchanged.

cataphoresis (kă-tă-fă-rē′sĭs): the forcing of substances into the deeper tissues, using the galvanic current from the positive toward the negative pole; the use of the positive pole to introduce an acid pH product such as an astringent solution into the skin.

cathode (kăth′ōd): the negative pole or electrode of a constant electric current; the negatively charged electrode from an outside source of current during electrolysis.

cathodermia (kăth′ō-dĕr′mē-ă): a process in which the skin acts as a cathode or negative electrode.

cation (kăt′ī′ŏn): an ion carrying a charge of positive electricity; the element which, during electrolysis of a chemical compound, appears at the negative pole or cathode.

cationic (kăt′ī-ŏn′ĭk): having a positive charge.

cationic detergent (kăt′ī-ŏn′ĭk dē-tĕr′-

jĭnt): a detergent, such as a quaternary ammonium salt, in which the cleansing action is inherent in the cation process.

catnip (kăt′nĭp): an aromatic, minty herb used in some cosmetic preparations to reduce puffiness around the eyes; also used as an antiseptic ingredient for dandruff control.

Caucasian (kô-kā′zhŭn): a member of the Caucasoid division of the human species; relating to the white race as defined by physical characteristics.

Caucasoid (kô′kă-soyd): pertaining to a major ethnic division of the human race; characterized by skin color ranging from light to brown and hair varying from light to dark and curly to straight.

caul (kôl): a type of netting with an open weave which is strong, soft and flexible; used in the crown area of some wigs.

causative (kôz′ă-tĭv): being or acting as a cause.

caustic (kôs′tĭk): an agent that damages tissues by burning; capable of eating away by chemical action.

caustic potash (kôs′tĭk pŏt′ăsh): potassium hydroxide.

caustic soda (kôs′tĭk sō′dă): sodium hydroxide.

cauterize (kô′tĕr-īz): to burn or sear with a caustic.

cautery (kô′tĕr-ē): pertaining to the destruction of growths on the skin by use of a caustic substance or a cauterizing implement.

cava (kā′vă); pl. **cavum:** vena cava; any cavity or hollow of the body.

cavity (kăv′ĭ-tē): a hollow space.

cayenne (kī-ĕn′): a biting powder made from seeds and fruit of a pepper plant; used as a condiment and in some medicine preparations.

celery seed (sĕl′ăr-ē sēd): seed of the celery plant noted for its diffusive power in the manufacture of perfume; also used in cookery.

cell (sĕl): a minute mass of protoplasm forming the structural unit of every organized body; capable of performing all the fundamental functions of life.

cell division (sĕl dĭ-vĭzh′ôn): the reproduction of cells by the process of each cell dividing in half and forming two cells.

cell membrane (sĕl mĕm′brān): a delicate protoplastic material that encloses a living plant or animal cell; cell wall.

cellular (sĕl′ĭ-lăr): consisting of or pertaining to cells; having a porous texture.

cellular pathology (sĕl′ū-lăr păth-ŏl′ô-jē): the study of changes in cells as the basis of disease.

cellular physiology (sĕl′û-lăr fĭz-ē-ŏl′ô-jē): the physiology of individual cells as compared with entire tissues or organisms.

cellulite (sĕl′û-līt): a word coined in European esthetics to describe the gel-like lumps composed of fat, water and residues of toxic substances beneath the skin, usually around the hips and thighs of overweight people.

cellulitis (sĕl′û-lī′tĭs): a diffuse inflammation of connective tissues, especially the subcutaneous tissues.

cellulose (sĕl′û-lōs): the principal carbohydrate constituent of the cell membranes of plants; absorbent cotton is a pure form of cellulose.

cellulose paper (sĕl′û-lōs pā′pĕr): a transparent, insoluble paper used to confine the ends of the hair in croquignole permanent waving.

Celsius (sĕl′sē-ûs): in metric measurement, a temperature scale in which the freezing point of water at normal atmospheric pressure is zero degrees and the boiling point is 100 degrees; the centigrade scale.

centigrade (sĕn′tĭ-grād): consisting of 100 divisions or degrees; pertaining to a temperature scale in which the freezing point of water is zero degrees and the boiling point is 100 degrees.

centigrade scale (sĕn′tĭ-grād skāl): a temperature scale in which the freezing point of water is zero degrees and the boiling point is 100 degrees.

centigram (sĕn′tĭ-grăm): in the metric system, the hundredth part of a gram.

centimeter (sĕn′tĭ-mē-tẽr): in the metric system, the hundredth part of a meter.

central nervous system (sĕn′trâl nür′vûs sĭs′tĕm): that part of the nervous system in vertebrates which consists of the brain and spinal cord.

centric (sĕn′trĭk): relating to or having a center; of or relating to a nerve center.

centrifugal movement (sĕn-trĭf′ă-gâl mo͞ov′mĕnt): movement directed away from a center part or point; in massage, the directing of massage movement away from the heart; moving outward from a nerve center.

centriole (sĕn′trē-ōl): a minute structure enclosed within the centrosome of the cell, considered to be the division center of the cell.

centripetal movement (sĕn-trĭp′ĭ-tâl mo͞ov′mĕnt): movement directed toward a center; in massage, a movement directed toward the heart; afferent; toward the central nervous system.

cephalic (sĕ-făl′ĭk): pertaining to the head; directed toward, at on, or near the head.

cephalic vein (sĕ-făl′ĭk vān): the vein of the upper arm.

cerebellum (sĕr-ê-bĕl′ûm): the posterior and lower part of the brain.

cerebral (sē-rē′brâl): pertaining to the brain or the cerebrum.

cerebral allergy (sĕr′ĕ-brâl ăl′ẽr-jē): symptoms of cerebral disturbances associated with certain allergies.

cerebral hemisphere (sē′rē-brâl hĕm′ĭ-sfĭr): one of the two halves of the brain.

cerebrospinal system (sĕr-ĕ-brô-spī′nâl sĭs′tĕm): consists of the brain, spinal cord, spinal nerves and the cranial nerves.

cerebrovascular (sĕr′ĕ-brô-vȧs′kū-lär): pertaining to the blood vessels of the cerebrum (brain).

cerebrum (sĕr-ē′brûm): the upper part of the brain, considered to be the seat of consciousness.

ceresin (sĕr′ē-sĭn): a white or yellow waxy substance made of naturally occurring hydrocarbons, soluble in alcohol, benzine, chloroform and naptha and insoluble in water; used in the manufacture of some cosmetics.

certificate (sẽr-tĭf′ĭ-kĭt): an official document certifying that one has fulfilled the requirements set forth and may practice or work in a particular field.

certification (sûr-tĭ-fĭ-kā′shûn): the act of certifying or guaranteeing certain facts; a written statement verifying something such as completion of a course of study.

certified color (sûr′tĭ-fīd kŭl′ẽr): a commercial coloring product permitted in foods, drugs and cosmetics by the FDA (Federal Food and Drug Administration).

cerumen (sĕ-ro͞o′mên): the waxy substance found within the ear; earwax.

cervical (sûr′vĭ-kâl): pertaining to the

C-D

neck or the neck of any organ or structure.

cervical artery (sûr′vĭ-kâl är′tĭr-ē): deep cervical artery which supplies blood to the deep muscles of the neck and the spinal cord.

cervical cutaneous nerve (sûr′vĭ-kâl kū-tā′nē-ûs nûrv): the nerve that receives stimuli from the front and sides of the neck.

cervical glands (sûr′vĭ-kâl glanz): the lymph nodes of the neck.

cervical nerves (sûr′vĭ-kâl nûrvz): motor sensory nerves affecting the neck muscles and skin, muscles and skin of the upper back, and diaphragm.

cervical vertebrae (sûr′vĭ-kâl vûr′tă-brē): the seven bones of the vertebral column.

cervico facial (sûr′vĭ-kō fā′shûl): pertaining to the face and neck.

cervix (sûr′vĭks): the neck; any neck-like structure.

cetyl alcohol (sēt′l ăl′kôhôl): a fatty alcohol soluble in water, used in lotions and ointments.

cetyl ammonium (sēt′l ă-mō′nē-ŭm): an ammonium compound, fungicide and germicide used in a wide range of cosmetic products, chiefly in creams and deodorants.

cetyl lactate (sēt′l lăk′tāt): cetyl alcohol and lactic acid; an emollient used in cosmetic preparations to improve their texture.

chafe (chāf): to irritate the skin by friction.

chamomile, camomile (kăm′ô-mīl): a plant having strongly scented foliage and flowers which are used in some skin care products; as a brightening rinse for hair and as a healthful tea.

chancre (shăn′kĕr): a sore; the primary lesion of syphilis (a venereal disease) or sporotrichosis; a fungus infection.

channel (chăn′ĕl): in anatomy: a passage for liquids such as blood and lymph channels.

chapped (chăpt): pertaining to a skin condition characterized by rough, red and cracked areas, generally caused by exposure to cold wind and moisture.

characterize (kăr′ăc-tĕr-īz): to indicate, delineate or describe the nature or qualities of a person or object.

character makeup (kăr′ăk-tĕr māk′ŭp): makeup and prosthetics used to create an appearance suitable for the portrayal of a certain character or personality type.

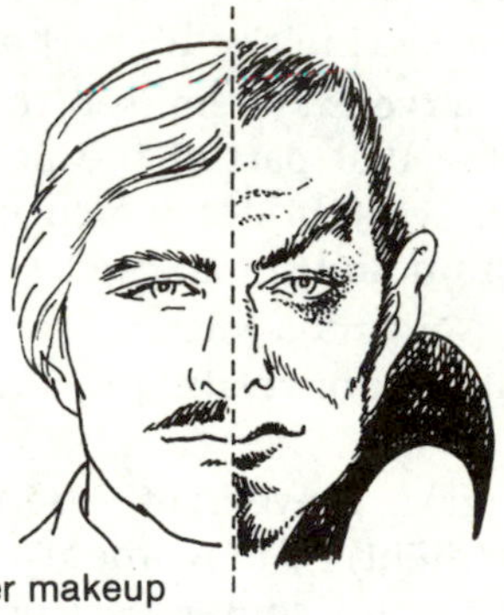

character makeup

charcoal (chär′kōl): a black, porous substance used in pencils or pieces for drawing; a term used to describe a color of lead used in cosmetic eye makeup.

chartreuse (shär-trōōz′): a bright, yellowish green color used in some articles of clothing and in decor.

check (chĕk): in cosmetology, to test, examine or compare; to give a final inspection or examination of a completed hairstyle, makeup or other service.

cheek (chēk): the fleshy part of the sides of the face, below the eyes and above the sides of the mouth.

cheekbone (chēk′bōn): zygomatic bone.

cheek color (chēk kŭl′ẽr): a cream or powder cosmetic used to color the cheek and the skin beneath the cheek bones; also called rouge.

cheilitis (kē′lī-tĭs): dermatitis of the lips usually caused by dyes found in lipsticks; dry, chapped lips.

cheiroplasty (kī′rō-plăs′tē): plastic surgery of the hand.

chemabrasion (kēm′ă-brā′zhûn): a medical process which removes superficial layers of the epidermis and upper layer of the dermis by applying a chemical agent to the skin; used to remove scars and other skin imperfections.

chemical (kĕm′ĭ-kâl): relating to chemistry; a substance of chemical composition.

chemical action (kĕm′ĭ-kâl ăk′shûn): the molecular change produced in a substance through the action of electricity, heat light or another chemical.

chemical blow-out (kĕm′ĕ-kâl blō-out): a chemical hair relaxing technique; a combination of chemical hair straightening and hairstyling for over-curly hair.

chemical bond (kĕm′ĭ-kâl bŏnd): the force exerted by shared electrons that holds atoms together in a molecule.

chemical cauterization (kĕm′ĭ-kâl kô′tẽr-ĭ-zā′shûn): the process by which tissue is destroyed by use of a caustic substance.

chemical change (kĕm′ĭ-kâl chānj): alteration in the chemical composition of a substance.

chemical composition (kĕm′ĭ-kâl kŏm-pō-zĭ′shûn): the balance and proportion of elements which make up a given substance; the formation of compounds.

chemical compound (kĕm′ĭ-kâl kŏm′-pound): a combination of elements chemically united in definite proportions; compounds formed by the chemical combination of the atoms of one element and the atoms of another element or elements.

chemical damage (kĕm′ĭ-kâl dăm′ĭj): the destruction of the protein structure of the hair produced by reactive chemicals during the process of permanent waving, coloring or bleaching of the hair.

chemical dye remover (kĕm′ĭ-kâl dī rē-mōōv′ẽr): a dye remover containing a chemical solvent.

chemical hair processing (kĕm′ĭ-kâl hâr prŏs′ĕs-ĭng): the process of straightening over-curly hair by the use of chemical agents.

chemical hair relaxer (kĕm′ĭ-kâl hâr rē-lăks′ẽr): also called straightener. A chemical agent which is employed to straighten over-curly hair.

chemical sterilizer (kĕm′ĭ-kâl stĕr′ĭ-lī-zẽr): an apparatus that contains chemical agents which sterilize implements by the destruction of living microorganisms.

chemistry (kĕm′ĭs-trē): the science which deals with the composition of substances; the elements and their mutual reactions, and the phenomena resulting from the formation and decomposition of compounds; the science that treats of structure, composition and properties of substances and their transformations.

cherry bark (chĕr′ē bärk): the bark of a cherry tree, used as a soothing astringent and as an ingredient in some hair conditioners to add body to the hair.

chestnut (chĕs′nŭt): a color resembling that of a chestnut; a reddish brown.

chevron (chĕv′răn): in hairstyling, the inverted "V" shape that forms the base curve of the hair shaping.

chiaroscuro (kē-är-ō-skū′rō): a technique of using contrasts of light and dark makeup to emphasize the contours of the face.

chic (shēk): stylish; a term used to describe a fashionable, well-groomed appearance.

chickweed (chĭk′wēd′): an herb used in some cosmetics for its strong cleansing qualities.

chigger (chĭg′ẽr): a red larva of mites that attach to the skin, and whose bites produce a painful, itching wheal.

chignon (shēn′yŏn): a knot or coil of hair worn at the crown of the head or nape of the neck.

chin (chĭn): the anterior prominence of the lower jaw below the mouth; the lower part of the face between the mouth and neck.

chin bone (chĭn bōn): the anterior part of the human mandible; the bone beneath the fleshy part of the chin.

chiropody (kī-rŏp′ô-dē): the art of treating minor diseases of the hands and feet.

chloasma (klô-ăz′mă): large brown irregular patches on the skin, such as liver spots.

Chlorazene (klō′ră-zēn): a trade name; a chemical used for preparing an antiseptic or disinfectant.

chloride (klôr′īd): a compound of chlorine with another element.

chlorinate (klôr′ĭ-nāt): to treat or combine with chlorine.

chlorine (klôr′ēn): greenish, yellow gas with a disagreeable, suffocating odor; used in combined form as a disinfectant and bleaching agent.

chlorophyll (klôr′ô-fĭl): the green coloring matter of plants by which photosynthesis is accomplished; preparations of water soluble chlorophyll derivatives are used in deodorants, in some medicinal preparations and as coloring agents.

cholesterin; cholesterol (kô-lĕs′tẽr-ĭn; -ol): a waxy alcohol found in human and animal tissues and their secretions and important in metabolism; present in lanolin and used as an emulsifier and ingredient in some cosmetics; a constituent of animal fats and oils.

choline (kō′lēn): a vitamin of the B complex group and a component of lecithin, found in animal and vegetable tissues; essential to proper liver function.

chop (chŏp): to cut hair in an irregular pattern; to cut abruptly so a line of demarcation can be seen.

choroid (kôr′oyd): the membrane of the eyeball lying between the sclera (outer membrane) and the retina.

chromatic colors (krō-măt′ĭk kŭl′ẽrs): all colors other than the achromatic (neutral) colors: black, white and gray.

chromatics (krō-măt′ĭks): the science of color.

chromatic vision (krō-măt′ĭk vĭzh-ôn): vision pertaining to the color sense.

chromatologist (krō′mă-tŏl′ô-jĭst): a person who specializes in the technology of hair coloring.

chromatology (krō′mă-tŏl′ô-jē): the science of colors; chromatics.

chromidrosis (krō-mĭ-drō′sĭs): the excretion of colored sweat (also see chromhidrosis).

chromosome (krō′mă-sōm): any of several bodies in the cell neucleus that transmit hereditary characteristics during cell division.

chromotherapy (krō′mō-thĕr′ă-pē):

treatment of disease by use of various colored lights or colors in the surroundings.

chronic (krŏn′ĭk): long continued; the opposite of acute.

chrysarobin (krĭs-ă-rō′bĭn): a powerful parasiticide indicated in various forms of tinea (skin disease).

chuck (chŭk): a term used in massage meaning to strike vigorously.

chucking (chŭck′ĭng): a massage movement (primarily for use on arms) accomplished by grasping the flesh firmly in one hand and moving the hand up and down along the bone, while the other hand keeps the arm in a steady position.

chunky (chŭnk′ē): a term used to describe a blunt haircut which creates weight; also called a club cut.

chyle (kīl): a creamy mixture of fat and lymph formed in the small intestine during digestion.

cicatrix (sĭk′ă-trĭks); pl., **cicatrices** (sĭk-ă-trī′sēz): the skin or film which forms over a wound, later contracting to form a scar.

cilia (sĭl′ē-ă): the eyelashes; microscopic hair-like extensions which assist bacteria in locomotion.

cinnamon oil (sĭn′ă-mŭn oyl): oil of cassia; yellowish brown oil from the leaves and stems of the cinnamon shrub; used as a flavoring and as a fragrance in cosmetics.

circle (sŭr′k'l): a geometric curvature shape, bounded by a circumference having equal radii from the point of origin.

circle design (sûr′k'l dê-zīn′): a design which is created by the equal distribution of straight or curved lines from a center point.

circle end (sûr′k'l ĕnd): the circular part of a pin curl, which determines the size and tightness of the curl.

circle technique (sûr′k'l tĕk′nēk): pertaining to inner and outer circles, a technique in hair setting of expanding a circle by a second row of rollers or pin curls.

circuit (sûr′kĭt): the path of an electric current.

circuit breaker (sûr′kĭt brāk′ẽr): a switch that automatically interrupts an electric circuit.

circuit, broken (sûr′kĭt brō′kĕn): a circumstance in which the current is diverted from its regular circuit.

circuit, closed (sûr′kĭt klōzd): a circuit in which current is continually flowing.

circuit, complete (sûr′kĭt, kôm-plēt′): the path of an electric current in actual operation.

circuit, short (sûr′kĭt, shôrt): a term used when electrical current is diverted from its regular circuit.

circular movements (sûr′kû-lär mōōv′-mênts): in massage: movements (circulatory friction) employed to increase circulation and glandular activity of the skin.

circulation (sûr-kû-lā′shûn): the passage of blood throughout the body.

circulation, general (jĕn′ẽr-âl): blood circulation from the heart throughout the body and back again.

circulation, pulmonary (sûr-kû-lā-shûn, pōōl′mă-nĕr-ē): blood circulation from the heart to the lungs and back to the heart.

circulatory system (sûr′kû-lă-tôr-ē sĭs′-tĕm): the system which carries blood from the heart to all parts of the body and back to the heart, circulating oxygen and nutrients for and wastes from the entire body.

circulatory vessels (sûr′kû-lă-tôr-ē

vĕs′'ls): the blood vessels of the circulatory system consisting of the large arteries (muscular), small arteries (arterioles), capillaries and veins.

circumference (sûr-kŭm′fĕr-ĕns): the outside boundary of a circle.

citral (sĭ′trăl): a liquid aldehyde, found in citrus fruits, oil of lemon, oil of lime and grapefruit; used in fragrances and cosmetic products for its pleasant odor.

citric acid (sĭt′rĭk ăs′ĭd): acid found in fruits such as lemons, limes, oranges and grapefruit, and often added to finishing rinses to smooth tangles and increase the sheen of the hair.

civet (sĭv′ĭt): the yellowish, fatty substance with a musk-like scent secreted by a gland of the genitalia of the civet cat; use as a fixative in perfumes.

civet cat (sĭv′ĭt kăt): a large cat-like animal with yellowish, spotted fur and valued for its civet; generally, the civet cat is found in Africa and India.

clamp (klămp): a small device used to hold a wave in place; in medicine, a surgical instrument for holding or compressing.

clamp (klămp), **table top:** a device employed to hold another object, such as a mannequin head, or for compressing something within its parts; used in wig styling to hold or steady the wood or canvas wig block.

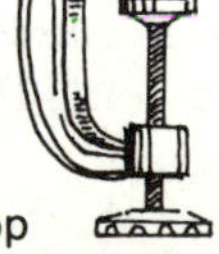

clamp, table top

clapping (klăp′ĭng): a movement in body massage accomplished by striking the area of skin with the palm of the hand slightly cupped.

clasp (klăsp): a bar with a catch or hook used to hold the hair in place, similar to a barrette; a catch or hook used to hold two parts together such as an opening in a garment.

classic (klăs′ĭk): belonging to a first class or highest rank; approved; accepted as in good taste; standard of excellence; as a classic hairstyle.

classic style (klăs′ĭk stīl): a hairstyle which is universally accepted and continues to be used.

clavicle (klăv′ĭ-k'l): collarbone joining the sternum and scapula.

clay (klā): an earthy substance containing kaolin; used for facial masks and packs.

clay mask (klā măsk): also called a clay pack; a colloidal clay preparation used in facial treatments to stimulate circulation and temporarily contract the pores of the skin; usually recommended for oily and blemished skin.

clean (klēn): the quality of being free from dirt, pollution or other offensive substances.

clean-cut (klēn-kŭt): neatly groomed; in hairstyling, hair that is sharply defined; to cut smooth and even.

cleaning solution (klēn′ĭng sô-lū′shûn): a liquid cleaning product especially formulated for wigs and hairpieces; both wet and dry cleaning solutions are used to clean various wig types.

cleanse (klĕnz): to clean or purify.

cleansing cream (klĕnz′ĭng krēm): a light-textured cream whose main purpose is to dissolve makeup and soil quickly.

cleansing lotion (klĕnz′ĭng lō′shûn): a lotion formulated to remove makeup and soil.

clear (klēr): free of blemishes; transparent or translucent; without cloudiness or murkiness.

cleido (klī′dô): a prefix meaning pertaining to the clavicle.

clinic (klĭn′ĭk): pertaining to an establishment where patrons can receive services, such as the cosmetology school clinic; medical clinic: an establishment where patients are received and treated.

clip (klĭp): a metal or plastic lever-type device used to secure pin curls, waves or hair rollers.

clipper (klĭp′ẽr): a haircutting implement with a fine, medium or coarse tooth cutting edge; hand or electric clippers.

clipper oil (klĭp′ẽr oyl): a lubricant which reduces friction, heat and wear when used between the two blades of a hair clipper.

clipping (klĭp′ĭng): the act of cutting split hair ends with the shears or the scissors; the operation of removing the hair by the use of hair clippers.

clockwise (klŏk′wīz): the movement of hair, in shapings or curls, in the same direction as the hands of a clock.

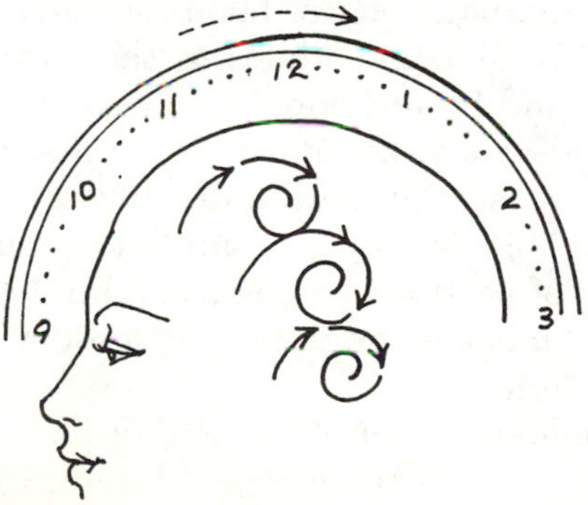

clockwise

clog (klŏg): to obstruct; to hamper; fill up; as a clogged pore.

closed end (klōz′d ĕnd): the rounded (convex) end of a shaping or wave.

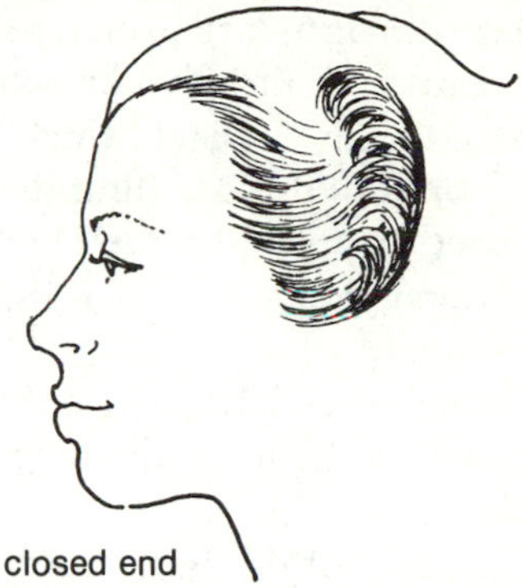

closed end

clot (klŏt): a mass or lump of coagulated blood.

clotting (klŏt′ĭng): forming into a mass of coagulated fluid or soft matter such as blood or cream; in blood, caused by exposure of the blood's fibrinogen to oxygen; in cream, the separating of the whey from the coagulated curd as certain bacteria colonies develop.

cloudy (klaů′dē): not clear; dull in color; murky.

clove (klōv): an herb used in some astringents and antiseptics; an herb (spice) used in cookery.

club cutting (klŭb kŭt′ĭng): cutting the hair straight off without thinning, slithering or tapering; a technique used to cut bangs and to cut ends the same length.

club hair (klŭb hâr): a condition caused by the root of the hair being surrounded by an enlarged substance made up of keratinized cells which occurs before normal hair loss.

cluster (klŭs′tẽr): to gather in a mass or group.

cluster curls (klŭs′tẽr kûrlz): artificial

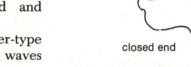

curls which can be pinned singly or in groups to the wearer's own hair.

coagulant (kô-ăg′û-lĕnt): a substance that produces coagulation.

coagulate (kô-ăg′û-lāt): to clot; to convert a fluid into a soft jelly-like solid.

coal tar (kōl tär): a black, thick, opaque liquid obtained from bituminous coal and used to make cosmetic colors.

coarse (kôrs): rough or thick in texture; not delicate.

coarse hair (kôrs hâr): a hair fiber that is relatively large in diameter or circumference.

coated hair (kōt′ĕd hâr): hair covered with a substance which interferes with and retards the action of chemicals upon the hair fiber.

coating (kōt′ĭng): residue left on the hair shaft; coating conditioner which does not penetrate into the hair but coats the hair shaft.

cocci bacteria (kŏk′sī băk-tē′rē-ă): a form of pathogenic bacteria; disease causing bacteria.

coccus (kŏk′ûs); pl., **cocci** (kŏk′sī): spherical cell bacterium appearing singly or in a group.

coccyx (kŏk′sĭks): the last bone in the vertebral column; tailbone.

cocoa butter (kō′kô bŭt′ĕr): a hard, yellowish fatty substance obtained from cocoa seeds; used in the manufacture of some soaps and cosmetics.

coconut oil (kō′kŏ-nŭt oyl): the oil extracted from the meat of the coconut, used in the manufacture of soaps and shampoos because of its high lathering quality.

coif (kwŏf): a close fitting cap; a hairstyle; to arrange or style the hair.

coiffeur (kwä-fūr′): French term; a male hairdresser.

coiffeuse (kwä-fūs′): French term: a female hairdresser.

coiffure (kwä-fūr′): an arrangement, styling or dressing of the hair; a finished hairstyle.

coil (koyl): to twist or wind the hair spirally: the spiral duct from the sweat (sudoriferous) gland to the epidermis.

cold cream (kōld krēm): a cleansing ointment for the skin.

cold pack (kōld păk): wet wrappings placed around the body as a form of therapy.

cold sore (kōld sôr): an eruption or sore around the mouth or nostril, often occurring during a cold or fever; medical name, herpes labialis.

cold waving (kōld wāv′ĭng): a system of permanent waving involving the use of chemicals rather than heating equipment.

cold waving lotion (kōld wāv′ĭng lō′-shûn): a chemical solution which breaks S-bonds (sulphur) so that curl may be formed in hair wrapped around rods.

collagen (kŏl′ă-jĕn): a protein forming the chief constituent of the connective tissues and bones; used in some cosmetics, such as face creams.

collapse (kô-lăps′): an abnormal sinking or retraction of the walls of an organ.

collarbone (kŏl′ĕr-bōn): the clavicle; the bone connecting the shoulder blade and breastbone.

collodion (kô-lō′dē-ôn): a thick viscous substance used to dress wounds.

colloid (kŏl′oyd): a substance consisting of particles having a certain degree of fineness and possessing a sticky consistency.

cologne (kă-lōn′): a toilet water consisting of alcohol scented with aromatic oils; a lighter fragrance than perfume.

color (kŭl′ẽr): any tint or hue distinguished from white; achromatic colors include black, white and the range of grays in between; chromatic colors are all other colors.

color blender (kŭl′ẽr blĕnd′ẽr): a preparation which cleanses, highlights and blends gray hair.

color blind (kŭl′ẽr blīnd): partial or total inability to distinguish one or more chromatic colors.

color builder (kŭl′ẽr bĭl′dẽr): a color filler employed on damaged or over-porous hair in order that it take and hold color evenly.

color catalyst (kŭl′ẽr kăt′ă-lĕst): a chemical preparation added to hair tint to aid penetration of the product and improve coverage; helps to eliminate a harsh, reddish, brassy cast.

color chart (kŭl′ẽr chärt): a chart of colors produced by manufacturers of hair-coloring products to serve as a guide in selecting appropriate colors; the color is shown as it would appear after application to white hair.

color developer (kŭl′ẽr dē-vĕl′ă-pẽr): an oxidizing agent, usually hydrogen peroxide, which is added to coloring agents before application to develop the color during processing.

color etching (kŭl′ẽr ĕch′ĭng): a technique of highlighting the hair by combing a frosting product through the hair.

colorfast (kŭl′ẽr-făst): resistant to fading or running.

colorfast shampoo (kŭl′ẽr-făst shăm-pōō′): a shampoo especially prepared to cleanse the hair and protect the color stability of hair that has been lightened or tinted.

color filler (kŭl′ẽr fĭl′ẽr): a preparation used to revitalize and correct abused or damaged hair, to equalize porosity and deposit a base color prior to tinting.

colorful (kŭl′ẽr-făl): vivid; full of color, especially constrating colors.

colorimeter (kŭl-ă-rĭm′ĕt-ẽr): an apparatus for determining color and color intensity.

colorist (kŭl′ẽr-ĭst): a cosmetologist who specializes in the application of hair color.

colorless (kŭl′ẽr-lĕs): lacking color; dull, uninteresting.

color lift (kŭl′ẽr lĭft): the amount of natural or artificial color pigment which is removed by some other substance.

color lifter (kŭl′ẽr lĭft′ẽr): a chemical designed to remove artificial color from the hair.

color, makeup (kŭl′ẽr, māk′ŭp): color used in makeup; eye color, lip color, cheek color; foundation color, etc.

color mixing (kŭl′ẽr mĭks′ĭng): mixing two or more colors together in order to obtain some in-between shade or tint.

color palette (kŭl′ẽr păl′ĕt): a selection of colors arranged on a kidney-shaped board or in a flat container; used by artists and makeup artists.

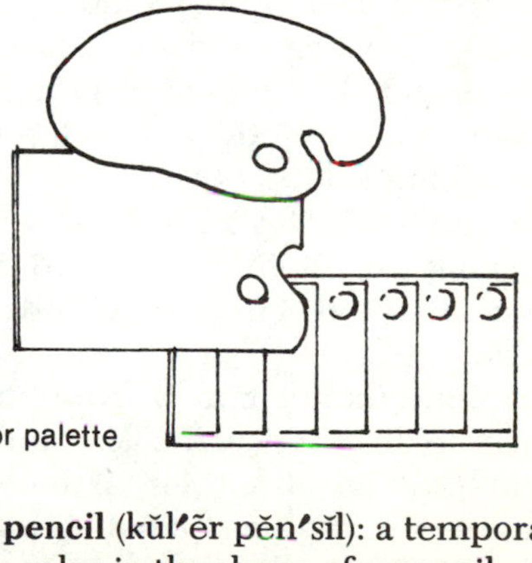

color palette

color pencil (kŭl′ẽr pĕn′sĭl): a temporary hair color in the shape of a pencil used to add color to the scalp where the hair is thin; a pencil with colored lead used as a makeup item.

color, personal (kŭl′ẽr, pẽr′sôn-âl): an individual's hair, eye and skin colors.

color pigment (kŭl′ẽr pĭg′mênt): the organic coloring matter of the body; substances that impart color to animal or vegetable tissues, as chlorophyll and melanin.

color pigment, hair (kŭl′ẽr pĭg′mênt, hâr): pigment found in the cortex layer of the hair.

color pigment, skin (kŭl′ẽr pĭg′mênt, skĭn): coloring matter of the skin: melanin, hemoglobin (oxygenated and reduced) and carotenes.

color psychology (kŭl′ẽr sī-kŏl′ô-jē): the science of color as it affects the emotions.

color remover (kŭl′ẽr rē-mo͞ov′ẽr): a prepared commercial product which removes tint from the hair.

color rinse (kŭl′ẽr rĭns): a rinse which gives a temporary tint to the hair.

color shampoo (kŭl′ẽr shăm-po͞o′): a preparation which colors the hair permanently without requiring presoftening treatment.

color stick (kŭl′ẽr stĭk): a crayon used to color new hair growth temporarily between permanent color treatments.

color swatch (kŭl′ẽr swŏch): a small sample of hair or cloth used to determine matching colors.

color test (kŭl′ẽr tĕst): a method of determining the action of a selected tint on a small strand of hair; also called strand test.

color tone (kŭl′ẽr tōn): a shade, tint or degree of a particular color, or a slight modification of a color, as blue with a green undertone or red with an orange tone.

color value (kŭl′ẽr văl′ū): the degree of shading, lightness or darkness of a color.

color vision (kŭl′ẽr vĭzh′ŭn): the ability to see and distinguish colors.

color wheel (kŭl′ẽr wēl): a chart, usually circular, used for selecting colors for hair, makeup, clothing and decorating; shows harmonizing and contrasting colors.

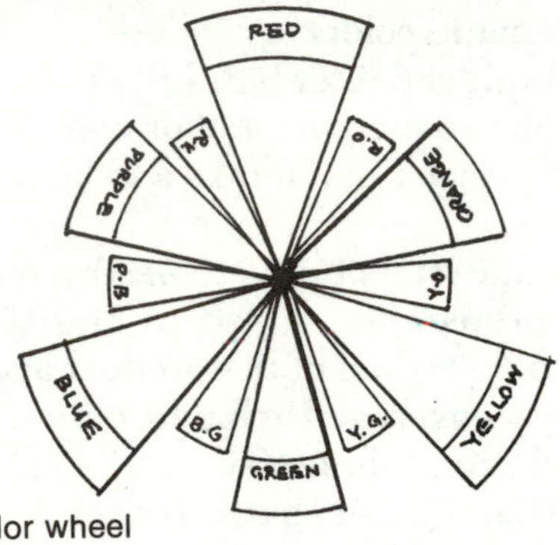

color wheel

coltsfoot (kōlts′fo͝ot): an herb bearing yellow flowers used for medicinal purposes.

comb (kōm): a toothed strip of plastic, metal, bone or other material used to groom and hold the hair in place; decorative combs are often used to enhance a hairstyle.

comb and brush cleaner (kōm and brŭsh klēn′ẽr): a powdered or liquid substance, usually diluted in water and used to clean combs and brushes.

comb out (kōm aůt): the opening and blending of the hair setting, curls or waves, into the finished style, using a hairbrush and/or comb.

combustion (kôm-bûs′chûn): the rapid oxidation of any substance, accompanied by the production of heat and light.

comedo (kŏm′ĕ-dō); pl., **comedones** (kŏm′ē-dōnz): blackhead; a worm-like mass in an obstructed sebaceous duct.

comedone extractor (kŏm′ĕ-dōn ĕks-străk′tẽr): an instrument sometimes used as an aid in removing blackheads.

comfrey (kŭm′frē): an herb whose root contains tannin; used as a tea to aid bodily functions, and in some cosmetic preparations for its astringent, soothing and healing qualities.

common carotid artery (kŏm′ûn kă-rŏt′ĭd är′tŭr-ē): the artery that supplies blood to the face, head and neck.

communicable (kă-mū′nĭ-kă-b'l): able to be communicated; transferable; as a communicable disease.

commutator (kŏm′û-tā-tẽr): an instrument for automatically interrupting or reversing the flow of electric current.

comose (kō′mōs): having soft hair.

compact (kŏm′păkt): closely united; dense; solid; a container, usually having a mirror on one side and a space for a cosmetic such as powder, eye or lip makeup.

compact bone (kŏm′păkt bōn): hard bone tissue that forms the outer covering of a bone.

compact tissue (kŏm′păkt tĭsh′ū): a dense, hard type of bony tissue.

complement (kŏm′plă-mĕnt): something that completes or makes perfect.

complementary (kŏm-plă-mĕn′tẽr-ē): serving as a complement; to fill out or complete.

complementary colors (kŏm-plă-mĕn′-tẽr-ē kŭl′ẽrz): any two colors of the spectrum which combine to form white or whitish light; two colors whose mixture produces a third color; colors that lie opposite on the color wheel.

complex (kŏm-plĕks′): complicated; intricate; difficult to analyze.

complexion (kôm-plĕk′shûn): hue or general appearance of the skin, especially the face.

compliment (kŏm′plĭ-mĕnt): an expression of admiration, praise or congratulation.

complimentary (kŏm-plĭ-mĕn′tẽr-ē): given free as a favor or courtesy.

component (kŏm-pō′nênt): one of the parts of a whole; a constituent part; an ingredient.

composition (kŏm-pô-zĭsh′ûn): the kind and number of atoms constituting the molecule of a substance.

compound (kŏm′paůnd): a substance formed by a chemical union of two or more elements, and different from any of them.

compound henna (kŏm′paůnd hĕn′ă): Egyptian henna to which has been added one or more metallic preparations.

comprehend (kŏm-prē-hĕnd′): to grasp mentally; to understand.

compress (kŏm′prĕs): a folded strip of cotton or cloth forming a pad which is pressed upon the face or a part of the body; cotton compress as used in facial treatments.

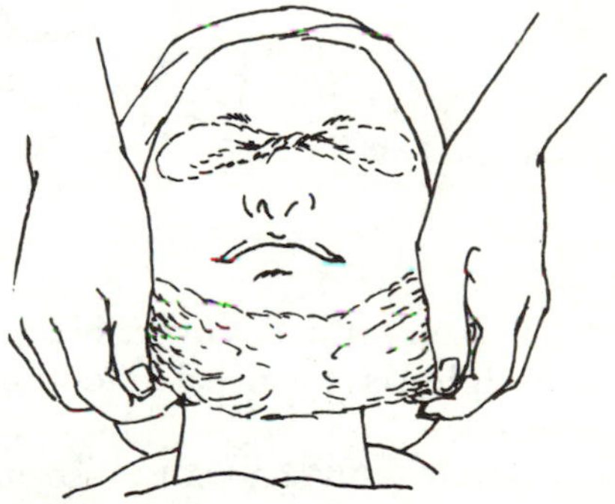

compress

compressor (kôm-prĕs′ẽr): a muscle that presses; an instrument for applying pressure on a blood vessel to prevent loss of blood.

compressor nasi (kôm-prĕs′ẽr nā′zī): the muscle which compresses the nostrils.

concave (kŏn-kāv′): hollow and round or curving inward; concave profile, a face having a prominent forehead and chin with other features receded inward; the opposite of convex.

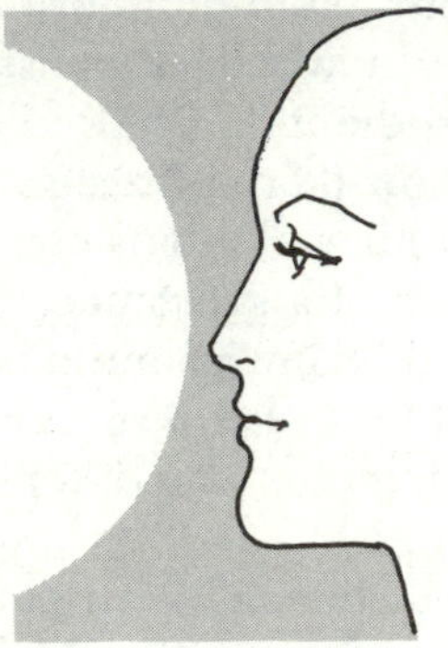

concave profile

concave rod (kŏn′kāv rŏd): a cold wave rod which has a smaller circumference in the center and increases to a larger circumference at both ends.

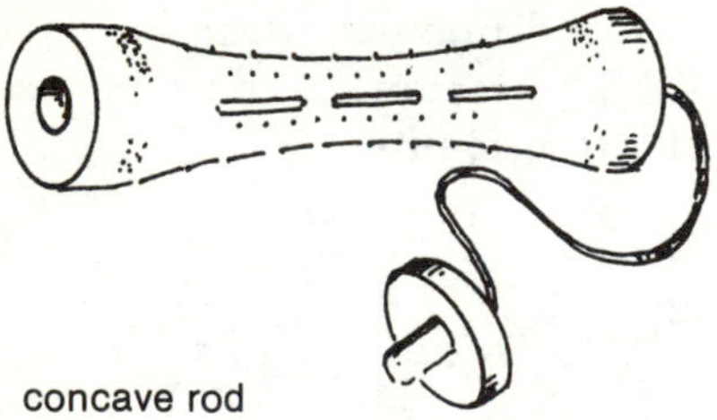

concave rod

conceal (kŏn-sēl′): to cover; hide; keep from sight; as to conceal a blemish with cosmetics.

concentrate (kŏn′sĕn-trāt): a strong or undiluted substance or solution; to make less dilute.

concentrated (kŏn′sĕn-trāt-ĕd): condensed; increased the strength by diminishing the bulk.

concentric (kŏn-sĕn′trĭk): having a common center, such as curls, waves and other movements of the hair that radiate from a common center.

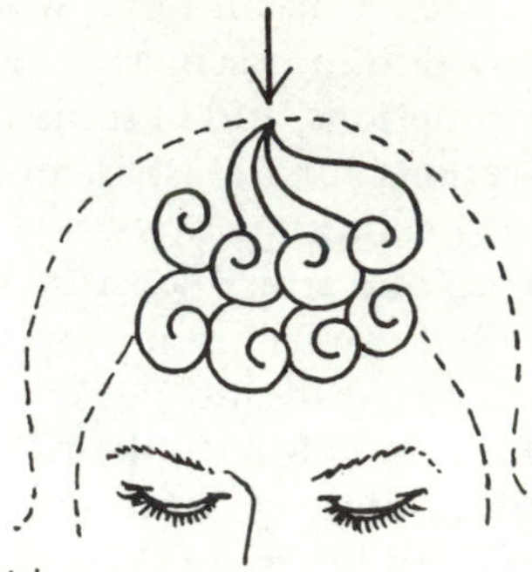

concentric

concha (kŏn′kă): a structure comparable to a shell in shape, as the auricle or pinna of the ear or a turbinated bone in the nose.

concise (kôn sīs′): brief and comprehensive.

condensation (kŏn-dĕn-sā′shûn): act of changing a gas or vapor to a liquid; reduction to a denser form.

condition (kŏn-dĭ′shûn): to protect or restore the natural strength and body of the hair; the state of health of the hair, such as too dry, too oily, damaged, normal, porous, etc.

conditioner (kŏn-dĭ′shûn-ẽr): a special chemical agent applied to the hair to help restore its strength and give it body to protect it against possible breakage.

condition filler (kŏn-dĭ′shŭn fĭl′ẽr): a cosmetic preparation used to recondition and correct damaged hair.

conditioning (kŏn-dĭ′shŭn-ĭng): the application of special chemical agents to the hair to help restore its strength and to give it body to protect it against possible breakage; descriptive of conditioning shampoos and rinses which help to normalize the condition of the hair.

conducting cords (kôn-dŭckt′ĭng kôrdz): insulated copper wires which convey the current from the wall plate to the patron and the cosmetologist who is performing the service.

conductivity (kôn-dŭk-tĭv′ĭ-tē): the capacity to transmit sound, heat or electricity.

conductor (kôn-dŭk′tẽr): any substance, material or medium that conducts electricity, heat or sound.

condyle (kôn′dĭl): a rounded articular surface at the extremity of a bone.

condyloid (kôn′dĭ-loyd): relating to or resembling a condyle.

cone-shaped curl (kōn-shāpt kûrl): a curl formed to be smaller at the end of the hair shaft and larger at the scalp.

congeal (kŏn-jēl′): to change from a fluid to a solid condition as by freezing or curdling to change to a jelly-like substance.

congenital (kŏn-jĕn′ĭ-tâl): pertaining to a condition existing at birth.

congestion (kŏn-jĕs′chŭn): excessive or abnormal accumulation of fluid in the vessels of an organ or body part; usually blood, but occasionally bile or mucus; this condition occurs in some diseases, infections or injuries.

conical (kŏn′ĭ-kâl): resembling the shape of a cone; as a cone-shaped curl or hairpiece.

conical hair roller (kōn′ĭ-kûl hâr rōl′ẽr): a cone-shaped hair roller.

connect (kôn-ĕkt′): to join or fasten together; link; associate.

connecting (kôn-ĕkt′ĭng): in fingerwaving; the joining of a ridge of wave from one side of the head with the ridge of a wave from the opposite side of the head.

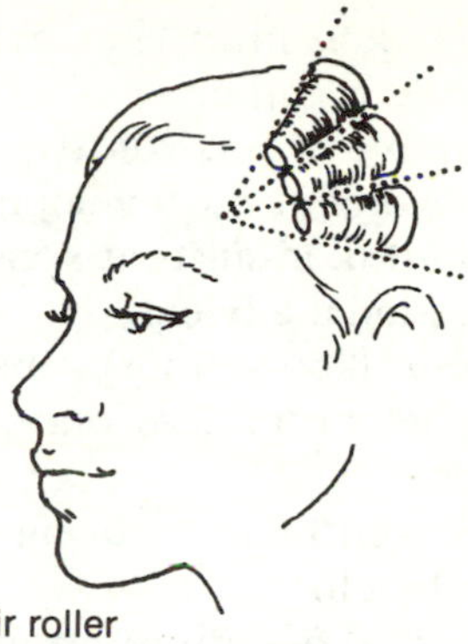

conical hair roller

connecting cords (kôn-ĕkt′ĭng kôrdz): the insulated strands of copper wires which join the apparatus and the commercial electric current.

connecting line (kôn-ĕkt′ĭng līn): a line blending two circular shapes of clockwise and counterclockwise forces; also referred to as a blending; connection between two or more shapes, referred to as blending, dovetailing and dividing.

connective tissue (kō-nĕk′tĭv tĭsh′o͞o): fibrous tissue that unites and supports the various parts of the body such as bone, cartilage or tendons.

consistency (kôn-sĭs′tĕn-sē): the degree of density, solidity or firmness of either a solid or a fluid.

constant base factor (kŏn′stănt bās făk′tẽr): in hair coloring: the factor that enhances warm tones and adds depth to dark shades; an ingredient in color formulation which neutralizes and balances color and prevents brassy tones.

constituent (kôn-stĭt′û-ênt): a necessary part or element of something; that which composes or makes up something.

constitutional (kŏn-stĭ-tū′shŭn-âl): belonging to or affecting the physical or vital powers of an individual.

C-D

constrict (kôn-strĭkt′): to make narrow; pressing together.

constructive (kôn-strŭk′tĭv): promoting improvement or development.

consultant (kôn-sŭl′tênt): one who gives professional advice.

consumer (kôn-sū′mẽr): one who uses materials or services; one of the buying public.

contact (kŏn′tăkt): to bring together so as to touch.

contagion (kôn-tā′jûn): transmission of specific diseases by direct or indirect contact.

contagiosa (kōn-tā-jē-ō′să): impetigo; a form of impetigo marked by flat vesicles that first become pustular, then crusted.

contagious (kôn-tā′jûs): transmittable by contact.

contagium animatum (kôn-tā′jē-ûm ăn′ĭ-mā-tûm): any living or animal organism that causes the spread of an infectious disease.

contaminate (kôn-tăm ĭ-nāt): to make impure by contact; to taint or pollute.

contamination (kôn-tăm-ĭ-nā′shûn): pollution; soiling with infectious matter.

contemporary (kôn-tĕm′pă-rĕr-ē): belonging to the same age; living or occurring at the same time.

contemporary style (kôn-tĕm′pă-rĕr-ē stīl): a current style in dress, hairstyle, makeup, etc., which is accepted and worn at the present time; modern.

contiguous (kôn-tĭg′û-ûs): in contact; touching; adjoining.

contour (kŏn′to͞or): the outline of a figure or body particularly one that curves; to shape the outline or shape something so as to fit the outline.

contour coloring (kŏn′to͞or kŭl′ẽr-ĭng): to shade or highlight the contours of a hairstyle with hair color; to use makeup to create shading or highlighting on the contours of the face.

contouring (kŏn′to͞or-ĭng): a makeup technique which utilizes the principles of light and shadow to sculpture or contour the face; used in theatrical and corrective makeup.

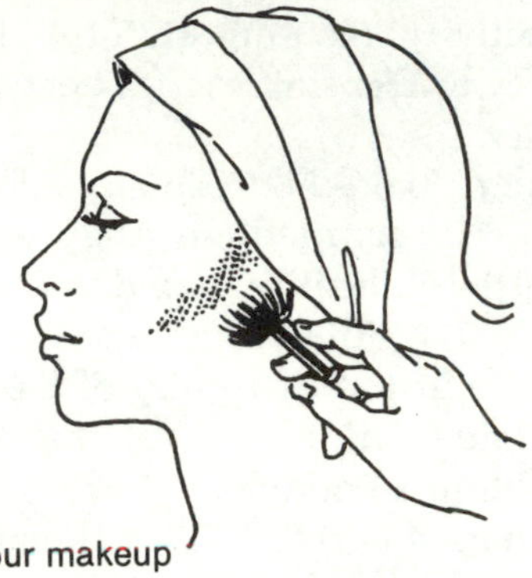

contour makeup

contour makeup (kŏn′to͞or māk′ŭp): a cream or powdered makeup used to create optical illusions by the shading and highlighting of facial features.

contour of hairstyle (kŏn′to͞or ŭv hâr′-stīl): the outline of the finished hairstyle.

contra (kŏn′tră): a prefix denoting against, opposite, contrary.

contract (kôn-trăkt′): to draw together; to acquire a disease by contagion.

contractible (kŏn-trăk′tĭ-b'l): having the ability to contract.

contractility (kŏn-trăk-tĭl′ĭ-tē): the property of contracting or shortening.

contraction (kôn-trăk′shûn): the act of shrinking or drawing together; the shortening and thickening of a functioning muscle.

contrary (kŏn′trâ-rē): in opposition.

contrast (kŏn′trăst): a striking difference which appears by comparison.

control (kôn-trōl′): to direct, regulate or influence; in experiments, a standard by which experimental observations may be studied and evaluated, as in determining safe or unsafe ingredients in products.

control brushing (kôn-trōl′ brŭsh′ing): in hairstyling: a comb-out technique to relax the setting pattern; hair is brushed with one hand while the palm of the other hand molds the hair into design lines.

controller (kôn-trōl′ẽr): a magnetic device for the regulation and control of an electric current.

convalesce (kôn-vă-lĕs′): to recover health and strength gradually after illness.

conventional (kôn-vĕn′shûn-âl): growing out of established customs; lacking in originality or spontaneity.

converge (kôn-vûrj′): to come together at a particular point.

conversion (kôn-vûr′shŭn): the act of converting or being converted in condition, substance, form or function.

conversion layer (kôn-vûr′zhŭn lā′ẽr): a cutting technique used to increase length; hair is directed opposite the area of the desired length increase.

converter (kôn-vûr′tẽr): an apparatus used to convert direct current to alternating current or alternating current to direct current.

convertible cut (kôn-vûr′tĭ-b'l kŭt): a haircut which can be styled in a variety of ways.

convex (kôn-vĕks′): curving outward like an exterior segment of a circle; in a convex profile, the forehead and chin recedes.

convolve (kôn-vŏlv′): to roll together; to coil, wind or twist as in braiding the hair.

convulsion (kôn-vŭl′shûn): an abnormal, violent, involuntary muscular contraction or series of contractions.

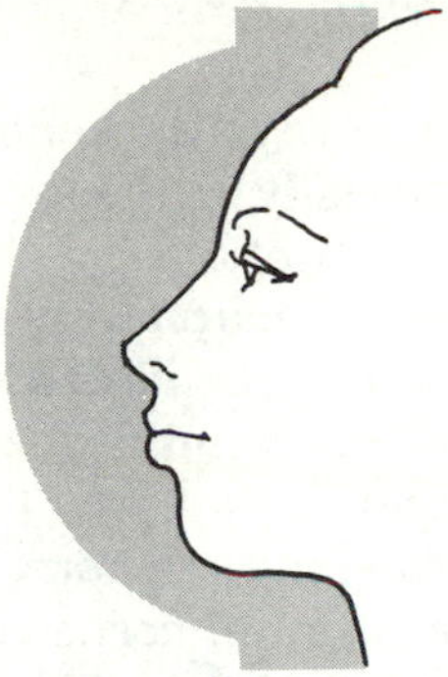

convex

coolant (ko͞ol′ênt): a substance, usually liquid, used as a cooling agent.

cool colors (ko͞ol kŭl′ẽrs): colors suggesting coolness; in hair colors, white, grey platinum, silver grey, steel gray, ash blond, blue grey; in clothing, blue, green and violet.

cooling period (ko͞ol′ĭng pĭr′ē-ŏd): a waiting period, generally ten minutes, before removing permanent wave rods from the hair following the neutralizing process.

coordinate (kō-ôr′dĭ-nāt): to bring into harmonious relationship, as to harmonize hair, makeup and clothing colors.

copious (kō′pē-ûs): large in amount.

copper (kŏp′ẽr): a metallic element that is a good conductor of heat and electricity.

copper color (kŏp′ẽr kŭl′ẽr): a reddish-gold color of hair resembling the color of copper.

coracoid (kŏr′ă-koyd): a projecting part of the shoulder blade.

core (kôr): the central or most vital part of anything.

corium (kō′rē-ûm): the dermis or true skin; the layer of the skin deeper than the epidermis, consisting of a dense bed of vascular connective tissue; also called cutis vera.

corkscrew curl (kôrk′skro͞o kûrl): strands

C-D

of hair having the form of a corkscrew spiral.

corn (kôrn): a horny, thickened, small area of skin, usually on the toes, caused by pressure or friction.

corner (kôr′nẽr): in haircutting and styling, a point where the direction or outline changes; the point formed where two lines meet.

corneum (kôr′nê-ûm): the horny layer of the skin; the stratum corneum.

cornflower (kôrn′flaü-ẽr): an herb used in some cosmetic preparations for its astringent, moisturizing and softening qualities.

cornification (kôr-nĭ-fĭ-kā′shûn): the process of becoming a horny substance or tissue.

corn oil (kôrn oyl): a concentrated oil from corn used in shampoo and in some skin preparations; also used in cookery.

corn rowing (kôrn′ rō-ĭng): a technique used in creating a hairstyle incorporating intricate braiding and braided patterns; strands of hair are woven to create narrow rows of braids which lie close to the scalp.

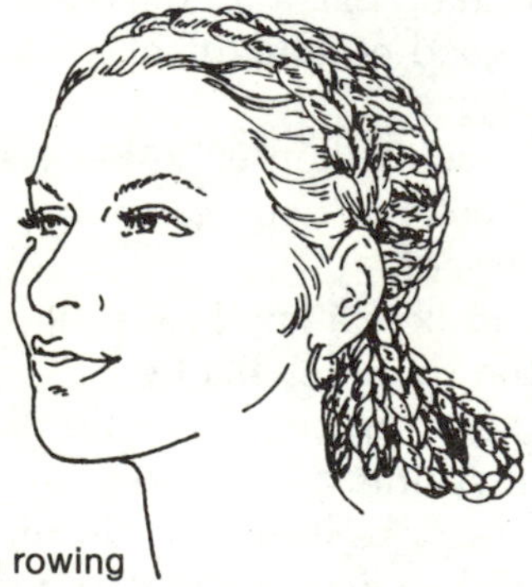
corn rowing

corn silk (kôrn′ sĭlk): the soft silky strands on an ear of corn which are commonly used in facial masks and powdered makeup.

cornstarch (kôrn′stärch): a very fine flour obtained from corn, used as a thickening agent in some cosmetics and foods.

corona (kă-rō′nă): a crown-like structure as the top of the head, or a crown-like braid of hair.

coronal suture (kôr′ô-nâl sū-chẽr): the line of junction of the frontal bone with the two parietal bones of the skull.

coronary (kŏr′ă-nĕr-ē): relating to a crown; a term applied to vessels, nerves or attachments that encircle a part or an organ; pertaining to either of two arteries of the aorta which supply blood to the heart muscle.

coronoid (kŏr′ô-noyd): crown-shaped, as the process of the large bone of the forearm or of the jaw.

corpus (kôr′pûs): a body; the human body.

corpuscle (kôr′pŭs′l): a small mass or body; a minute cell; a cell found in the blood.

corpuscle, red (kôr′pŭs′l, rĕd): cells in blood whose function is to carry oxygen to the cells.

corpuscle, white (kôr′pŭs′l, whīt): cells in the blood whose function is to destroy disease germs.

corrective makeup (kă-rĕk′tĭv māk′ŭp): a procedure using a makeup product such as a cream or stick to cover blemishes or birthmarks and to bring uneven facial features into balance.

corrode (kô-rōd): to eat away or destroy gradually, usually by chemical action.

corrosive (kô-rō′sĭv): having the power to corrode; a substance that eats away or destroys.

corrugated (kŏr′ōō-gāt-ĕd): formed or shaped in wrinkles or folds or alternate ridges and grooves.

corrugator supercilli (kŏr′ōō-gā′tẽr sū′-

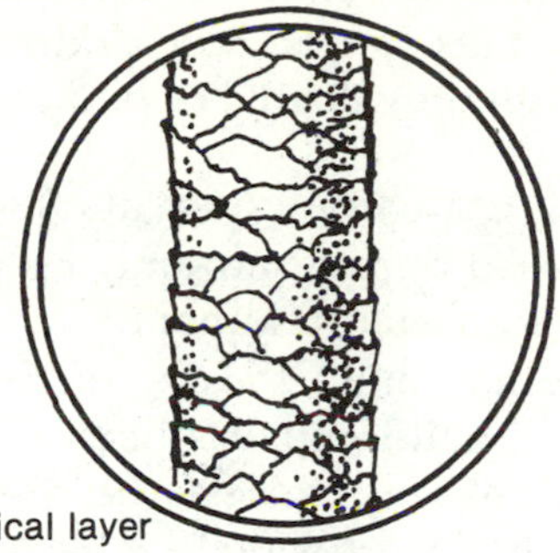

pĕr-sĭl′lē): muscle that draws eyebrows inward and downward.

cortex (kôr′tĕks): the second or middle layer of the hair shaft; the external portion of the adrenal glands.

cortical (kôr′tĭ-kâl): pertaining to or consisting of the outer portion; the bark or rind, or outer layer (cortex) of the hair.

cortical fibers (kôr′tĭ-kâl fī′bĕrz): fibers that make up the cortex of the hair.

cortisone (kôr′tĭ-sōn): a powerful hormone extracted from the cortex of the adrenal gland and also made synthetically: used in the treatment of disease and some diseases of the skin.

corynebacterium (kŏ′rĭ-nē-băk-tē′rē-ûm): pathogenic bacterium which spreads infection and is usually present in acne lesions along with other bacteria.

coryza (kô-rū′ză): an acute condition affecting the nasal mucous membranes associated with the common cold, causing a discharge from the nostrils.

cosmetic (kŏs-mĕt′ĭk): any external preparation intended to beautify the skin, hair or other areas of the body.

cosmetic acne (kŏz-mĕt′ĭk ăk′nē): a skin disorder caused by hormonal changes in the body during puberty; acne that becomes activated by improper cleansing and improper use of cosmetics.

cosmetic dermatology (kŏz-mĕt′ĭk dûr-mă-tŏl′ô-jē): a branch of dermatology devoted to improving the health and beauty of the skin and its appendages.

cosmetician (kŏz-mĕ-tĭsh′ăn): one trained in the use and/or art of selling and demonstrating the application of cosmetics.

cosmetic surgery (kŏz-mĕt′ĭk sûr′jă-rē): plastic surgery performed to correct and beautify the face or body.

cosmetic therapy (kŏz-mĕt′ĭk thĕr′ă-pē): a term used by some state boards to designate the practice of cosmetology; cosmetic treatments for skin, hair or nail disorders.

cosmetologist (kŏz-mĕ-tŏl′ô-jĭst): one skilled in the science and practice of cosmetology.

cosmetology (kŏs-mĕ-tŏl′ô-jē): the art or science of beautifying and improving the skin, nails and hair: the study of cosmetics and their application.

cosmopolitan (kŏz-mă-pŏl′ĭt'n): common to all the world; not limited to one area or locality.

costal (kŏs′tâl): pertaining to a rib or rib-like structure.

cotton (kŏt′'n): a soft, fibrous material, usually white or light yellow, of high cellulose content, from the seed of the cotton plant; used widely as a textile.

cotton cleansing pads (kŏt′'n klĕnz′ĭng pădz): small round or square pads made of beautician's cotton; used as eye pads and for cleansing during facial treatments.

cotton compress mask (kŏt′'n kŏm′prĕs măsk): strips of cosmetologist's cotton moistened in water and applied to the face to aid in the removal of a treatment mask.

C-D

cotton mitts (kŏt′'n mĭtz): strips of cotton wrapped around the fingers and used to remove cosmetic products following cleansing or a facial treatment.

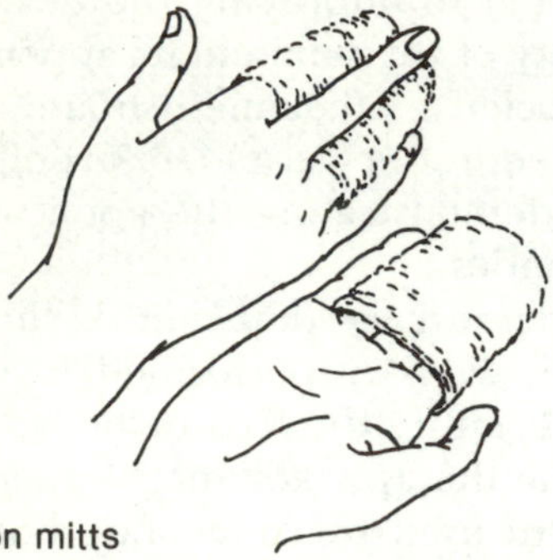

cotton mitts

cottonseed oil (kŏt′'n sēd oyl): a pale yellow, odorless, oily liquid pressed from the seed of the cotton plant; used in creams, lotions, soaps, lubricants and polish remover.

counteract (kaůn-tẽr-ăkt′): to neutralize or make ineffective; to act in opposition.

counterclockwise (kaůn′tẽr-klŏk′wīz): the movement of hair, in shapings or curls, in the opposite direction to the hands of a clock.

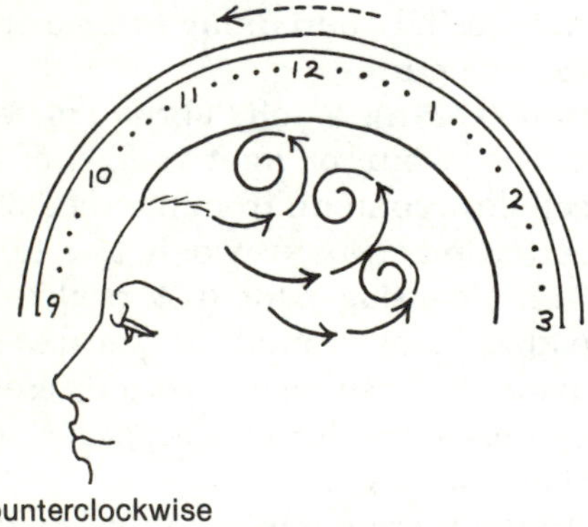

counterclockwise

counter-irritant (kaůn′tẽr ĭr′-ĭ-tênt): a substance that produces inflammation of the skin to relieve a more deep-seated inflammation.

couperose (ko͞o′pẽr-ōs): a word used by estheticians to describe a skin condition caused by dilated or broken capillaries.

couvette (ko͞o-vĕt′): a specially designed bowl used during the spraying procedure of a facial treatment.

coverage (kŭv′ẽr-âj): the degree to which gray or white hair has been covered by the coloring process; the degree of concealment provided by a cosmetic product, foundation or coverage stick.

cowlick (kaů′lik): a tuft of hair that stands up.

cradle cap (krā′d'l kăp): an oily type of dandruff characterized by heavy, greasy crusts on the scalp of an infant.

cranial (krā′nē-âl): of or pertaining to the cranium.

cranial index (krā′nē-âl ĭn′dĕks): a method of measuring the skull.

cranial nerves (krā′nē-âl nûrvz): any pair of nerves arising from the lower surface of the brain.

cranium (krā′nē-ûm): the bones of the head, excluding the bones of the face; bony case of the brain.

crayon (krā′ôn): a temporary hair coloring, massaged or brushed on with a lipstick-like applicator.

cream (krēm): a semi-solid cosmetic preparation such as cleansing cream and other skin care creams.

crease (krēs): a line or slight depression in the skin, such as grooves across the palms of the hands, at the wrist or where there are folds of skin.

create (krē-āt′): to bring into being, specifically to produce something that has not existed before, such as a new hairstyle or work of art.

creme (krēm): a thick liquid or lotion.

creme bleach (krēm blēch): a chemical

preparation of thick consistency, used to remove color from hair.

creme rinse (krēm rĭns): a colorless, usually acidic preparation applied to the hair to neutralize the effects of the shampoo; it assists in removing tangles from the hair and increases its manageability.

creosol (krē′ô-sōl): a colorless, oily liquid obtained from creosote.

creosote (krē′ô-sōt): an oily liquid obtained from beechwood tar and used in antiseptics.

crepe wool (krāp wōōl): in wiggery, wool made from sheep wool and used to confine ends in winding or to fill in bulk.

crepey skin (krāp′ē skĭn): skin resembling a thin fabric, usually silk, and having a crinkled surface.

crepon (krāp′ŏn): a woven hairpiece frontlet; usually dressed in pomadour style and extending in length to the top of the ears.

crescent shape (krĕs′ĕnt shāp): in manicuring, a term referring to the small, white area at the base of the nail; a shape like that of the moon when less than half of it is visible.

cresol (krē′sōl): a liquid obtained from coal tar and used as a powerful antiseptic and disinfectant; used to sterilize instruments and other objects.

crest (krĕst): in hairdressing, tuft of hair; the high ridge of a finger wave; a line or thin mark made by folding or doubling over, as the crest between two waves, where one begins and the other ends.

crew cut (krōō kŭt): a very short men's haircut that leaves a bristle-like surface over the entire head.

crimping rod (krĭmp′ĭng rŏd): a flat, plastic clamp-like rod, designed to produce hairstyles that have a tightly waved, fluffy appearance.

crimp perm (krĭmp pûrm): a perm given with a unique crimping tool to produce small waves resembling waves created by braiding the hair.

crimpy (krĭm′pē): having a crimped, frizzy appearance; very curly or wavy.

crimson (krĭm′zĕn): a deep red color having a tinge of blue.

crinkle (krĭng′kâl): to form wrinkles; a wrinkle or fold.

crisscross (krĭs′krôs): to pass back and forth, through or over; to mark with intersecting lines, as the crisscross movement of the fingers while giving a facial.

criterion (krī-tĭr′ē-ŭn): a standard on which a judgment may be based; a rule or test.

croquignole (krō′kĭ-nōl): winding of hair strands from the ends to the scalp.

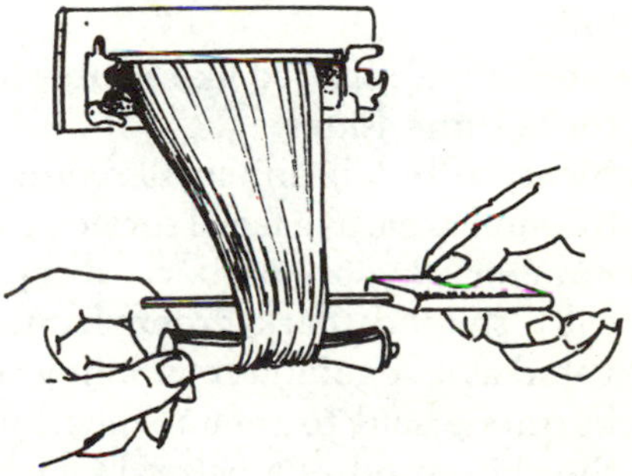

croquignole

croquignole curl (krō′kĭ-nōl kûrl): any curl that is wound from the ends of the hair toward the scalp.

croquignole heat curling (krō′kĭ-nōl hēt kûrl′ĭng): the process of curling the hair with a hot iron by winding the hair under in a special manner, as the hair strand is clicked into the iron until the ends disappear.

croquignole marcel wave (krō′kĭ-nōl

mär′sĕl wāv): a wave in the hair produced by the use of a marcel iron and winding the hair croquignole fashion.

croquignole winding (krō′kĭ-nōl wīnd′-ĭng): the process of winding the hair from hair ends toward the scalp.

cross bonds (krôs bŏndz): the bonds holding together the long chains of amino acids which compose hair.

crown (kraûn): the topmost part of the skull or head.

crude (kro͞od): in a natural or unrefined state; imperfect; unfinished.

crust (krŭst): a coating of dried blood; dead cells which form over a wound or blemish while it is healing; also called a scab.

cryosurgery (krī-ô-sûr′jĕr-ē): a skin treatment done with the use of liquid nitrogen, usually in case of nodular and cystic forms of acne.

crypt (krĭpt): a small cavity on the skin; a small sac or follicle; a glandular tubule.

cubic (kū′bĭk): shaped like a cube; having three dimensions.

cubical (kū′bī-k'l): any small room or partitioned area, as a facial service cubical.

cucumber (kyo͞o′kŭm-bĕr): a cylindrically shaped, dark green fruit, cultivated as a vegetable; contains a certain hormone said to retain smoothness of the skin; used as a natural facial mask and as an ingredient in some cosmetics.

cuneiform (kū′nê-ĭ-fôrm): wedge-shaped; a bone of the wrist or corpus.

cupful (kŭp′fo͞ol): a measure of eight ounces; a half pint; in metric measure, one metric cup liquid equals approximately 236 milliliters.

curative (kūr′ă-tĭv): having the power to cure.

curd (kûrd): a soap residue found on the hair after an unsatisfactory shampoo, usually as the result of nonlathering of soap in hard water.

curd soap (kûrd sōp): a white soap of curdy texture, usually containing free alkali.

cure (kūr): to heal or restore to a sound, healthy condition.

curl (kûrl): to form hair into curves, spirals or ringlets; a lock of hair that curves or coils.

curl, barrel (kûrl, băr′ĕl): a curl made in a similar manner to the standup curl and used where there is insufficient room to place a roller.

curl base (kûrl bās): the stationary or immovable foundation of the curl, which is attached to the scalp.

curl, cascade (kûrl, kăs′kād): a stand-up curl which is wound from the hair ends to the scalp.

curl clip (kûrl klĭp): a pronged device used to secure a curl in place.

curl direction (kûrl dī-rĕk′shûn): the placement of the hair so that it moves or curls toward or away from a certain point.

curler (kûrl′ĕr): that which curls anything.

curler, electric iron (kûrl′ĕr, ê-lĕk′trĭk): a curling iron heated by electricity; thermal iron; electric vaporizing thermal iron.

curling (kûrl′ĭng): a process of hair waving.

curling, brush (kûrl′ĭng, brŭsh): tightly winding a damp strand of hair around the index finger, brushing with a stiff brush, pinning to the scalp with wire pins, and drying the hair with artificial heat.

curling iron (kûr′lĭng ī′ûrn): an implement with a long tube-like base over which a top piece can be raised, the hair placed between the two and curled while it is dry; thermal iron.

curling, paper (kûr′lĭng pā′pēr): produced by dividing the hair into small strands which are formed into flat ringlets and held in place by means of a folded piece of paper and heated between the prongs of a pressing iron.

curling pin (kûr′lĭng pĭn): the forming of hair ringlets by winding the hair in a series of concentric circles, fastened in place with hair pins.

curling, round (kûr′lĭng round): curls produced by twisting the hair tightly and evenly around a heated curling iron.

curl, overlapping (kûrl, ō-vēr-lăp′ĭng): a strand of wet hair wound around the finger in a spiral movement with the hair ends on the outside; also known as maypole or post curl.

curl paper (kûrl pā′pēr): a fine porous tissue paper around which a lock of hair is wound for curling.

curl placement (kûrl plās′mênt): the positioning of a curl in a location which has been predetermined.

curl, ridge (kûrl, rĭdj): a curl placed behind and close to the ridge of a finger wave and pinned across its stem.

curl, roller (kûrl, rōl′ēr): a curl formed over a specially made roller.

curl stem (kûrl stĕm): that part of the pin curl between the base and the first arc of the circle.

curl styles (kûrl stīlz): various kinds of curls such as pin curl, sculptured curl, standup curl, cascade curl, etc.

curl, thermal (kûrl, thûr′mâl): a curl formed with thermal irons.

curly (kûr′lē): tending to curl; full of curves, twists, ripples, ringlets.

curly hair (kûr′lē hâr): hair that has a curved or spiral shape; the opposite of straight.

curly head (kûr′lē hĕd): pertaining to a person who has curly hair.

current, alternating (kûr′ênt, ôl′tēr-nāt-ĭng): an interrupted current of electricity.

current D'arsonval (kûr′ênt där-sôn-vâl′): a high frequency current of low voltage and high amperage.

current, direct; D.C. (kûr′ênt dī-rĕkt′): an uninterrupted and even flowing current of electricity.

current, electric (kûr′ênt ê-lĕk′trĭk): electricity in motion or moving within a conductor.

current, foradic (kûr′ênt, fă-răd′ĭk): an induced, interrupted current whose action is mechanical.

current, galvanic (kûr-ênt, gâl-văn′ĭk): a direct, constant current, having a positive and negative pole and providing a chemical action.

current, high frequency; tesla (kûr′ênt hī-frē′kwĕn-sē; tĕs′lă): an electric current of medium voltage and medium amperage.

current, sinusoidal (kûr′ênt sī′nû-soy′-dâl): an induced interrupted current somewhat similar to faradic current.

current strength (kûr′ênt strĕngth): the relation of the electromotive force to the resistance of the circuit.

current style (kûr′ênt stīl): a style which is worn or in favor at the present time.

curriculum (kă-rĭk′û-lŭm): the course of study in a college or university; a particular course of study.

curvalinear (kûr′vă-lin′ē-är): in hairdressing, formed, bounded, or characterized by curved lines.

curvature (kûr′vă-chēr): the state of being curved.

curvature lines (kûr′vă-chēr līnz): shaping of the hair and combing out into a series of curved lines running inward and outward.

curve (kûrv): the continuous bending of a line as an arc or circle.

cushioning (ko͞osh′ŭn-ĭng): a form of back combing or back brushing in the scalp area in order that the tapered hairs interlock and form a foundation to support the longer lengths of hair.

cushion wrap (ko͞osh′ŭn răp): end paper used to prevent hair from expanding against a perm rod during the processing procedure of permanent waving.

custom made (kŭs′tŭm mād): a wig or hairpiece which has been specially measured and constructed for a specific individual.

cut (kŏt): in hair cutting, to reduce or shorten by removing the ends with an instrument such as a scissor or razor; a haircut; to style the hair by cutting.

cutaneous (kû-tā′nē-ûs): pertaining to, involving or affecting the skin and its appendages.

cutaneous appendage (kû-tā′nē-ûs ă-pĕn′dâg): an organ or structure of ectodermal origin attached to or embedded in the skin; examples are: hair, nails, sebaceous and sudoriferous glands.

cutaneous colli (kû-tā′nē-ûs kŏl′ī): a nerve of the skin of the neck.

cutaneous diphtheria (kû-tā′nē-ûs dĭf-thēr′ē-ă): an ulcer-like infection of the skin.

cutaneous gland (kû-tā′nē-ûs glănd): any gland of the skin.

cutaneous horn (kû-tā′nē-ûs hôrn): a small growth resembling a miniature horn commonly found on the face, scalp or chest.

cutaneous muscle (kû-tā′nē-ûs mŭs′l): a muscle having an insertion into the skin or origin and insertion in the skin.

cutaneous nerves (kû-tā′nē-ûs nûrvz): nerves affecting the skin.

cutaneous reaction (kû-tā′nē-ûs rē-ăk′-shûn): any reaction of the skin such as a rash or change in appearance as the result of disease, drugs, sunburn, allergy, etc.

cutaneous reflex (kû-tā′nē-ûs rē′flĕx): the response of the skin to irritation or sensations, such as goose bumps on the skin as a reaction to cold.

cutaneous sensation (kû-tā′nē-ûs sĕn-sā′shûn): pertaining to the skin's receptors for sensing touch, temperature changes, pain or irritation.

cutaneous test (kû-tā′nē-ûs tĕst): a test involving the skin; skin test.

cuticle (kū′tĭ-k'l): the very thin outer layer of the skin or hair; the epidermis; the cresent of toughened skin around the base of fingernails and toenails; any fine covering.

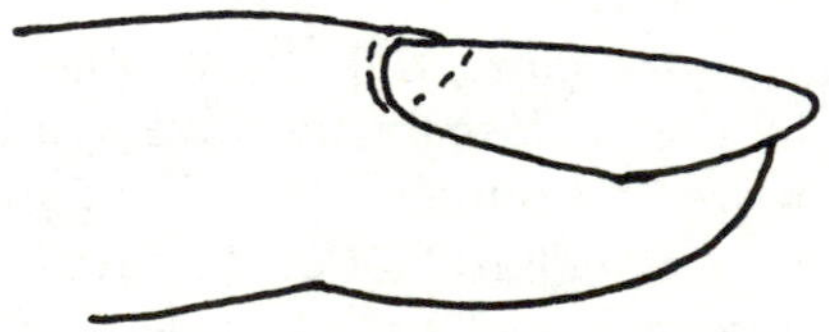

cuticle

cuticle nippers (kū′tĭ-k'l nĭp′ĕrs): a small cutting tool used in manicuring or pedicuring to nip or cut excess cuticle (epidermis); the tool is characterized by its double handle and short clipping blades.

cuticle of hair (kū′tĭ-k'l of hâr): the outer keratinized layers of the hair shaft which surround the polypeptide chain.

The cuticle layers of hair may differ in various ethnic groups. Example: It is thought that Caucasian hair has approximately 6 layers, Negroid (black) hair 12 layers and Oriental hair approximately 15 to 20 cuticle layers.

cuticle oil (kū′tĭ-k'l oyl): a special oil used to soften and lubricate the cuticle (epidermis) around fingernails and toenails.

cuticle pusher (kū′tĭ-k'l pōōsh′ĕr): an implement used in manicuring or pedicuring to loosen and push back the cuticle around the fingernails or toenails; the implement is shaped to conform with the shape of the nails.

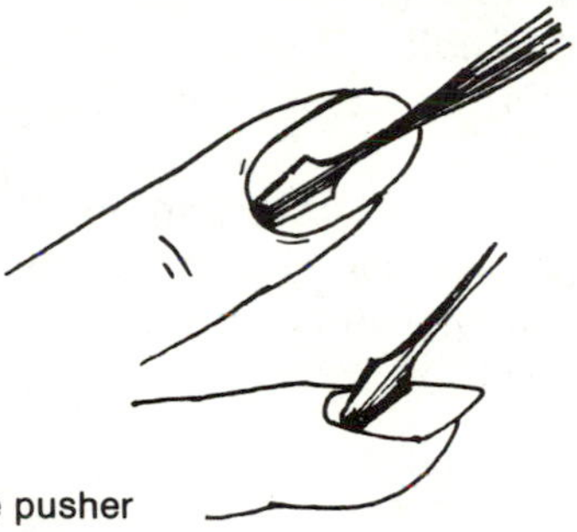

cuticle pusher

cuticle remover (kū′tĭ-k'l rē-mōōv′ĕr): a solution of alkali, glycerine and water used to soften and remove dead cuticle from around the nail.

cuticle scales (kū′tĭ-k'l skālz): the overlapping formation of the outer layer of the hair (the cuticle); also referred to as imbrications.

cuticle scissors (kū′tĭ-k'l sĭz′orz): a small implement designed to trim excess cuticle (epidermis) around the fingernails or toenails. It is distinguished by the long shank and short, sharp cutting blades.

cuticle softener (kū′tĭ-k'l sŏ′fĕ-nĕr): a substance used in manicuring and pedicuring to soften the cuticle (epidermis) around the fingernails and toenails prior to removing the excess cuticle.

cuticolor (kū′tĭ-kŭl′ĕr): simulating the color of the skin as color in some cosmetics and medicines.

cuticularization (kū-tĭk′ū-lär-ī-zā′shŭn): the growth of new skin over a wound or blemish.

cutis (kū′tĭs): the derma or deeper layer of the skin.

cutis marmorata (kū′tĭs mär′mō-rā′tă): blue or purple spots on the skin due to exposure to cold air.

cutis rhomboidalis muchae (kū′tĭs rŏm′-boy-dā′lĭs nû-kē): a skin condition characterized by furrows and a leathery appearance; usually caused by over-exposure to the sun, wind and weather.

cutis verticis gyrata (kū′tĭs vĕr′tĭ-sĭs jī-rā′tă): hypertrophy and looseness of the skin or scalp resulting in folds.

cutting lotion (kŭt′ĭng lō′shûn): a wetting agent used to control the hair during a haircut.

cuvette (kū′vĕt): a specially designed bowl used to protect the client's body from spray during a facial treatment.

cyanosis (sī′ă-nō′sĭs): a condition of circulation due to inadequate oxygenation of the blood, causing the skin to take on a bluish cast.

cycle (sī′k'l): a complete wave of an alternating current.

cyclical (sī′klĭ-k'l): pertaining to or moving in a circle; having parts arranged in a ring or closed chain structure.

cycloid (sī′kloyd): arranged in circles; something circular.

cylinder (sĭl′ĭn-dĕr): a long circular body, solid or hollow, uniform in diameter.

C-D

cylindrical (sĭ-lĭn′drĭ-kâl): pertaining to, or having the form of a cylinder.

cylindrical hair roller (sĭ-lĭn′drĭ-kâl hâr rōl′ĕr): a roller made of lightweight metal or plastic, in various sizes, lengths and circumferences, around which strands of hair are wound to create a specific style.

cylindrical shaped curl (sĭ-lĭn′drĭ-kâl shāpt kûrl): a curl which is formed to be about the same circumference along its entire shaft from the ends to the scalp.

cypress oil (sī′prĕs oyl): oil from the buds of the cypress tree, used in astringent preparations and in some fragrances.

cyst (sĭst): a closed, abnormally developed sac, containing fluid, semi-fluid or morbid matter.

cysteic acid (sĭs′tē-ĭk ȧs′ĭd): a crystalline amino acid formed as the result of oxidation of cystine.

cystic acne (sĭs′tĭk ăk′nē): acne that is distinguished by cysts.

cystine (sĭs′tēn): sulfur containing amino acid which is present in hair in the form of cross bonds (links) joining adjacent polypeptide chains; an amino acid component of many proteins, especially keratin.

cystine links (sĭs′tēn lĭnks): the cross bonds formed from the amino acid, cystine.

cystoma (sĭs-tō′mă): a tumor containing cysts of pathogenic origin.

cytochemistry (sī′tō-kĕm′ĭ-strē): the science dealing with the chemistry of cells.

cytocrine theory (sī′tô-krĭn thē′ă-rē): the theory that pigment granules are transferred from melanocytes directly into the cells of the epidermis.

cytogenesis (sī′tō-jĕn′ĕ-sĭs): the formation of cells.

cytolysis (sī-tōl′ĭ-sĭs): the dissolution of cells.

cytoplasm (sī-tô-plăz′ĕm): all the protoplasm of a cell except that in the neucleus; the watery fluid which nourishes the cell.

D

dab (dăb): to pat or apply with a light towel; a small amount.

damage (dăm′ĭj): to injure or harm; loss.

damaged hair (dăm′ăjd hâr): a hair condition characterized by one or more of the following: high porosity, brittleness, split ends, dryness, rough, lifeless feeling, matting, sponginess when wet, lacking gloss and elasticity.

damp (dămp): moist, not saturated with liquid.

dandelion (dăn′dē-lī-ŏn): a green plant which provides high vitamin A and C in cosmetic substances for skin and hair.

dander (dăn′dẽr): scales from animal skin, hair of feathers; may act as an allergen.

dandricide (dăn′drĭ′sīd): a chemical substance; counteracts the effects of dandruff.

dandruff (dăn′drăf): pityriasis; scurf or scales formed in excess upon the scalp; greasy or dry keratotic material shed from the scalp.

dandruff conditioner (dăn′drăf kôn-dĭ′shûn-ẽr): a product containing ingredients formulated to improve or eliminate a dandruff condition of the scalp.

dandruff lotion (dăn′drăf lō shûn): a lotion applied to the scalp to aid in loosening and removing dandruff scales.

dandruff ointment (dăn′drăf oynt′mênt): a specially formulated salve or unguent to be applied to the scalp to treat a dandruff condition.

dandruff rinse (dăn′drăf rĭns): a liquid applied to the hair and scalp following a treatment or shampoo to control and eliminate a dandruff condition.

dandruff shampoo (dăn′drăf shăm-pōō′): a commercially prepared product designed to control and eliminate dandruff.

dark (därk): a deep shade of color; dark skin; brunette in complexion, not fair; dark hair; almost black.

darken (därk′ĕn): to make a deeper color; to darken hair; to use a darker shade of makeup in contour shading of the face.

dark skin spot (därk skĭn spŏt): commonly called "age" or "liver" spots; spots or splotches on the skin indicative of melanosis or melanoderm, a condition in which dark pigment is deposited in the skin and tissues.

D'arsonval current (d'är′sŏn-vâl kûr′-ênt): high frequency of low voltage and high amperage; a biterminal current.

dart (därt): the folding and sewing together a curved section of material to form a tapered seam; used in wiggery to reduce the size of a wig cap.

data (dā′tă): facts, figures and various forms of information from which measurements and statistics can be drawn; record keeping.

data processing (dā′tă prŏs′ĕs′ĭng): the converting by computers of information into a form for use or storage; a technique for keeping and storing all kinds of records and for ease in retrieving information when needed.

daub (dôb): to smear or coat with a greasy

or sticky substance without exercising skill.

daylight bulb (dā′līt bŭlb): an electric bulb made of special glass that produces light similar to daylight.

daylight makeup (dā′līt māk′ŭp): a choice of colors in makeup products to give the face a natural appearance for daylight wear.

de (dē): a prefix denoting from; down or away.

deacidify (dē′ă-sĭd-ĭ-fī): to remove acid from a substance.

dead (dĕd): lacking life; not responsive; lacking sensation; in skin care, dead surface cells; in hair care, hair that is dull, dead, lifeless.

debility (dê-bĭl′ĭ-tē): weakness; loss of strength.

debris (dê′-brē): remains; rubbish; excess matter.

decade (dĕk′ād): a period of ten years.

decalvant (dĕ-kâl′vănt): a substance used to remove or destroy hair.

decay (dē-kā): decomposition of matter by the action of bacteria.

decimeter (dĕs′ă-mē′tĕr): in the metric system, the tenth part of a meter.

decolorization (dē-kŭl′ĕr-ĭ-zā′shûn): the removal of color from the hair.

decolorize (dē-kŭl′ĕr-īz): to remove color; to lighten.

decompose (dē-kôm-pōz′): to decay or rot; to separate into constituent parts; to bring to dissolution.

decomposition (dē-kŏm-pōz-zĭ′shûn): to separate or disintegrate into constituent parts or elements.

decreasing graduation (dĕ-krēs′ĭng grăj′-ōō-wā′shûn): graduation found within two nonparallel lines; it diminishes as it moves back from the face.

decrustation (dē′krŭs-tā′shûn): the detachment or removal of a crust.

decurved (dē-kûrvd′): curved or bent downward.

deep (dēp): extending below or far from the surface; a color of intense or dark hues; high saturation.

deep cervical artery (dēp sûr′vĭ-kâl är′tĭr-ē): the artery which supplies blood to the deep muscles of the neck.

deep kneading (dēp nēd′ĭng): a massage movement in which the flesh is lifted and squeezed with the hand.

deep temporal artery (dēp tĕm′pâ-râl är′tĭr-ē): the artery which supplies blood to the temporal (temple) muscle and skull.

defect (dē′fĕkt): an imperfection.

defective (dê′fĕk′tĭv): imperfect; lacking in some physical quality.

deficiency (dê-fĭsh′ĕn-sē): a lacking; something wanted.

deficiency disease (dê-fĭsh′ĕn-sē dĭz′ēz): a disease such as pellagra or scurvy, etc. caused by the lack of essential vitamins and other nourishment in the body.

define (dĕ′fīn): to outline; to fix with precision an outline or boundary.

defluvium (dê-flōō′vē-ŭm): to flow down; to lose something.

defluvium capilorum (dê-flōō′vē-ŭm kăp-ĭ-lō′rŭm): complete loss of hair.

defluvium unguium (dê-flōō′vē-ŭm ŭng′gwē-ŭm): complete loss of nails.

deformed (dê′fôrmd): disfigured; misshaped; abnormal.

deformity (dê-fôr′mĭ-tē): abnormal shape of a part of the body.

deft (dĕft): skilled, dexterous.

degenerate (dê-jĕn′ĕr-āt): to pass to a lower level of mental or physical qualities.

degenerative (dê-jĕn′ĕr-ă-tĭv): a biochemical change caused by injury or disease and leading to loss of vitality, of function, etc; prone to deteriorate.

degrease (dê-grēs): to remove grease or a greasy substance.

degree (dĕ′grē′): to do in steps or stages; extent or amount; gradually.

dehumidifier (dē′hū-mĭd′ĭ-fī′ẽr): an apparatus designed to reduce moisture in the air.

dehydrate (dē-hī′drāt): to deprive of water or to suffer loss of water; to dry out.

dehydrator (dē′hī-drā′tôr): an agent that removes or reduces water in the tissues of the body.

delicate (dĕl′ĭ-kĭt): exquisite and fine workmanship; fragile.

deltoid (dĕl′toyd): a triangular muscle covering the shoulder joint which allows the arm to be extended outward and to the side of the body.

demarcation (dē′mär-kā′shûn): a line setting bounds or limits; in makeup, to blend colors to avoid a line of demarcation.

demi (demĭ): less in size; partial.

demiwig (demĭ′wĭg): a small hairpiece; smaller than a full wig usually designed to be blended with the patron's own hair.

demonstration (dĕm-ĕn′strā-shûn): to point out or prove; to describe by examples and experiments; a display; a teaching or performing technique.

denature (dē-nā′chẽr): to change the nature of something by chemical or physical means.

dendrites (dĕn′drīts): a tree-like branching of nerve fibers extending from a nerve cell; short nerve fibers that carry impulses toward the cells.

dense (dĕns): close; thick; heavy.

density (dĕn′sĭ-tē): the quality or condition of being close; thick; heavy.

dental (dĕn′tâl): pertaining to the teeth.

dentifrice (dĕn′tĭ-frĭs): a powder, paste or liquid used to clean the teeth.

denude (dē-nōōd′): to remove overlying matter or material; to expose to view; to clear the face of makeup.

deodorant (dē-ō′dẽr-ânt): a substance that conceals or removes offensive odors.

deodorize (dē-ō′dẽr-īz): to free from odor.

depigment (dē-pĭg′mênt): to cause the loss of pigment.

depilate (dĕp′ĭ-lāt): to remove hair from the surface of the skin.

depilation (dĕp′ĭ-lā′shûn): removal of superfluous hair.

depilatory (dê-pĭl′ă-tôr-ē): a substance, usually a caustic alkali, used to destroy the hair.

deplete (dē-plēt′): to reduce; lessen; use up.

depleted (dê-plēt′ĕd): that which is exhausted; reduced.

depletion (dē-plē′shûn): reduction or exhaustion in number or by draining away strength, power or value.

depot (dēp′ō): the site of an accumulation, as depot fat which occurs in certain regions of the body as: hips, buttocks, abdominal walls, thighs, etc.

depress (dê-prĕs′): to press down.

depression (dê-prĕsh′ŭn): a hollow or sunken area; in psychiatry, a state of dejection, sadness or melancholy.

depressor (dê-prĕs′ẽr): that which presses or draws down; a muscle that depresses.

depressor alae nasi (dê-prĕs′ẽr ā′lē nā′zī): depressor septi; a muscle which contracts the nostril.

depressor anguli oris (dê-prĕs′êr ăng′û-lī ô′rĭs): a muscle that depresses the angle of the mouth.

depressor area (dê-prĕs′ẽr âr′ē-ă): the vasomotor center which, when stimulated, can cause a drop in blood pressure and result in a slower heart rate.

depressor labii inferioris (dê-prĕs′ĕr lā′bē-ī ĭn-fēr-ē-ô′rĭs): quadratis labii inferioris; a muscle that depresses the lower lip.

depressor septi nasi (dê-prĕs′ĕr sĕp′tē nā′zī): a muscle which contracts the nostril.

depressor supercilii (dê-prĕs′ĕr sū′pĕr-sĭl′ē-ī): the portion of the orbicularis oculi muscle which draws the eyebrows downward.

depth (dĕpth): distance from top to bottom; distance; in hairdressing, the degree of intensity and saturation of color.

depth of side section (dĕpth of sīd sĕk′-shûn): in hairstyling, the amount of hair in sectioning from the hairline to the back of the ear.

depth of top section (dĕpth of tŏp sĕk′-shûn): in hairstyling, the amount of hair sectioned from the hairline at the forehead to the crown of the head.

derivative (dê-rĭv′ă-tĭv): that which is derived; anything obtained or deduced from another.

derm, derma, dermo (dûrm, dûr′mă, dûr′mō): pertaining to the skin.

derma (dûr′mă): the true skin; the corium; the sensitive layer of the skin below the epidermis.

dermabrasion (dûr′mă-brā′zhûn): the removal of skin in varying amounts and depths by such mechanical means as revolving wire brushes or sandpaper, for the purpose of correcting scars.

dermafat (dûr-mă-făt): the adipose tissue of the skin.

dermal (dûr′mâl): pertaining to the skin.

dermal graft (dûr′mâl grăft): a skin graft using split or full thickness of skin for the grafting procedure.

dermal papilla (dûr′mâl pă-pĭl′ă): an elevation of the projecting corium into the overlying epidermis.

dermal sense (dûr′mâl sĕns): the perception of cold, heat, pain, pressure or other sensations through the receptors of the skin.

dermatalgia (dûr′mă-tâl′jē ă): pain accompanied by a burning sensation of the skin when no injury or other changes can be observed.

dermatherm (dûr′mă-thĕrm): an apparatus designed to measure skin temperature.

dermatician (dûr-mă-tĭsh′ân): one skilled in the treatment of the skin.

dermatitis (dûr′mă-tī′tĭs): an irritation of the skin; resulting either from the primary irritant effect of a substance or more frequently from the sensitization to a substance coming in contact with the skin.

dermatitis combustiones (dûr′mă-tī′tĭs kŏm-bŭs-tĭ-ō′nēs): a type of dermatitis produced by extreme heat.

dermatitis, cosmetic (dûr′mă-tī′tĭs, kŏz-mĕ′tĭk): an inflammation of the skin caused by contact with some cosmetic product to which the individual may be allergic.

dermatitis, medicamentosa (dûr′mă-tī′-tĭs, mĕd′ĭ-kă-mĕn-tō′să): a type of dermatitis caused by the internal use of medicines such as bromides.

dermatitis, occupational (dûr′mă-ti′tĭs ŏk-û-pā′shûn-âl): an inflammation of the skin caused by the kind of employment in which the individual is engaged and by substances used on the job.

dermatitis seborrheica (dûr′mă-tī′tĭs sĕbō-rē′ĭ-kă): a type of dermatitis found co-existing with seborrhea.

dermatitis venenata (dûr′mă-tī′tĭs vĕn-ĕ-nāy′tă): inflammation of the skin caused by the action of an irritating substance such as hair dye.

dermatodysplasia (dûr′mă-tô-dĭs-plā′zē-ă): a condition characterized by abnormal development of the skin.

dermatologist (dûr′mă-tŏl′ô-jĭst): a skin specialist; a physician who understands the science of treating the skin, its structures, functions and diseases.

dermatology (dûr′mă-tŏl′ă-jē): the science which deals with the skin and its diseases.

dermatomycosis (dûr′mă-tō-mī-kō′sĭs): a superficial infection of the skin or its appendages caused by pathogenic fungus.

dermatoneurology (dûr′mă-tō-nū-rŏl′ă-jē): the study of the nerves of the skin in health and disease.

dermatopathic (dûr′ma-tō-păth′ĭk): pertaining or attributable to disease of the skin.

dermatophyte (dûr′mă-tô-fīt): a fungus parasitic on the skin.

dermatophytosis (dûr′mă-tō-fī-tō′sĭs): commonly called athlete's foot.

dermatoplasty (dûr′mă-tō-plăs′tē): the science of skin grafting; an operation in which flaps of skin are used from another part of the body to replace lost or damaged skin.

dermatotherapy (dûr′mă-tō-thĕr′ă-pē): the treatment of the skin and its diseases.

dermatosis (dûr′mă-tō′sĭs): any disease of the skin; usually a disease not characterized by inflammation.

dermatotrophic (dûr′mă-tō-trōf′ĭk): affecting, infesting or infecting the skin.

dermis, derma (dûr′mĭs, dûr′mă): the layer below the epidermis; the corium or true skin.

dermoid (dûr′moyd): resembling skin.

desensitize (dē-sĕn′sĭ-tīz): deprive of sensation; to cause the paralysis of a sensory nerve by blocking.

desiccate (dĕs′ĭ-kāt): to deprive a substance of moisture; to dry.

desiccation (dĕs-ĭ-kā′shûn): the process of drying.

design (dê-zīn′): arrangement of shapes, lines and ornamental effects which create an artistic unit, as in hairstyling, makeup application and the creation of fashions.

design component (dê′zīn kăm-pō′nênt): one of four elements; texture, form, structure and direction that make up a hair design.

design line (dê-zīn līn): the artistic concept of a finished hairstyle as expressed in its lines and shapes; a line used as a guide in creating the form of a design.

design, three dimensional (dê-zīn′, thrē dĭ-mĕn′shûn-âl): a sculpturing effect with hair, creating volume and/or indentation into a shape.

design, two dimensional (dê-zīn′, to͞o dĭ-mĕn′shûn-âl): a pattern effect on a flat surface.

desmosine (dĕs′mō-sĭn): one of two amino acids found in elastin; the other is isodesmosine.

desquamate (dĕs′kwă-māt′): to shed in scales; to shed the superficial layer of the skin.

desquamation (dĕs-kwă-mā′shûn): scaling of the cuticle.

destructive (dê-strŭk′tĭv): tending to destroy.

detergent (dē-tûr′jênt): a compound or

C-D

solution used for cleansing; an agent that cleanses the skin and hair.

deteriorate (dê-tēr′-ē-ă-rāt): to grow worse; to become impaired in quality; to degenerate.

deterrent (dê-tĕr′ênt): that which hinders or prevents.

detoxification (dē-tŏk′sĭ-fĭ-kā′shŭn): reduction of toxic poisons; ridding the body of toxic substances.

detriment (dĕ′trĭ-mênt): a cause of injury or damage.

detumescence (dē′tū-mĕs′ĕns): the subsiding of swelling; to go down.

develop (dē-vĕl′ŏp): take effect; as during the process of a hair tint or lightener.

developer (dê-vĕl′ŏp-ēr): an oxidizing agent, such as 20-volume hydrogen peroxide solution; when mixed with an oxidation dye, it supplies the necessary oxygen gas.

developing time (dê-vĕl′ŏp-ĭng tīm): the period required for the hair lightener or tint solution to act upon the hair.

device (dê-vīs′): an invention or contrivance of a simple nature for a particular use and purpose.

dewy (dōō′ē): to appear moist; fresh; unblemished.

dexterity (dĕks-tĕr′ĭ-tē): skill and ease in using the hands; expertness in manual acts.

dextral (dĕks′trâl): right-handed; right as opposed to left.

di (dī): a prefix denoting two fold; double; twice; separation or reversal.

dia (dī′ă): a prefix denoting through; apart; asunder; between.

diabetic (dī′ă-bĕt′ĭk): one who has diabetes, a disease associated with deficient insulin secretion.

diagnose (dī′ăg-nōs′): to determine the nature of a condition from the symptoms.

diagnosis (dī′ăg-nō′sĭs): the determination of the nature of a disease from its symptoms.

diagonal (dī-ăg′ă-n'l): a line with a slanting or sloping direction.

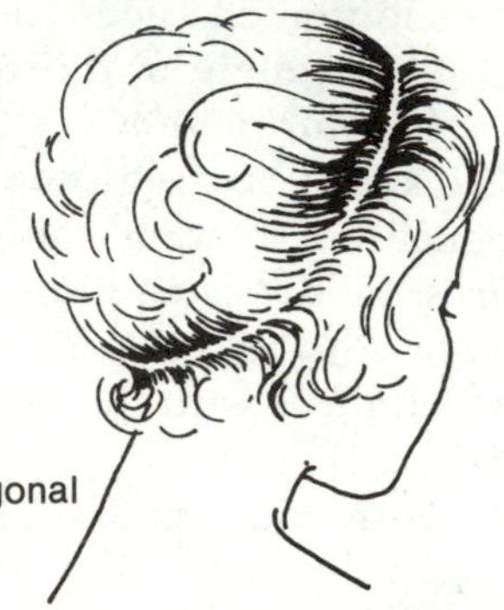

diagonal back design (dī-ăg′ă-n'l băk dē-zīn′): a design resulting in a backward flow of hair from the face.

diagonal forward design (dī-ăg′ă-n'l fôr′-wärd dē-zīn′): a design resulting in a forward movement of hair onto the face.

diagonal left (dī-ăg′ă-n'l lĕft): a diagonal line that travels to the left.

diagonal right (dī-ăg′ă-n'l rīt): a diagonal line that travels to the right.

diagram (dī′ă-grăm): a figure for ascertaining or exhibiting certain relations between objects under discussion; an outline, figure or scheme of lines, spaces, points; used in demonstrations, etc.

dialysis (dī-ăl′ĭ-sĭs): the process of separating different substances in solution by diffusion through a moist membrane or septum; separation.

diameter (dī-ăm′ĕ-tēr): the length from one border to another of a straight line that passes through the center of an object.

diamond mesh (dī′ă-mûnd mĕsh): a method of sewing up wefts into a diamond-shaped mesh.

diamond shape (dī′ă-mûnd shāp): a figure bounded by four equal straight lines, having two angles acute and two obtuse.

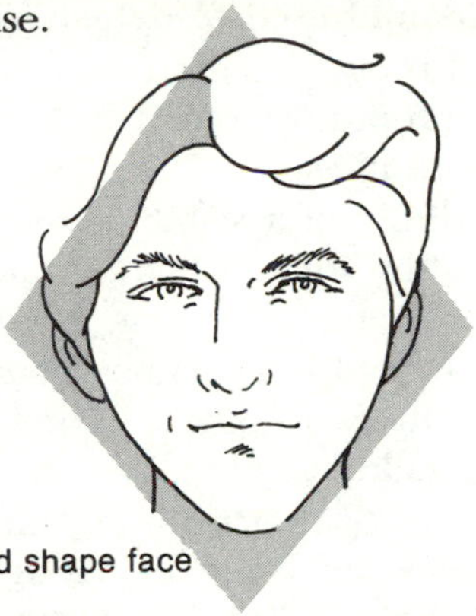

diamond shape face

diamond shape face (dī′ă-mûnd shāp fās): a face with a narrow forehead and chin, with the greater width across the cheekbones.

diaphoretic (dī′ă-fō-rĕt′ĭk): producing perspiration.

diaphragm (dī′ă-frăm): a muscular wall which separates the thorax from the abdominal region and helps to control breathing.

diathermy (dī′ă-thûr′mē): the method of raising the temperature in the deep tissues by using high frequency current.

dichromatic (dī-krō-māt′ĭk): having two colors.

dielectric (dī′ĕ-lĕk′trĭk): a nonconductor of direct electric current.

diet (dī′ĕt): a selection of foods in a regulated course of eating and drinking, especially for health reasons; to regulate kinds and amounts of food and drink for specific reasons.

dietetics (dī′ĕ-tĕt′ĭks): the science of regulating the diet for hygenic or therapeutic purposes.

diffuse (dĭ-fūz′): to pour out; to spread in every way; scattered; not limited to one spot.

diffusion (dĭ-fū′zhûn): a spreading out; dialysis.

digest (dī-jĕst′): to prepare for absorption; to change food chemically in the alimentary canal for assimilation by the body.

digestion (dī-jĕs′chûn): the process of converting food into a form which can be readily absorbed; the breaking down of substances into simple forms, as food into simpler chemical compounds.

digestive system (dī-jĕs′tĭv sĭs′tĕm): the internal organs that change food into nutrients and wastes; the alimentary canal with its associated glands.

digit (dĭj′ĭt): a finger or toe.

digital (dĭj′ĭ-tâl): pertaining to the fingers or toes.

digital artery (dĭj′ĭ-tâl är′tĭr-ē): the artery that supplies blood to the fingers and toes.

digital function (dĭj′ĭ-tâl fŭnk′shûn): a massage technique using the fingertips in a rotating motion; pressing and rotating the fingers on the skin.

digitalis (dij′ĭ-tâl′ĭs): a drug used as a stimulant.

digital nerves (dĭj′ĭ-tâl nûrvs): sensory nerves of the fingers and toes; nerves that receive stimuli from the fingers or toes.

digital stroking (dĭj′ĭ-tâl strōk′ĭng): a massage movement in which the fingertips are used to lightly glide over the face and neck.

digital tapotement (dĭj′ĭ-tâl tă-pōt-män′): a massage movement to promote stimulation of blood to the skin surface;

C-D

consists of light, tapping movements with the tips of the fingers.

digital vibration (dĭj′ĭ-tâl vī-brā′shûn): a massage movement using the tips of the fingers pressed on a pressure point such as the temples, then using a rapid shaking movement for a few seconds duration.

digiti manus (dĭj′ĭ-tī măn′ûs): the digits of the hand.

digiti pedis (dĭj′ĭ-tī pĕd′ĭs): the digits of the foot.

digitus (dĭj′ĭ-tûs): finger.

digitus anularis (dĭj′ĭ-tûs ăn-û-lär′ĭs): the ring finger, or second finger from the little finger, or third finger from the thumb side of the hand.

digitus demonstrativus (dĭj′ĭ-tûs dê-mŏn′strā-tē′vûs): the index finger.

digitus medius (dĭj′ĭ-tûs mē′dē-ûs): the middle finger.

digitus minimus (dĭj′ĭ-tûs mĭn′ĭ-mûs): the last finger on the hand opposite the thumb.

dilate (dī′lāt): to enlarge; expand; distend.

dilator (dī-lā′tĕr): that which expands or enlarges; an instrument for stretching or enlarging a cavity or opening.

dilute (dī-lo͞ot′): to make less concentrated, thinner or more liquid by mixing with another substance, especially water.

dimension (dĭ-mĕn′shûn): a measurement of width, height, thickness, or circumference.

dimensional coloring (dĭ-mĕn′shûn-âl kŭl′ĕr-ĭng): two or three different shades of the same color on the same head of hair.

dimensional design (dĭ-mĕn′shûn-âl dê-zīn′): three-dimensional sculpturing effect with hair, creating volume or indentation into a shape and silhouette.

dimensional styling (dĭ-mĕn′shŭn-âl stīl′ĭng): hairstyling achieved by creating volume or indentation.

dimethylglyoxime (dī-mĕth′ĭl-glī-ŏk′-sēm): compound used in ash testing; a compound used to detect nickle in a hair dye.

diminish (dĭ-mĭn′ĭsh): to make smaller or less; to reduce.

dimple (dĭm′p'l): a slight depression or indentation on the body, usually the cheeks or chin.

dioxide (dī-ŏk′sīd): a chemical compound containing two atoms of oxygen to one of a metallic element.

diphtheria (dĭf-thēr′ē-ă): an infectious disease in which the air passages, and especially the throat, become coated with a false membrane, caused by specific bacillus.

diplococcus (dĭp′lō-kŏk′ûs): a bacterium that occurs in groups of two.

diplomacy (dĭ-plō′mă-sē): the practice of negotiations; skill and tact when dealing with others.

direct current (dī-rĕkt′ kŭr′ênt): an electric current constant in direction, as distinguished from an alternating current; the movement or flow of electricity in one direction.

directional iron (dī-rĕk-shûn-âl īm′ûrn): a curling iron with an oversized rod and groove used for the formation of straight, smooth lines.

directional roller (dī-rĕk′shûn-âl rōl′ĕr): a roller used to direct the hair forward or backward to create a specific style.

direct point (dī-rĕkt poynt): in hairstyling, parting of curved or straight lines from a point to the outline of a circular shape.

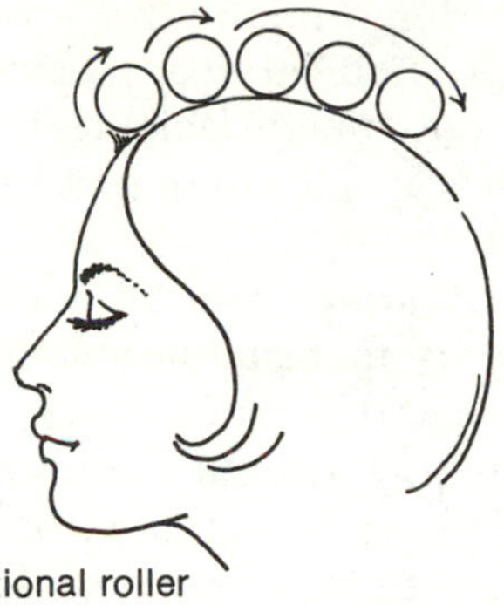

directional roller

dis (dĭs): a prefix denoting apart; away; asunder; between.

disarray (dĭs-ă-rā′): lacking orderly arrangement; in a state of confusion.

disassemble (dĭs-ă-sĕm′b'l): to take apart.

disc (dĭsk): a circular plate or surface.

discard (dĭs-kärd): to cast aside; to throw away.

discharge (dĭs-chärj′): to set free; to remove the contents or load; to relieve of responsibility (dĭs′chärj) the escape or flowing away of the contents of a cavity.

discharger (dĭs-chärj′ĕr): an instrument for setting free electricity.

discolor (dĭs-kŭl′ĕr): to change or destroy the color.

discoloration (dĭs-kŭl′ĕr-ā′shŭn): the development of an undesired color.

discomfort (dĭs-kŭm′fôrt): to make uncomfortable or uneasy.

disconnect (dĭs-kŏ-nekt′): to sever or to terminate a connection.

discretion (dĭs-krĕsh′ŭn): good judgment; the ability to make responsible decisions.

disease (dĭ-zēz′): a pathological condition of any part or organ of the body or of the mind.

disease carrier (dĭ-zēz′ kăr′ē-ĕr): a healthy person who carries and may transmit disease germs to another person.

disentangle (dĭs′ĕn-tăng'l): to free from clumping together; to straighten out snarls in hair.

disfigure (dĭs-fĭg′yĕr): to impair or destroy the beauty of a person or object.

disincrustation (dĭs-ĭn′kră-stā′shŭn): a process used during a facial treatment to soften and emulsify grease deposits and blackheads in the follicles.

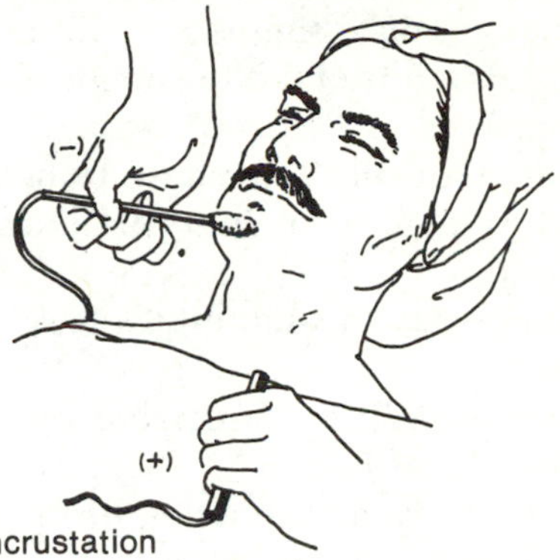

disincrustation

disinfect (dĭs′ĭn-fĕkt′): to free from infection.

disinfectant (dĭs-ĭn-fĕk′tânt): an agent used to destroy germs.

disinfection (dĭs-ĭn-fĕk′shŭn): the act of freeing one from infection.

disintegrate (dĭs-ĭn′tĕ-grāt): to separate or decompose a substance into its component parts; to reduce to fragments or powder.

dispensary (dĭs-pĕn′să-rē): a place where supplies are prepared and dispensed (given out).

dispersion (dĭs-pûr′zhŭn): the act of scattering or separating; the incorporation of the particles of one substance into the body of another, comprising solutions, suspensions, and colloid solutions.

displacement (dĭs-plās′mênt): volume or

weight of fluid displaced by submerging something of equal weight into the fluid.

display (dĭs-plā′): to exhibit products to encourage sales.

disposable (dĭs-pō′ză-b'l): designed to be discarded after use, as disposable products.

dissipate (dĭs′ĭ-pāt): to dissolve.

dissociation (dĭ-sō′sē-ā′shŭn): the process by which combined chemicals are changed into simpler constituents.

dissoluble (dĭs-ŏl′û b'l): capable of being dissolved or decomposed.

dissolve (dĭ-zŏlv′): to cause to become a solution; to break into parts; to disintegrate.

dissymmetry (dĭs-sĭm′ĕ-trē): lack of symmetry.

distal (dĭs′tâl): farthest from the center or median line.

distance (dĭs′tâns): the degree or amount of separation between two objects or points.

distend (dĭs-tĕnd′): to expand; to swell.

distill (dĭs-tĭl′): to extract the essence or active principle of a substance.

distillation (dĭs-tĭ-lā′shŭn): the process of distilling.

distilled water (dĭs-tĭld′ wô′tẽr): purified or refined water.

distribute (dĭs-trĭb′yo͞ot): to disperse through space or over an area; to arrange; in hairdressing and design, distribution refers to the direction hair is combed in relation to its base parting.

disulfide (dī-sŭl′fīd): a chemical compound in which two sulphur atoms are united with a single atom of an element, i.e., carbon.

disulfide links (dī-sŭl′fīd lĭnks): bonds or cross linkages between the polypeptide chains of the hair cortex.

dominant (dŏm′ĭ-nênt): the prominent part or position; large or more impressive, as a dominant facial feature.

dorsal (dôr′sâl): pertaining to the back of a part.

dorsal nasal artery (dôr′sâl nā′zâl är′-tĭr-ē): artery that supplies blood to the dorsum of the nose.

dorsal vertebrae (dôr-sâl vûr′tă-brē): the bones of the vertebral or spinal column located in the midsection of the back.

dorso, dorsi (dôr′sō, dôr′sī): pertaining to the back of the body; denoting relationship to a dorsum or to the posterior aspect of the body.

double (dŭb′l): combined with another; repeated; having two parts.

double adhesive plaster (dŭb′l ăd-hē′sĭv plăs′tẽr): plaster which is adhesive on both sides, used on the adhesive patch to hold a hair piece in position.

double application tint (dŭb′l ăp-lĭ-kā′-shŭn tĭnt): a product requiring two separate applications to the hair, a softener or lightener followed by a penetrating tint; also called a two-process tint.

double bond (dŭb′l bŏnd): a chemical bond consisting of two bonds between two atoms of a molecule, each bond formed by shared electrons.

double chin (dŭb′l chĭn): a fleshy fold under the chin giving the appearance of two chins.

double flat wrap (dŭb′l flăt răp): a hair wrap in which one end paper is placed under, and one paper over, the strand of hair that is being wrapped for permanent waving.

double halo (dŭb′l hā′lō): in permanent waving, a technique using two rows of rods around the face area.

double knotting (dŭb′l nŏt′ĭng): the

method employed to attach the hair to the netting in the formation of hairpieces.

double prong clips (dŭb′l prŏng klĭps): small clips with short prongs used to hold pin curls flat; also used in other shaping, rolling and setting of hair.

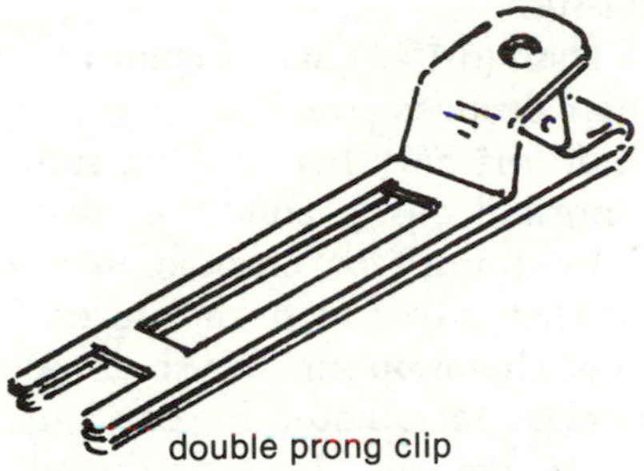

double prong clip

dove tail (dŭv tāl): a connecting line in a style between two or more shapes.

downblending (daůn′ blĕnd′ĭng): blending the hair down from the crown.

down elevation (daůn ĕl′ĕ-vā-shûn): downward angle cutting of hair.

down stroke (daůn strōk): a stroke made with a razor while shaving; in facials, stroking lightly upward and downward with the tips of fingers.

downward (daůn′wôrd): in hairdressing, toward the shoulder down from a part in the hair; in facials, strokes and movements from top to bottom as from cheeks to chin.

downward angle cutting (daůn′wôrd ăng′âl kŭt′ĭng): a technique in haircutting; hair cut in graduating lengths from short to long.

downy hair (daůn′ē hâr): soft, lightweight hair growth; fine hair.

drab (drăb): a shade which has no red or gold tones; usually a dull yellowish brown or gray color.

drabber (drăb′ẽr): a coloring agent designed to reduce the presence of red or gold tones.

drabbing agent (drăb-ĭng ā-jênt): a chemical used to eliminate red or gold tones from the hair color.

drab color (drăb kŭl′ẽr): a hair color lacking red and gold tones; colors such as ash, gray, silver, white, platinum, smoky or steel gray.

drag (drăg): a term to describe a feeling of resistance when a product is applied; the opposite of slip or ease of application.

drape (drāp): a cape or covering placed on a customer to protect clothing while receiving salon services; a coverlet placed over a customer during a facial treatment.

draped hair (drāp′t hâr): to arrange a section of hair in a curved or draped effect; to allow a portion of hair to fall into a curved design.

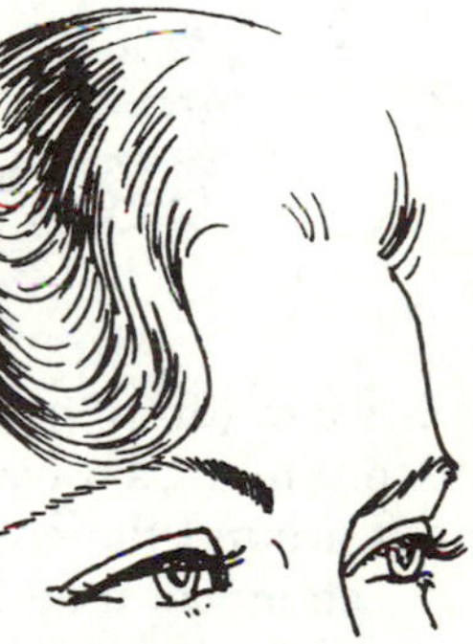

draped hair

draw (drô): in haircutting, to bring the section of hair through the fingers to hold it taut while cutting and shaping.

drawing cards (drâw′ĭng kärdz): in the manufacture of wigs, two identical pieces of leather with steel prongs, used to disentangle and properly arrange hair.

drawn through parting (draůn thro͞o

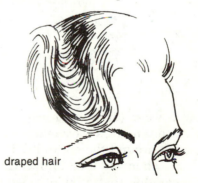

C-D

pärt′ĭng): in the manufacture of wigs, a specially prepared portion of a wig in which the hair, after being knotted, is drawn through a fine silk material, which gives the appearance of the natural scalp.

drench (drĕnch): to saturate; to soak; to wet thoroughly.

dressing (drĕs′ĭng): arranging hair in a style; a substance applied to the hair; a salve or pomade.

droop (dro͞op): to hang downward; be limp; lifeless; lacking bounce or elasticity.

drop crown (drŏp craŭn): permanent waving technique for long hair using crown rods on extended stems to achieve a smooth crown effect.

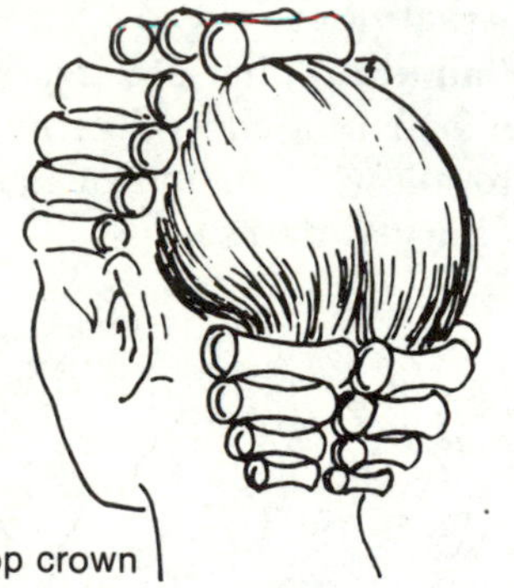

drop crown

dropping a wave (drŏp′ĭng ă wāv): the act of discontinuing a wave rather than carrying it around the entire head.

drug (drŭg): chemical used in dyeing; a substance other than food intended to affect the structure or function of the body; a chemical compound or substance used in some medications.

dry cell (drī sĕl): a battery; a direct (DC) current source.

dry clean (drī-klēn′): to clean with a substance or with a solvent, other than water, such as tetrachloride.

dry cleaner (drī klēn′ĕr): one who cleans clothing; a solution for cleaning fabric or wigs.

dry cut (drī kŭt): a technique for cutting the hair while it is dry; to cut hair before it is shampooed, or after it has been shampooed and dried.

dryer (drī′ĕr): an apparatus for drying the hair; hair dryer; a device to absorb moisture.

dryer chair (drī′ĕr châr): a chair to which a hair dryer is attached.

dry hair (drī hâr): hair lacking sufficient or normal oils; a condition that may be temporary or chronic in nature; hair that is free from moisture.

dry hair shampoo (drī hâr shăm-po͞o′): a shampoo formulated for dry hair.

dry heat (drī hēt): heat produced in a dry airtight cabinet containing an active fumigant; used to sanitize implements and keep them clean until ready for use.

drying lamp (drī′ĭng lămp): an infrared lamp used to dry wet hair during a haircutting procedure.

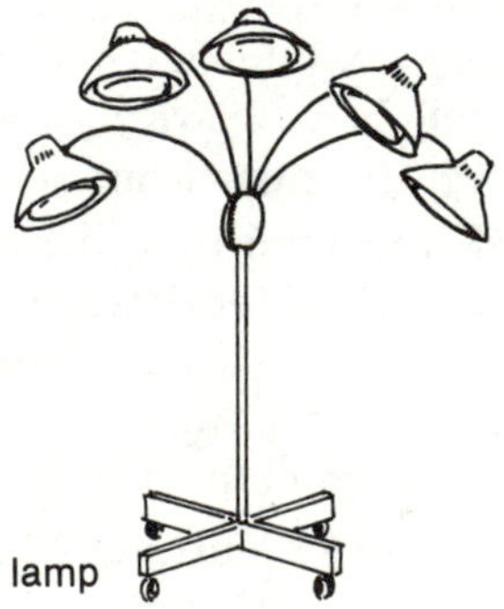

drying lamp

dry sanitizer (drī săn′ĭ-tīz-ĕr): an airtight, specially constructed cabinet containing a disinfectant such as formalin; used to keep implements sanitary.

dry shampoo (drī shăm′po͞o′): a substance used to cleanse the hair without the use of soap and water.

dry skin (drī skĭn): skin that is deficient in oil and/or moisture.

ducktail (dŭk′tāl): in hairstyling, a style popular during the 1950s and revived in the 1980s; the hair is cut short and brushed to a center point at the back of head and napeline.

duct (dŭkt): a passage or canal for fluids.

duct gland (dŭkt glănd): gland that produces a substance that travels through small tubelike ducts; examples are the sudoriferous (sweat) glands and sebaceous (oil) glands.

ductless gland (dŭkt′lĭs glănd): a gland that has no excretory duct but releases secretions directly into the blood or lymph.

duodenum (dû′ô-dē′nûm): the part of the small intestines just below the stomach.

durability (dûr-ă-bĭl′ĭ-tē): the quality of being able to last for a long time without significant wear or deterioration.

dusky (dŭs′kē): somewhat dark in shade or coloring, especially dark skin.

dye (dī): to stain or color; a chemical compound or mixture formulated to penetrate the hair and effect a permanent change in hair color; made from plants, metals, or synthetic compounds.

dye brush (dī brŭsh): a small, flat, long-handled brush designed for the application of hair coloring or hair treatment products.

dye remover (dī rē-mo͞ov′ẽr): a prepared commercial product which removes tint from the hair; also called color remover.

dye solvent (dī sŏl′vênt): a chemical solution which is employed to remove artificial color from the hair.

dye stain remover (dī stān rē-mo͞ov′ ẽr): a chemical substance used to remove tint stains from the skin following the hair tinting procedure.

dynel (dī-nĕl): a synthetic fiber, resembling wool, which is employed in the manufacture of machine-made wigs and hairpieces.

dyschromia (dĭs-krō′mē-ă): abnormal pigmentation of the skin.

dyskeratoma (dĭs′kĕr ă tō′mă): a skin tumor; warty growth; a brownish, red nodule with a soft, yellowish keratotic plug appearing on the face or scalp.

dysvitaminosis (dĭs′vĭ-tă-mĭn-ō′sĭs): a disorder due to an excess of or a deficiency of a particular vitamin or vitamins.

E

ear (ēr): the organ of hearing and equilibrium.

earlap (ēr′lăp): the external ear, especially the ear lobes.

ear lobe (ēr′lōb): the soft, fleshy lower part of the external ear.

earphone (ēr′fōn): a listening device held near or inserted into the ear as a hearing aid.

ear protector (ēr prō-tĕk′tẽr): a plastic ear-shaped shell used over the ears as a protection during the hair drying procedure.

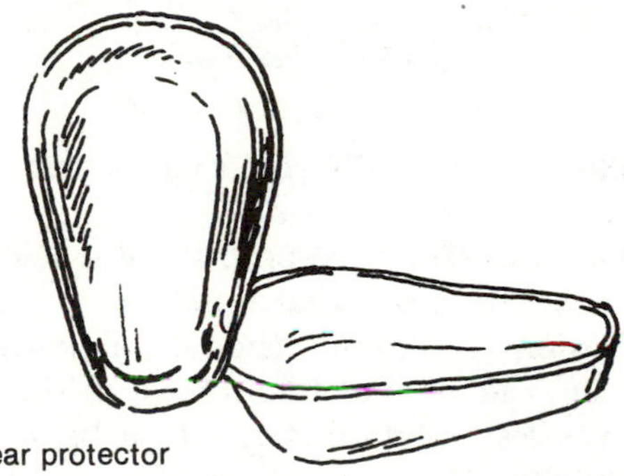
ear protector

earth color (ûrth kŭl′ẽr): any of several pigments or paints prepared from materials found in the earth; examples are: umber, chalk, clay, ocher, and charcoal.

earwax (ēr′wăks): a yellowish-brown substance secreted by the glands lining the passages of the external ear; also called cerumen.

eau de cologne (ō dē kă-lōn′): a fragrant toilet water.

ebony (ĕb′ăn-ē): a hard dark, almost black wood used for fine furnishings; a term used to describe a deep, dark skin tone.

ecchymosis (ĕk′ĭ-mō′sĭs): a discoloration such as a bluish spot caused by the rupture of a small blood vessel beneath the surface of the skin; a bruise.

eccrine (ĕk′rĭn): pertaining to the eccrine glands and their secretions.

eccrine glands (ĕk′rĭn glăndz): small sweat glands distributed over the surface of the skin of the human body; the glands that produce secretions important for heat regulation and hydrating the skin.

ecderon (ĕk′dẽr-ŏn): the epithelial, outermost layer of the skin and mucous membrane.

eclectic (ĕk-lĕk′tĭk): selecting from various sources; composed of elements or methods drawn from various sources.

ecology (ē-kŏl′ă-jē): the study of the environmental relations of organisms.

ectal (ĕk′tâl): external; outer.

ecthyma (ĕk-thī′mă): a virus disease which forms ulcerating pustules on the skin.

ecto (ĕk′tô): a prefix denoting without; outside; external.

ectoderm (ĕk′tô-dûrm): the outermost layer of the three primary germ layers in an embryo that develops into skin, the nervous system and sense organs.

ectodermic (ĕk-tô-dûr′mĭk): pertaining to the outer layer of cells formed from the inner cell mass in the embryonic cell.

ectomorph (ĕk′tô-môrf): a person who is characterized by a lean, lanky body structure.

E-F

ectothrix (ĕk′tō-thrĭks): a fungal parasite that affects the hair shaft.
ectylotic (ĕk′tĭ-lŏt′ĭk): describing an agent that removes warts.
eczema (ĕk′zĕ-mă): an inflammatory, itching disease of the skin.
eczematization (ĕk′zē-mă-tĭ-zā′shûn): the presence or formation of eczema or like irritation by allergic reaction or physical or chemical irritants.
eczematoid reaction (ĕk-zē′mă-toyd rē-ăk′shûn): a dermal and epidermal inflammatory condition characterized by edema and scaling.
eczematosis (ĕk′zē-mă-tō′sĭs): any eczematous skin disease.
eczematous (ĕk-zē′mă-tûs): having the characteristics of eczema.
edema, oedema (ĕ-dē′mă): an abnormal accumulation of clear watery fluid in the lymph spaces of the tissues; dropsy; hydrops.
edge (ĕj): the cutting side of a blade.
edging (ĕj′ĭng): the process of cutting the sideburn and nape area; feathering.
effect (ĕ-fĕkt′): consequence; result.
effector (ĕ-fĕk′tôr): a gland or muscle that responds to stimulation.
efferent (ĕf′ĕr-ênt): conveying outward, as efferent nerves conveying impulses away from the central nervous system.
efferent lymphatic (ĕf-′ĕr-ênt lĭm-făt′ik): a vessel conveying lymph away from a lymph node.
efferent neuron (ef′ĕr-ênt nū′rŏn): a neuron conducting impulses away from a nerve center.
effete (ĕ-fēt′): worn out; incapable of further vital use; exhausted of energy.
efficacious (ĕf-ĭ-kā′shûs): possessing the quality of being effective.
efficiency (ĕ-fĭsh′ên-sē): usefulness; quality or degree of being able to produce results; economic productivity.
efficient (ĕ-fĭsh′ênt): characterized by energetic and useful activity.
effilate (ĕf′ĭ-lāt): to cut the hair strand by a sliding movement of the scissors.
effilating (ĕf′ĭ-lāt-ĭng): a method of cutting and tapering hair in the same operation by a sliding movement of the scissor.
effleurage (ĕf-lo͞o-răzh): a stroking movement in massage.

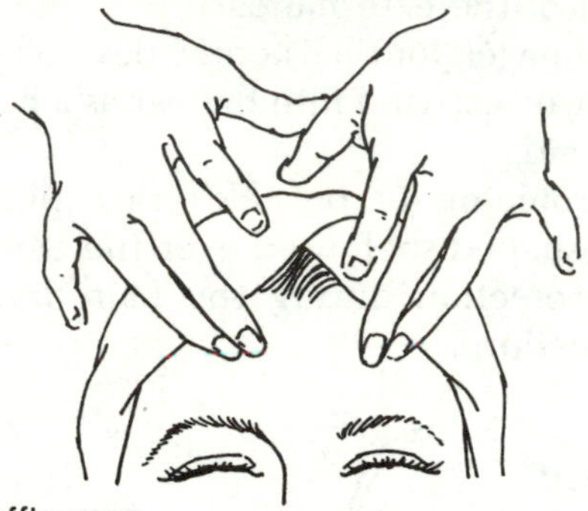

effleurage

efflorescence (ĕf′lô-rĕs′ĕnts): a rash or eruption of the skin.
effluvium (ĕf-lo͞o′vē-ûm): an ill smelling emanation or exhalation.
effusion (ĕ-fū′zhûn): the act of pouring out; the escape of fluid from the blood vessels or lymphatics into a tissue or cavity.
egg (ĕg): ovum; a round or oval reproductive body produced by female birds, fish, etc.; used primarily as a food and in some products such as shampoos and facial masks.
egg oil (ĕg oyl): fatty oil extracted from the yolk of eggs; used in some types of cosmetic creams and ointments.
egg powder (ĕg poù′dĕr): pulverized egg shell; used in many cosmetics including bath preparations, shampoos, facial masks, and creams.
eggshell nails (ĕg′shĕl nâlz): nails which are abnormally thin, translucent and

blue-white; onychotrophic condition.

Egyptian henna (ê-jĭp′shân hĕn′ă): a cosmetic used for dyeing the hair; a color varying from reddish orange to coppery brown.

elastic (ê-lăs′tĭk): capable of returning to the original form after being stretched; having the ability to stretch and return to the original form.

elastic band (ê-lăs′tĭk bănd): a flexible band used in wigs to make them adjustable; a band of elasticized material used to hold hair off the face during a facial treatment or makeup; a fastening band on a perm wave rod.

elasticity of hair (ê-lăs′tĭs′ĭ-tē ŏv hâr): property of the hair enabling it to retain curl formation and spring back into curled shape after being extended; important in the ability of hair to retain curl.

elastin (ê-lās′tĭn): a protein base similar to collagen, which forms elastic tissue.

elastoma (ê-lăs-tō′mă): a tumor formed by an excess of elastic tissue fibers or abnormal collagen fibers of the skin.

elastosis senilis (ĕ-lăs-tō′sĭs sĕ-nī′lĭs): degeneration of the elastic connective tissues in advanced age.

elbow (ĕl′bō): the joint of the arm between the upper arm and the forearm.

elder (sambucus) (ĕl′dĕr): a shrub of the honeysuckle family, the oil from which is used to soften the skin; provides mineral salts and amino acids which help reduce hardening effects of keratinization and aging of skin cells.

electrical (ē-lĕk′trĭ-kâl): consisting of, containing, producing, or operated by electricity.

electrical sterilizer (ê-lĕk′trĭ-kâl stĕr′ĭ-lī′zĕr): a cabinet electrically heated and used to keep implements sanitized.

electric comb (ê-lĕk′trĭk kōm): a comb heated electrically and used in blow-dry styling of the hair.

electric clippers (ê-lĕk′trĭk klĭp′ĕrs): an electrically powered implement used to cut and trim hair, especially on the neck area.

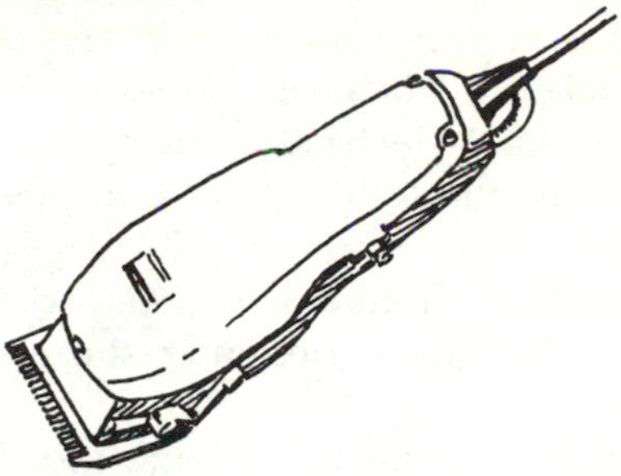

electric clippers

electric current (ê-lĕk′trĭk kûr′ênt): the flow of electric charge.

electric facial mask (ê-lĕk′trĭk fā′shâl măsk): a contoured pad heated electrically and placed over the face to soften grease deposits and to induce deep penetration of beneficial products into the skin.

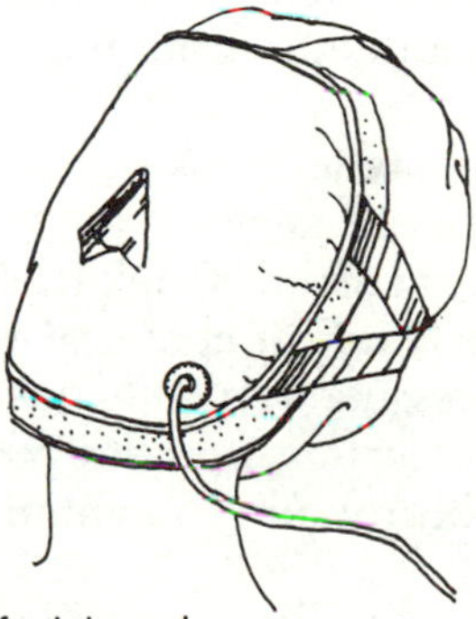

electric facial mask

electric hair roller (ê-lĕk′trĭk hâr rō′lĕr): a cylindrical roller designed to retain heat and used to style hair while it is dry.

electric heater (ê-lĕk′trĭk hē′tĕr): as used

E-F

in permanent waving, a heating device connected to a permanent wave machine.

electricity (ê-lĕk-trĭs′ĭ-tē): a form of energy, which when in motion, exhibits magnetic, chemical or thermal effects.

electricity, animal (ê-lĕk-trĭs′ĭ-tē, ăn′ĭ-mâl): the free electricity in the body.

electricity, chemical (ê-lĕk-trĭs′ĭ-te kĕm′ĭ-kâl): electricity which is generated by chemical action in a galvanic cell.

electricity, franklinic (ê-lĕk-trĭs′ĭ-tē, frănk-lĭn′ĭck): a friction or static electricity.

electricity, frictional (ê-lĕk-trĭs′ĭ tē, frĭk′-shûn-âl): electricity produced by friction.

electricity, galvanic (ê-lĕk-trĭs′ĭ-te, găl-văn′ĭk): electricity which is generated by chemical action in a galvanic cell.

electricity, induced or inductive (ê-lĕk-trĭs′ĭ-tē, ĭn-dūst′ or ĭn-dŭk′tĭv): electricity produced by proximity to an electrified body.

electricity, magnetic (ê-lĕk-trĭs′ĭ-tē măg-nĕt′ĭk): electricity developed by bringing a conductor near the poles of a magnet.

electricity, static (ê-lĕk-trĭs′ĭ-tē, stăt′ĭk): frictional electricity.

electricity, voltaic (ê-lĕk-trĭs′ĭ-tē, vōl-tā′ĭk): galvanic or chemical electricity.

electric pressing iron (ê-lĕk′trĭk prĕs′ĭng ī′ûrn): a curling iron designed with a larger barrel for straightening curly hair.

electric sanitizer (ê-lĕk trĭk săn′ĭ-tī-zĕr): a dry sanitizer unit containing an ultraviolet lamp which keeps implements sanitary.

electric shaver (ê-lĕk′trĭk shāv′ĕr): an electrically powered device used to remove facial and body hair.

electric straightening comb (ê-lĕk′trĭk strāt′n-ĭng kōm): a comb with a wooden handle and metal teeth designed with a heating element and used to straighten curly hair.

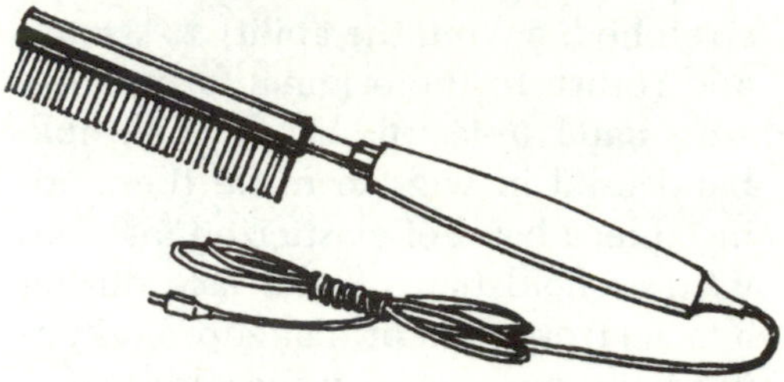

electric straightening comb

electric styling brush (ê-lĕk′trĭk stī′lĭng brŭsh): an implement which combines a hand-held dryer with a brush; used to style hair.

electrification (ê-lĕk′trĭ-fĭ-kā′shûn): the process of applying electricity to the body by holding an electrode in the hand and charging the body with electricity.

electrocoagulation (ê-lĕk′trō-kō-ăg-û-lā′shûn): the single needle shortwave method of electrolysis; the use of high frequency current to remove superfluous hair.

electrode (ê-lĕk′trōd): a pole of an electric cell; an applicator for directing the use of electricity on a customer.

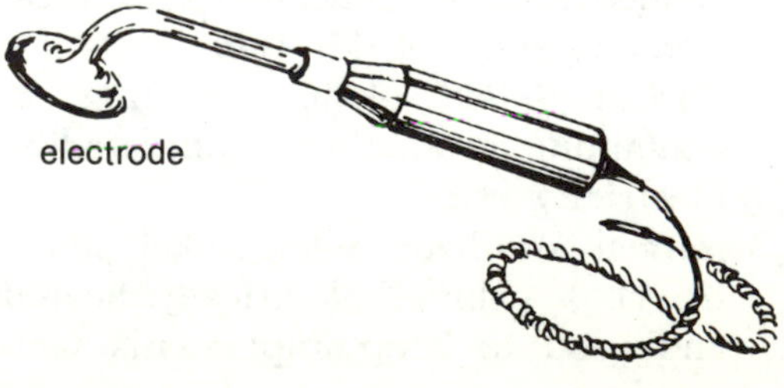

electrode

electrode jel (ê-lĕk′trōd jĕl): a jel used to improve contact between the electrode and the skin when the electrode is used in a specific treatment.

electrologist (ê-lĕk-trŏl′ô-jĭst): one who removes hair and various skin imperfections by means of an electric current applied to the body with a needle shaped electrode.

electrology (ê-lĕk-trŏl′ô-jē): the science of electricity.

electrolysis (ê-lĕk-trŏl′ĭ-sĭs): decomposition of a chemical compound or body tissues, particularly hair roots, by means of electricity.

electrolyte (ê-lĕk′trô-līt): any compound which, in solution conducts a current of electricity.

electrolytic (ê-lĕk-trô-lĭt′ĭk): pertaining to electrolysis.

electrolytic cup (ê-lĕk-trô-lĭt′ĭk kŭp): an appliance used to cleanse the skin before giving a facial or body massage.

electrolytic rebonding (ê-lĕk′trô-lĭt′ĭk rē-bŏnd′ĭng): chemical process involving reformation of electromagnetic or ionic bonds.

electromagnet (ê-lĕk′trô-măg′nĕt): a mass of soft iron surrounded by a coil of wire; a current passing through the wire will make the iron core magnetic.

electromotive force (ê-lĕk′trô-mō′tĭv fôrs): something that moves or tends to move electricity.

electron (ê-lĕk′trŏn): a basic negatively charged particle found outside the nucleus of an atom, arranged in orbits or shells.

electronic tweezing (ê-lĕk-trŏn′ĭk twē′-zĭng): the use of high frequency current in removal of superfluous hair.

electrophobia (ê-lĕk′trô-fō′bē-ă): a morbid fear of electricity.

electropositive (ê-lĕk′trô-pŏz′ĭ-tĭv): relating to or charged with positive electricity.

electrostatic (ê-lĕk′trô-stăt′ĭk): pertaining to static electricity.

electrotherapeutics (ê-lĕk′trô-thĕr-ă-pū′tĭks): the application of electricity for therapeutic purposes.

element (ĕl′ĕ-mênt): the simplest form of basic matter; a substance that cannot be broken down into a simpler substance without loss of identity; of the more than 100 elements, examples are: iron, sulfur, hydrogen, mercury, carbon.

elementary (ĕl-ĕ-mĕn′tă-rē): basic introductory; relating to the simplest elements or principles of something.

elements in hair (ĕl′ĕ-mênts in hâr): elements commonly found in hair are: nitrogen, oxygen, carbon, sulfur, hydrogen and phosphorus.

elevate (ĕl′ĕ-vāt): to raise; to make higher.

elevation (ĕl′ĕ-vā′shûn): a term employed in hair shaping (cutting) and styling to indicate the angle or degree hair is held from the head.

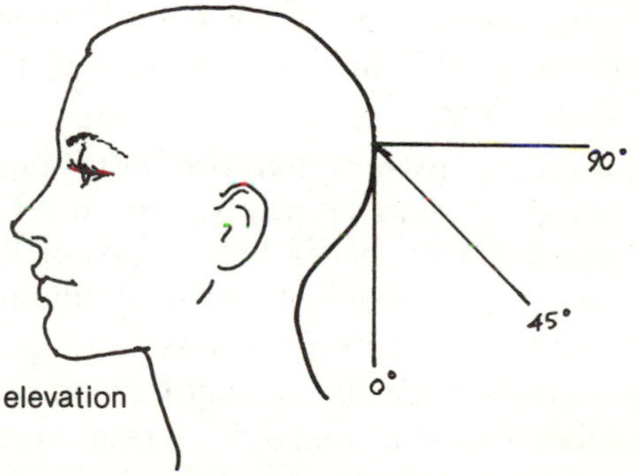

elevation

elevation, high (ĕl-ĕ-vā′shûn, hī): when hair is approximately the same length when extended at right angles from

E-F

the scalp; in high elevation hair is held 90 degrees from the headform.

elevation, low (ĕl-ĕ-vā′shûn, lō): hair is held 15 degrees from the headform creating a slight amount of layering.

elevation, medium (ĕl-ĕ-vā′shûn, mē-dĭ′ŭm): the hair is held 45 degrees from the headform.

eliminate (ê-lĭm′ĭ-nāt): to rid the body of; to excrete; to set aside.

elimination (ê-lĭm′ĭ-nā′shûn): act of expelling or excreting.

eliminative (ê-lĭm′ĭ-nă-tĭv): relating to or tending to eliminate.

ellipse (ê-lĭps′): a wide oval curve.

elutriate (ê-lo͞o′trē-āt): purify by washing, separating and straining.

emaciation (ê-mā′shē-ā′shûn): the state of being wasted away physically; loss of fat of the body; extreme leanness.

embed (ĕm-bĕd′): to fix firmly in surrounding matter.

embellish (ĕm-bĕl′ĭsh): to decorate; to add something to adorn.

embryo (ĕm′brē-ō): an organism in the early stages of development; a developing human from the moment of conception to the end of the eighth week after fertilization.

embryology (ĕm-brē-ŏl′ô-jē): science dealing with the development of the embryo.

embryonic extract (ĕm′brē-ŏn′ĭk ĕks′-trăct): substances taken from any living thing in the earliest stages of life and used in some types of medicinal and cosmetic preparations.

emerald (ĕm′ĕ-râld): a bright green precious stone; a deep, rich green color.

emery board (ĕm′ẽr-ē bôrd): a disposable manicuring instrument having rough cutting ridges; used to file or remove the free edge of the nail.

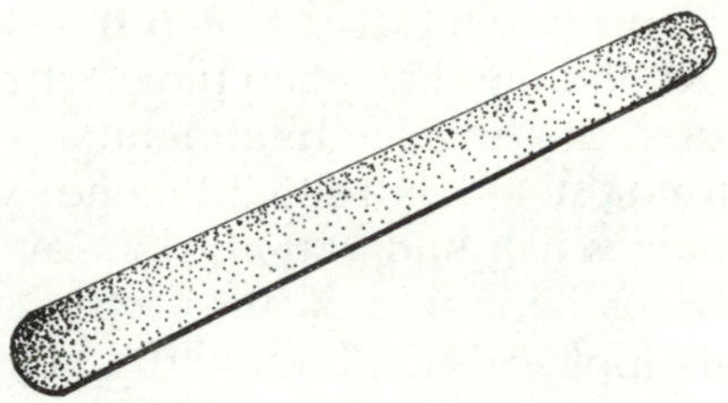
emery board

emit (ê-mĭt′): to send out; to give off light, heat, sound.

emollient (ē-mŏl′yênt): an agent that softens or smooths the surface of the skin.

emollient cream (ē-mŏl′yênt krēm): a specially prepared cream used in facial and body massage.

emphasize (ĕm′fă-sīz): to give importance or prominence to; to enhance facial features by use of cosmetics.

emphysema (ĕm-fĭ-zē′mă): abnormal presence of air or gas in body tissues; a disease of the lungs marked by swelling of air spaces and destructive changes in the alveolar walls.

emulsified (ê-mŭl′sĭ-fīd): made into an emulsion.

emulsifier (ê-mŭl′sĭ-fī-ẽr): a substance, as gelatin, gum, etc., which helps to keep oils and liquids in suspension to prevent separation of ingredients.

emulsion (ê-mŭl′shûn): substantially permanent mixture of two or more liquids that are normally nonsoluble, and are held in suspension by emulsifiers.

enamel (ē-năm′ĕl): gloss; polish.

encephalic (ĕn-sĕ-fâl′ĭk): pertaining to the brain.

enclose (ĕn-klōz′): to close in; confine.

end (ĕnd): termination.

end bonds, peptide bonds (ĕnd bŏndz, pĕp′tīd bŏndz): the chemical bonds which join amino acids to form the long chains which are characteristic of all proteins.

endepidermis (ĕnd-ĕp-ĭ-dûr′mĭs): the inner layer of the epidermis.

endermic (ĕn-dûr′mĭk): acting through the skin by absorption, as a product applied to the skin.

endermosis (ĕn′dẽr-mō′sĭs): the application of a product to the skin by rubbing.

enderon (ĕn′dẽr-ŏn): the deeper part of the skin or mucous membrane; as distinguished from the epidermis or epithelium.

endo (ĕn′dô): a prefix denoting inner; within.

endocrine (ĕn′dô-krĭn): secreting directly into the bloodstream as a ductless gland; secreting internally.

endocrine gland (ĕn′dō-krĭn glănd): one of several ductless glands, as the thyroid or pituitary and suprarenal glands, whose secretions are released directly into the blood stream.

endocrine obesity (ĕn′dō-krĭn ô-bē′sĭ-tē): a condition causing weight gain due to dysfunction of the endocrine glands.

endocrinology (ĕn′dō-krĭ-nŏl-ă-jē): the study of the endocrine glands and their function.

endomorph (ĕn′dô-môrf): an individual having a body build characterized by roundness, large viscera and fat accumulation; large of trunk and thighs.

end organ (ĕnd ôr′găn): the termination of nerve fiber in the skin, muscle, mucous membranes, etc.

endosteum (ĕn-dŏs′tê-ŭm): the membrane covering the inner surface of bone in the medullary cavity.

endothelial (ĕn′dô-thēl′ē-âl): a thin lining of the interior of the heart, blood vessels, lymphatics, etc.

endotoxin (ĕn′dō-tŏk′sĭn): a toxic substance found in some forms of bacteria.

end papers (ĕnd pā′pẽrz): absorbent papers used to control the ends of hair in wrapping and winding hair on rods or rollers.

end permanent (ĕnd pẽr′mă-nênt): a permanent wave applied only to the ends of the hair.

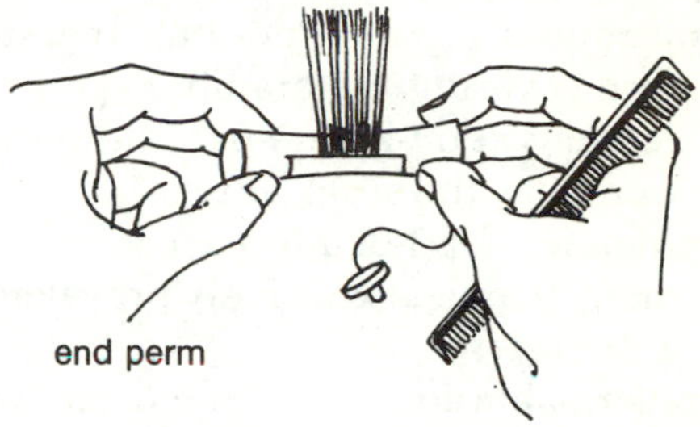

end perm

ends, hair (ĕndz, hâr): the last inch of the hair furthest away from the scalp.

energy (ĕn′ẽr-jē): internal or inherent power or capacity for performing work.

enfleurage (än-flĕ-razh′): a process of extracting perfume by placing blossoms in glass trays lined with odorless fat: the fat takes up the fragrance and when mixed with alcohol then distilled, provides the essential oils used in fine perfumes.

enhance (ĕn-hăns′): to increase beauty or attractiveness; to add value and desirability.

enlarged pores (ĕn-lärg′d pôrz): follicles (pores) that have been stretched due to accumulation of sebum and dead surface cells.

entangle (ĕn-tâng′l): to intertwine the hair in a confused manner.

environment (ĕn-vī′rûn-mênt): the surrounding conditions; influences or forces which influence or modify.

enzyme (ĕn′zīm): an organic compound, frequently a protein, capable of accelerating or producing high catalytic action that will promote a chemical change.

eosin (ē′ō-sĭn): a synthetic, organic red dye used in cosmetics, especially in lip and cheek coloring.

epi (ĕp′ĭ): a prefix denoting upon, beside.

epicranium (ĕp′ĭ-krā′nē-ûm): the structure covering the cranium.

epicranius (ĕp′ĭ-krā′nē-ûs): the occipito frontailis; the scalp muscle.

epidemic (ĕp′ĭ-dĕm′ĭk): common to many people; excessively prevalent, as a disease.

epidermabrasion (ĕp-ē-dûrm′ă-brā-zhûn): cosmetic skin peeling achieved with chemicals or special machines; sloughing off the outermost layer of the skin.

epidermal (ĕp′ĭ-dûr′mâl): pertaining to or arising from the outer layer of the skin.

epidermin (ĕp-ĭ-dûr′mĭn): a regenerating substance; an extract of animal tissues which has been used in the renewal of destroyed skin, such as in wounds and burns.

epidermis (ĕp-ĭ-dûr′mĭs): the outer epithelial portion of the skin.

epilate (ĕp′ĭ-lāt): to remove hair from below the skin surface; to uproot hair.

epilation (ĕp′ĭ-lā′shûn): the removal of hair by the roots.

epilatory (ĕ-pĭl′ă-tô-rē): a substance used to remove hair from the face.

epilepsy (ĕp′ĭ-lĕp′sē): a chronic nervous disease characterized by sudden loss of consciousness and convulsions.

epileptic (ĕp′ĭ-lep′tĭk): one affected by epilepsy.

epinephrine (ĕp′ĭ-nĕf′rĭn): a hormone secreted by the medulla of the adrenal glands in response to emergency; used as an injection for the relief of some allergic reactions.

epithelial (ĕp′ĭ-thēl′ē-âl): having the nature of epithelium.

epithelial cell (ĕp′ĭ-thēl′ē-âl sĕl): one of various kinds of cells that form the epidermis and lines hollow organs, such as the stomach and all passages.

epithelial tissue (ĕp-ĭ-thēl′ē-âl tĭsh′o͞o): pertaining to cells that form the epidermis.

epithelioma (ĕp′ĭ-thēl-ē-ō′mă): a malignant growth consisting of epithelial cells.

epithelium (ĕp′ĭ-thēl′ē-ŭm): a cellular tissue or membrane, with little intercellular substance, covering a free surface or lining of a cavity.

eponychium (ĕp′ô-nĭk′ē-ŭm): the extension of cuticle at base of nail; the quick of the nail.

equal (ē′kwâl): uniform; even; exactly the same in measurement or amount.

equal blending (ē′kwâl blĕnd′ĭng): in hair styling, the blending of hair that is one length at an equal distance from the scalp.

equation (ê-kwā′zhûn): a method of expressing a chemical reaction by using chemical formulas and symbols.

equilibrium (ē-kwĭ-lĭb′rē-ŭm): the state of balance between two or more forces acting within or upon a body in such a way that stability is maintained.

equipment (ê-kwĭp′mênt): supplies and instruments required to perform a particular service.

equivalent (ê-kwĭv′ă-lĕnt): a state of being or having equal values; equal in volume, area, force, etc.

eradicate (ê-răd′ĭ-kāt): to destroy thoroughly.

eradication (ê-răd-ĭ-kā′shûn): act of plucking by the roots; destroying utterly.

erecter pilae (ê-rĕk′tẽr pē′lī): minute muscles located at the base of each hair that contract when the skin becomes cold, causing the hair to stand erect; compression of skin glands; gooseflesh.

erector (ê-rĕk′tẽr): an elevating muscle.

erector muscle (ê-rĕk′tẽr mŭs′l): a muscle that produces erection; for example, the arrector pili, fan-like muscles attached to hair follicles which contract, especially when cold, causing the hair to stand up in a "gooseflesh" manner.

erosion (ê-rō′zhûn): the eating away of tissue.

eructation (ē-rŭk-tā′shûn): belching; that which is forced out.

eruption (ê-rŭp′shûn): a visible lesion of the skin due to disease; marked by redness or papular condition or both.

erysipelas (ĕr-ĭ-sĭp′ê-lûs): an acute infectious disease accompanied by a diffused inflammation of the skin and mucous membrane.

erythema (ĕr′ĭ-thē′mă): a superficial blush or redness of the skin.

erythematous (er′ĭ-thēm′ă-tûs): pertaining to or characterized by abnormal redness of the skin caused by a congestion of capillaries.

erythrasma (ĕr′ĭ-thrăz′mă): eruption of reddish brown patches in the axillae and groin, especially due to the presence of a fungus.

erythrism (ĕr′ĭ-thrĭzm): exceptional redness of the hair, beard and skin.

erythrocyte (ĕ-rĭth′rô-sīt): a red blood cell; red corpuscle.

erythrosis (ĕr′ĭ-thrō′sĭs): a reddish or purple discoloration of the skin and mucous membranes.

eschar (ĕs′kär): a dry crust of dead tissue or a scab caused by heat or a corrosive substance.

esophagus (ĕ-sŏf′ă-gûs): the canal leading from the pharynx to the stomach.

essence (ĕs′âns): the extract of a plant or food containing the distinctive properties of the plant or food such as might be used in perfumes.

essential (ĕ-sĕn′shâl): important in the highest degree; necessary; indispensable.

essential fatty acid (ĕ-sĕn′shâl făt′ē ă′sĭd): any of the polyunsaturated fatty acids that are required in the diet, including lionleic, linolenic and arachidonic acids.

essential oils (ĕ-sĕn′shâl oyls): any class of volatile oils that impart the characteristic odors to plants; in perfumes and flavorings.

ester (ĕs′tẽr): an organic compound formed by the reaction of an acid and an alcohol.

esthetic, aesthetic (ĕs-thĕt′ĭk): of or relating to beauty; describing beauty in art and nature; appreciation of beauty.

esthetician, aesthetician (ĕs-thē′tĭsh-ĕn): a specialist in or devotee of esthetics; one whose occupation is in the cleansing, preservation of health and beautification of the skin and body; one who gives therapeutic facial treatments.

esthetics, aesthetics (ĕs-thĕt′ĭks): the branch of cosmetology which deals with the health and beautification of the skin and the entire body.

estrogen (ĕs-′trō-ǰen): any of various substances that influence estrus or produce changes in the sexual characteristics of female mammals.

ether (ē′thẽr): a substance obtained from

distilling alcohol with sulphuric acid, used as an anesthetic.

etheric oils (ĭ-thĕr′ĭk oylz): oils from the leaves of certain plants (rosemary, sage, thyme); used in herbal essence therapy.

ethics (ĕth′ĭks): principles of good character and proper conduct.

ethmoid (ĕth′moyd): resembling a sieve; a bone forming part of the walls of the nasal cavity.

ethmonasal (ĕth-mō-nā′zâl): pertaining to the ethmoid and nasal bones.

ethnic (ĕth′nĭk): belonging to or distinctive of a particular racial or cultural division.

ethyl acetate (ĕth′ĭl ăs′ĕ-tāt): a colorless liquid with a fruity odor that occurs in fruits and some berries; used as a solvent in nail polish and polish remover.

ethyl alcohol (ĕth′ĭl ăl′kô-hôl): the basis of some alcoholic beverages; used in cosmetic products such as astringents, antiseptics and fragrances.

etiology (ē′tē-ŏl′ă-jē): the science of the causes of disease and their mode of operation.

eucalyptus (ū′kă-lĭp′tûs): an oil from the eucalyptus plant; used for its stimulating properties and often called "blue gum."

eukeratin (û-kĕr′ă-tĭn): a true keratin found in hair, nails, feathers, hoofs, horns, etc.

European hair (yōōr-ă-pē′ên hâr): fine quality human hair, usually from European countries, used in constructing wigs and hairpieces.

evaporate (ê-văp′ô-rāt): to disburse in the form of vapor.

evaporation (ê-văp-ô-rā′shûn): the product of changing from liquid to vapor form.

evascularization (ê-vas′kū-lär-ĭ-zā′shûn): the destruction of a vessel or a duct which conveys blood to a part of the body.

ex (ĕks): a prefix denoting out of; from; away from.

exaggerate (ĕg-zăj′ĕr-āt): to delineate extravagantly; to enlarge or increase beyond the normal.

excess (ĕk′sĕs): more than a normal amount.

excitation (ĕk-sī-tā′shûn): the act of stimulating or irritating.

excoriate (ĕks-kō′rē-āt): to wear away scrape, or strip off the skin.

excoriation (ĕks-kō-rē-ā′shûn): act of stripping or wearing off the skin; an abrasion.

excrement (ĕks′kră-mênt): waste material expelled from the body; also called feces.

excrescence (ĕks-krĕs′ĕns): a disfiguring outgrowth.

excrete (ĕks-krēt): to eliminate from the blood or tissue from the body as through the kidneys or sweat glands.

excretion (ĕks-krē′shûn): that which is thrown off or eliminated from the body; a substance that is produced by some cells, but in itself is of no further use to the body; the act or process of excreting.

excretory (ĕks′krê-tô-rē): pertaining to or serving for excretion.

exercise (ĕk′sĕr-sīz): a putting into action, use or practice; exertion for the sake of improvement.

exfoliation (ĕks-fō′lē-ā′shûn): peeling and shredding of the horny layer of the skin; a process that normally follows inflammation or occurs in some skin diseases.

exfoliative dermatitis (ĕks-fo′lē-ă-tĭv dûr-mâ-tī′tĭs): any dermatitis where there is excessive hair loss and denudation of the skin.

exhalation (ěks-hă-lā′shûn): the act of breathing outward.

exhaustion (ěq-zôs′chûn): loss of vital and nervous power from fatigue or protracted disease.

exocrine gland (eks′ô-krĭn glănd): a gland that secretes to an epithelial surface directly or through ducts.

exothermic (ěk′sō-thẽr′mĭk): characterized by or formed with the giving off of heat.

exotic (ĕg-zŏt′ĭk): unusual, striking or different.

expansion (ěks-păn′shûn): distention, dilation or swelling; the distance a completed sculptured form extends into space.

expel (ěks-pĕl′): to force out; to eject or dislodge; to remove a blackhead from a follicle.

experiment (ěk-spĕr′ĭ-mênt): to test; discover or illustrate a truth, principle or effect; to try.

expert (ěks′pûrt): an experienced person; one who has special knowledge in a particular subject.

expertize (ěk′spẽr-tēz′): knowledge or skill in a particular field.

expiration (ěk-spĭ-rā′shûn): the act of breathing out; expelling air from the lungs.

expire (ěk′spī-ẽr): to breathe out air from the lungs; to exhale; to die.

exposure (ěks-pō′zhûr): state of being open to view or unprotected, as from the weather.

exquisite (ěk′skwĭ-zĭt): rare; delicate; showing a high degree of excellence of craftmanship.

extend (ěk-stěnd′): to open or stretch more or to full length.

extensibility (ěks-těn-sĭ-bĭl′ĭ-tē): capable of being extended or stretched.

extension (ěks-těn′shûn): a type of fantasy hairpiece in which the hair is sewn to a wire covered with tubular ribbon; the extension is used to add space but not density to a coiffure.

extensor (ěks-těn′sôr): a muscle which serves to extend or straighten out a limb or part.

extensor carpiradialis (ěks-těn′sôr kär′pī-rā-dē-ā′lĭs): a strong muscle in the wrist which operates with other muscles to bend the hand backward.

extensor digitorum longus (ěks-těn′sôr dĭj-ĭ-tō′rŭm lông′ûs): a muscle which bends the foot upward and enables the toes to be extended.

exterior (ěks-tē′rē-ẽr): outside.

external (ěks-tûr′-nâl): pertaining to the outside.

external carotid artery (ěks-tûr′nâl kă-rŏt′ĭd är′tĭr-ē): artery that supplies blood to the anterior parts of the scalp, ear, face, neck and side of the head.

external jugular vein (ěks-tûr′nâl jŭg-û-lăr vān): the vein located on the side of the neck.

external maxillary artery (ěks-tûr′nâl măk′sĭl-ẽr-ē är′tĭr-ē): the artery which supplies blood to the mouth and the lower region of the face.

external respiration (ěks-tûr′nâl rěs′pĭ-rā′shûn): the exchange of gases between the air in the atmosphere and air in the lungs: then the exchange of air in the lungs and the pulmonary capillaries.

external verterbral plexuses (ěks-tûr′nâl vûr′tě-brâl plěk′să-sěs): veins located anterior and posterior to the vertebral column.

externus (ěks-tûr′-nûs): external; pertaining to the outside.

E-F

extracellular (ĕk′stră-sĕl′û-lăr): outside of a cell or cells.

extract (ĕks′-trăkt): a solid obtained by evaporating a solution of a drug; to draw out; to extract a blackhead.

extracurricular (ĕk′stră-kă-rĭk′û-lăr): pertaining to activities or studies that are in addition to a regular course of study; supplementary.

extraocular muscle (ĕk′stră-ŏk′û-lăr mŭs′l): the six small voluntary muscles that control the movement of the eyeball within its orbit.

extravagant (ĕk-străv′ă-gănt): overly lavish; excessive.

extreme (ĕks-trēm′): to a very great or to the greatest degree; to the farthest point.

extremity (ĕk-strĕm′i-tē): the distant end or part of any organ; a hand or foot.

extricate (ĕks′trĭ-kāt): to disentangle.

extrusion (ĕk-strōō′zhûn): a forcing out or expulsion as the expelling of a blackhead.

exudation (ĕks-û-dā′shûn): act of discharging sweat, moisture, or other liquid from a body through pores or incisions; oozing out.

exudative eczema (ĕks′û-dā-tĭv ĕk′zē-mă): an acute form of dermatitis in which serum is exuded; also called "weeping eczema."

exude (ĕks′ūd, ĕqz-ūd′): to discharge slowly from a body through pores or incisions, as sweat.

exuviate (ĕg-zōō′vē-āt): to cast off; to shed; as to shed skin.

exuviation (ĕg-zōō′vē-ā′shûn): the shedding of epidermal structures; the act of shedding.

eye (ī): the organ of vision.

eyeball (ī′bôl): the ball-shaped part of the eye; the globe of the eye.

eyebrow (ī′brau̇): the bony ridge upon which hair grows in an arch above the eye.

eyebrow arching (ī′brau̇ ärch′ĭng): the plucking, trimming or waxing of the brow hair to create a neat arched effect.

eyebrow brush (ī′brau̇ brŭsh): a small, short handled brush used to groom the eyebrows.

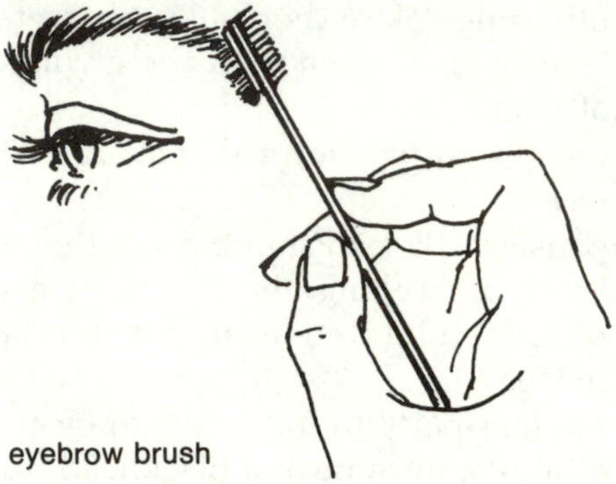
eyebrow brush

eyebrow comb (ī′brau̇ kōm): a small comb with a short handle used for grooming the eyebrows.

eyebrow pencil (ī′brau̇ pĕn′sĭl): a pencil used to add color and shape to the eyebrows.

eyebrow remover (ī′brau̇ rē-mōō′vĕr): the product, such as wax, or implement, such as tweezers or a shaver, used to remove superfluous hair from the eyebrows.

eyebrow tint (ī′brau̇ tĭnt): a metallic salt dye formulated to be used in tinting eyebrows and eyelashes.

eye color (ī kŭl′ĕr): the color of the iris of the eye; color in eye makeup products.

eye cream (ī krēm): a cream or emollient formulated for the delicate skin around the eyes; some of the ingredients used in eye creams are: beeswax, cholesterol, lanolin, sodium benzoate, boric acid, mineral oil, almond oil, ascorbyle palmitate and lecithin.

eye cup (ī kŭp): a small cup with a curved rim to fit the eye; used when washing or applying lotion or liquid to the eye.

eyedrops (ī′drŏps): a specially formulated cleansing wash for the eyes that is dispensed with an eyedropper.

eyehole (ī′hōl): an opening for the eyes, as in a gauze mask.

eyelash adhesive (ī′lăsh ăd-hē′sĭv): a product that is used to make artificial eyelashes adhere to the natural lash line; surgical adhesive.

eyelash brush (ī′lăsh brŭsh): a small, long-handled brush with short bristles used to groom the eyelashes and to apply mascara to the lashes.

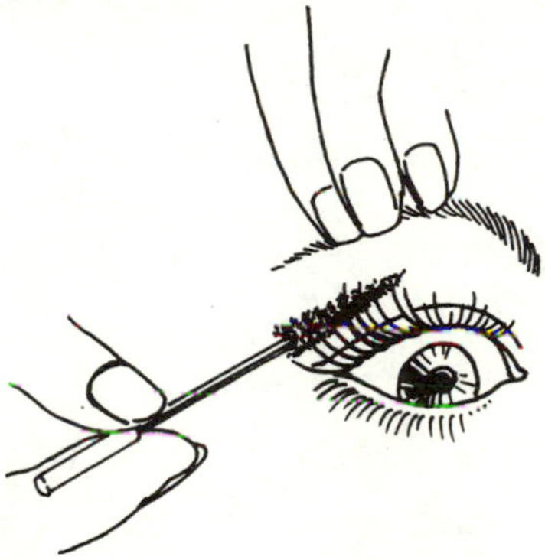

eyelash brush

eyelash comb (ī′lăsh′ kōm): a small comb with a long handle designed to comb and curl the eyelashes.

eyelash curler (ī′lăsh′ kûr′lĕr): an implement designed to fit the curve of the eyelid so that when lashes are pressed between two parts, they will be curled upward.

eyelashes (ī′lăsh-ĕz): the hair of the eyelids.

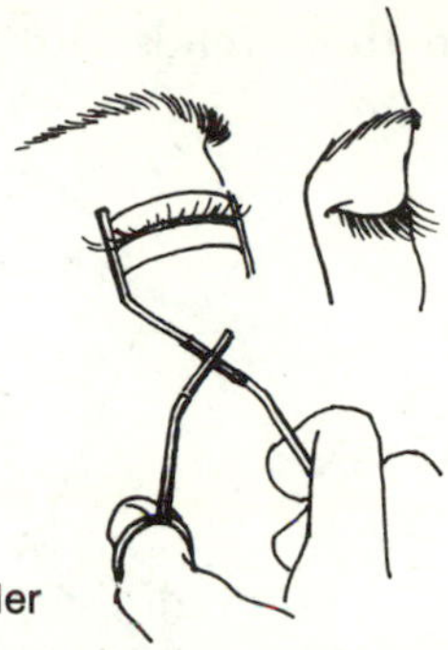

eyelash curler

eyelashes, artificial (ī′lăsh-ĕz, är-tĕ-fĭsh′-âl): individual lash hair on a strip, applied with adhesive to the natural lash line.

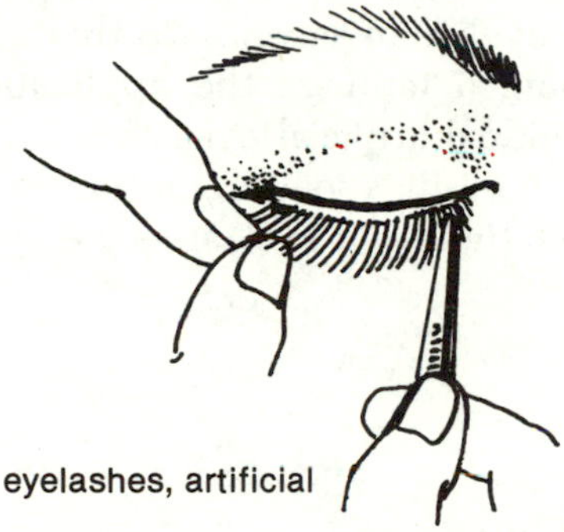

eyelashes, artificial

eyelash remover (ī′lăsh rē-mōōv′ĕr): a liquid used to remove artificial eyelashes by dissolving the adhesive which fastens the lashes to the natural lash line.

eyelash tint (ī′lăsh′ tĭnt): a metallic salt dye formulated to be used in dyeing eyelashes and eyebrows.

eyelid (ī′lĭd): the movable fold of skin over the eye; the protective covering of the eyeball.

eyeliner (ī′līn-ĕr): a pencil or liquid makeup used to outline the eyes.

eye makeup (ī māk′ŭp′): cosmetics created especially for the enhancement of brows, lashes and eyelids.

eye pads (ī pădz): cotton pads shaped to

E-F

fit over the eyelids during a facial treatment.

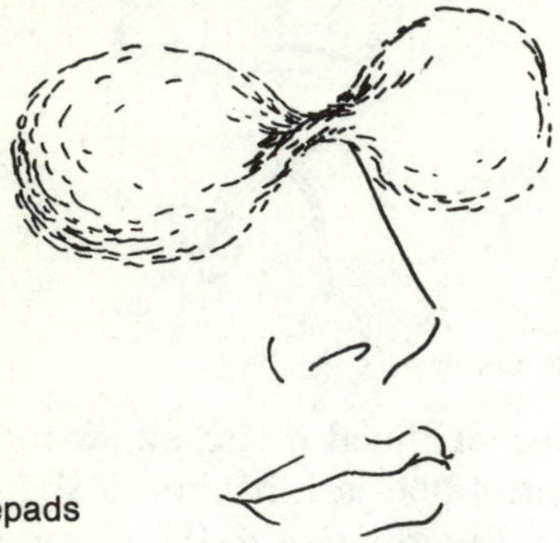

eyepads

eye shadow (ī shăd′ō): a cosmetic applied on the eyelids to accentuate them.

eye tabbing (ī tăb′ĭng): the application of individual artificial eyelashes.

eyewash (ī′wäsh): a soothing lotion to alleviate fatigue and to cleanse the eyes.

F

face (fās): the front portion of the head comprising the area from forehead to chin and ear to ear; the forehead, eyes, nose, mouth, cheeks and chin.

face framing (fās frā′ĭng): a frame formed by lightening (one or two shades) a narrow section of hair around the face.

face lift (fās lĭft′): in cosmetic surgery, rhytidectomy, the removal of excess skin to correct sagging areas of the face.

face powder (fās′ paù′dẽr): a fine cosmetic powder sometimes tinted and scented which is used to add a matte or dull finish to the face.

facial (fā′shâl): pertaining to the face; also, the seventh cranial nerve.

facial arteries (fā′ shâl är-tĭr′ēz): the arteries that supply blood to the face.

facial bowl (fā′ shâl bōl): a specially designed bowl used during the spraying procedure of a facial treatment; also called a couvette.

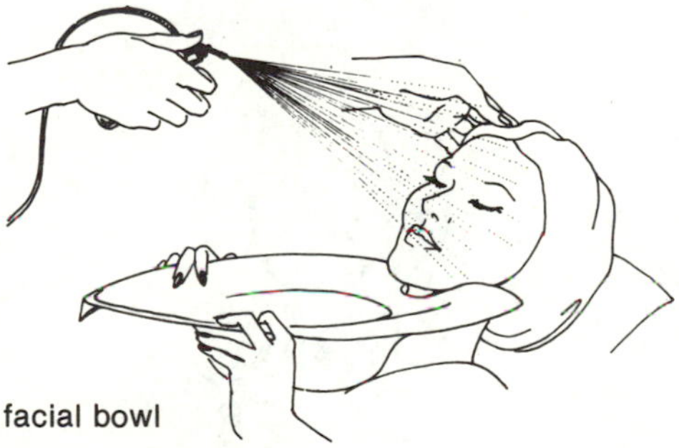

facial bowl

facial chair (fā′ shâl châr): a reclining chair with a headrest.

facial cream (fā′shâl krēm): a product in cream form used during a facial treatment for specific purposes, such as cleansing and hydrating.

facial feature (fā′shâl fē ′chẽr): a distinctive part of the face, such as the eyes, nose, mouth cheeks or chin.

facial hair (fā′shâl hâr): any hair on the face; whiskers, beard, mustache, eyebrows; superfluous facial hair, usually found on upper lip and between the eyebrows.

facial index (fā′shâl ĭn′ dĕks): a number which expresses the ratio of the breadth of the face to the length multiplied by 100.

facial machines (fā′shâl mă-shēnz′): specially constructed apparatus, appliances and equipment used to give facial treatments.

facial mask (fā′shâl măsk): a mask of gauze or wax with openings for eyes and nose, used with products to benefit specific skin conditions; types include oil mask and wax mask.

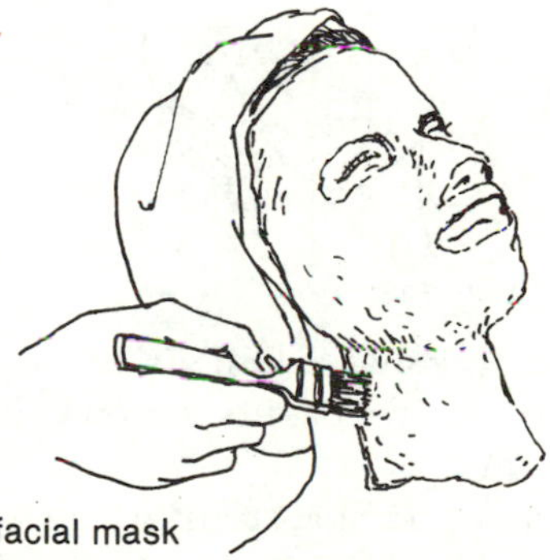

facial mask

facial massage (fā′shâl mă-säzh): a series of movements designed to benefit the facial muscles, skin and tissues; a procedure given by a trained esthetician

E-F

to stimulate, tone, cleanse and beautify the skin.

facial movements (fā′shâl mo͞ov′mênts): a massage procedure where certain manipulation and movements are used in facial treatment to benefit the skin.

facial muscles (fā′shâl mŭs′ĕlz): pertaining to the muscles of the face; see muscles.

facial nerve (fā′shâl nûrv): the seventh cranial nerve, one of a pair that serve to activate the muscles which control facial expressions.

facial pack (fā′shâl păk): a product placed on the face for beneficial purposes, such as tightening the skin, cleansing the follicles, and removing impurities from the skin.

facial proportions (fā′shâl prō-pôr′-shûnz): the dimensional relationship of one facial feature to another, to be considered in makeup artistry and hairstyling.

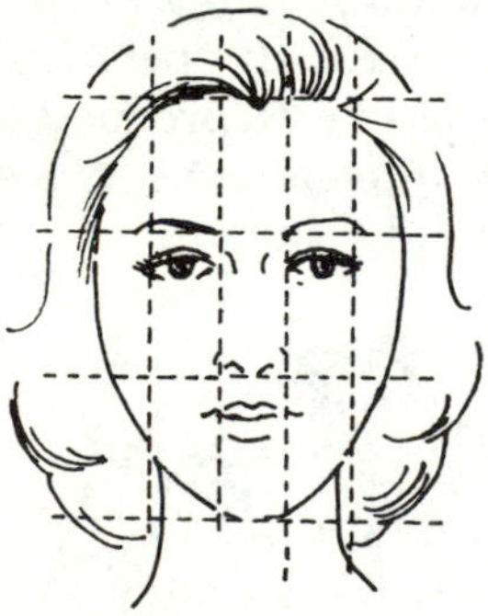

facial proportions

facial salon (fā′shâl să-lŏn; săl′ŏn): a salon or shop where clients receive facial treatments.

facial steamer (fā′shâl stēm′ĕr): an apparatus used to apply steam at a comfortable temperature to the face during a facial treatment.

facial towel (fā′shâl taů′ĕl): a small towel, usually of white cotton terry cloth about 16 × 24 inches (40.64 cm by 60.96 cm) used to apply warm, moist steam to the face during a facial treatment or a shaving procedure.

facial treatment (fā′shâl tret′mênt): a cosmetic treatment applied to the face and neck generally for preventive or corrective purposes and for the general enhancement of skin and muscle tone.

facial veins (fā′shâl vānz): veins located on the anterior side of the head; see veins.

facioplasty (fă′shē-ō-plăs-tē): plastic surgery of the face.

fad (făd): a style which is accepted for a short period of time and then disappears.

fade (fād): to become indistinct; to gradually disappear.

Fahrenheit (fă′rên-hīt): pertaining to the Fahrenheit thermometer or scale; water freezes at 32°F and boils at 212°F.

fair (fâr): light in color; pleasing to the eye.

fake (fāk): artificial; false; such as hair or eyelashes.

fall (fôl): an artificial section of hair placed across the back of the head.

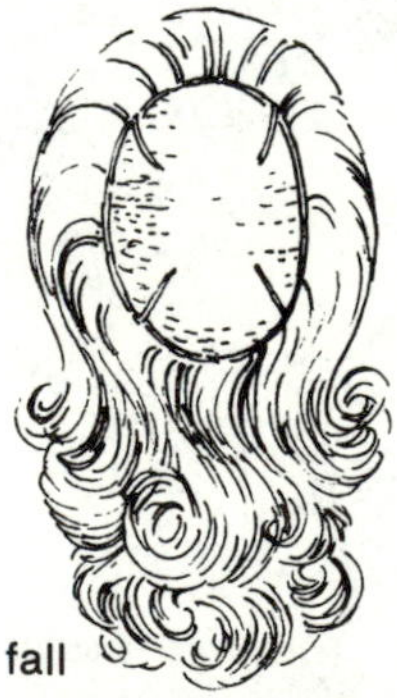

fall

fall point (fâl poynt): point at crown of head from which hair grows in a circular direction.

false (fôls): artificial, such as hair or eyelashes; to deceive or pretend.

fancy (făn′sē): extravagant; elaborate; not ordinary.

fantail comb (făn′tāl kōm): a comb with a tapering tail used for sectioning and parting hair, and for use in wrapping and smoothing; also called a rattail comb.

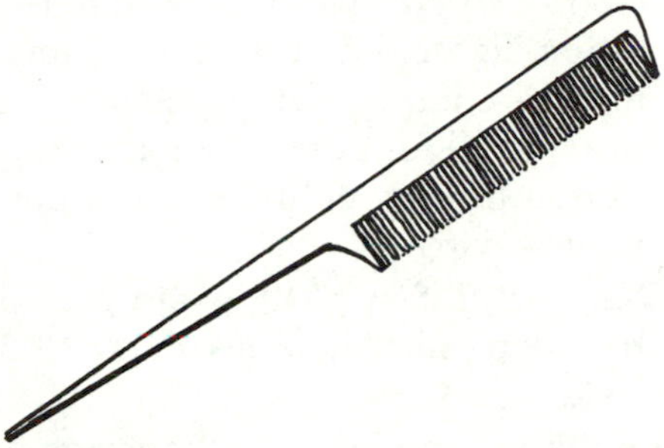

fantail comb

fantasy (făn′tă-sē): a type of hairpiece which is intended only as a form of art and not for practical usage.

faradic (fâ-răd′ĭk): relating to an induced interrupted current.

faradic current (fă-răd′ĭk kŭr′ênt): an induced interrupted current.

faradism (făr′ă-dĭz′m): a form of electrical treatment used for stimulating activity of the tissues.

fascia (făsh′ē-ă): a sheet of connective tissue covering, supporting, or binding together internal parts of the body.

fascial (făsh′ē-âl): relating to a fascia.

fascicle (făs′ĭ-k'l): a small band or a bundle of muscle or nerve fibers; fasciculus.

fashion (făsh′ên): the prevailing style during a particular period of time.

fashionable (făsh′ên-ă-b'l): conforming to the mode of dress; behavior or lifestyle prevailing in a society at a given time.

fat (făt): adipose tissue; a greasy, soft solid material found in animal tissues; plump; obese.

fatigue (fă-tēg): physical or mental exhaustion.

fatty acid (făt′ē ăs′ĭd): an acid derived from the saturated series of open chain hydrocarbons.

fatty alcohols (făt′ē ăl′kô-hŏl): cetyl, lauryl, myristye, stearyl; these are solid alcohols used in creams and lotions.

favus (fā′vûs): a contagious parasitic disease of the skin, characterized by yellowish crusts.

feather cut (fĕ′thẽr kŭt): a basic hair shaping consisting of a smooth crown surrounded by tapered ends.

feather edge (fĕth′ẽr ĕj): a very thin fringe of hair resembling the edge of a feather.

feathering (fĕ′thẽr-ĭng): shortening the hair in a graduated effect; see tapering.

feature (fē′chẽr): distinctive parts of the face (nose, mouth, chin, lips, cheeks, etc.).

fecal (fē′kăl): relating to the discharge from the bowel during defecation.

feel (fēl): to examine with the hands; to explore to determine or to get an impression through the sense of touch; as to examine the texture of the hair.

felon (fĕl′ûn): paronychia of the nail; a painful inflammation of a fingernail or toenail.

felt (fĕlt): an unwoven, matted type of fabric.

feminine (fĕm′ê-nĭn): pertaining to the female sex; womanly.

femur (fē′mûr): the thigh bone; the long bone extending from the pelvis to the knee; also called the femoral bone.

fennel (fĕn′êl): an herb used in cookery and in medical and aromatic preparations.

E-F

ferment (fẽr-mĕnt): to cause or undergo fermentation.

fermentation (fûr-mĕn-tā′shûn): a chemical decomposition of organic compounds into more simple compounds, brought about by the action of an enzyme.

ferrous sulfate (fĕr′ûs sŭl′fāt): a salt of sulfuric acid derived from iron.

fertilization (fûr′tĭ-lĭ-zā′shûn): the union of the male and female reproductive cells.

fester (fĕs′tẽr): to develop inflammation and pus.

fetid (fĕt′ĭd): having a foul odor.

fever (fē′vẽr): rise of body temperature above normal which is 98.6°F or about 37°C.

fever blister (fē′vẽr blĭs′tẽr): an acute skin disease characterized by the presence of vesicles over an inflammatory base; herpes simplex.

fiber (fī′bẽr): a slender, threadlike structure that combines with others to form animal or vegetable tissue.

fiber rod (fī′bẽr rŏd): a rod composed of fibrous material, not metal.

fiber tape (fī′bẽr tāp): a type of self-sticking tape made with nonwoven fibers; it is well suited for protection from wire endings.

fibrillar (fī′brĭ-lâr): having a fibrous form or structure.

fibrin (fī′brĭn): the active agent in coagulation of the blood.

fibrinogen (fī-brĭn′ô-jĕn): a substance capable of producing fibrin.

fibroma (fī-brō′mă): a tumor composed mainly of fibrous or fully developed connective tissue.

fibrous (fī′brûs): containing, consisting of, or like fibers.

fibula (fĭb′ū-lă): the outer and smaller of two bones forming the lower part of the human leg from the knee to the ankle.

filament (fĭl′ă-mênt): a thread-like structure.

file (fīl): a hardened steel instrument having cutting ridges, for the removal of portions of anything; nail file; used to remove portion of the free edge of the nail.

filler (fĭl′ẽr): a preparation used to recondition lightened, tinted or damaged hair; a commercial product used to provide fill for porous spots in the hair during tinting, lightening and permanent waving.

fill-in curl (fĭl′-ĭn kûrl): a pin curl used between roller shapings for continuous style.

film (fĭlm): a membranous covering causing opacity; thin skin.

filter (fĭl′tẽr): anything porous through which liquid is passed to cleanse or strain it.

fine (fīn): being of small diameter, not coarse or thick.

fine hair (fīn hâr): a hair fiber that is relatively small in diameter or circumference.

finesse (fĭ-nĕs′): delicate skill.

finger (fĭn′gẽr): one of the digits of the hand; little or fourth finger, ring finger, middle finger, forefinger or index finger; the thumb is sometimes called the first finger.

finger air waving (fĭn′gẽr âr-wāv′ĭng): a technique of rolling the hair over the fingers while air waving, as opposed to using a brush.

finger bowl (fĭn′gẽr bōl): a small bowl used to hold water for soaking the fingers during a manicure procedure; a small bowl used to cleanse the fingers following the serving of food.

finger breadth (fĭn′gẽr brĕdth): the width of a finger, about ¾ to one inch.

finger curls (fĭn′gẽr kûrlz): elongated, spiral wound curls resembling the fingers; long curls.

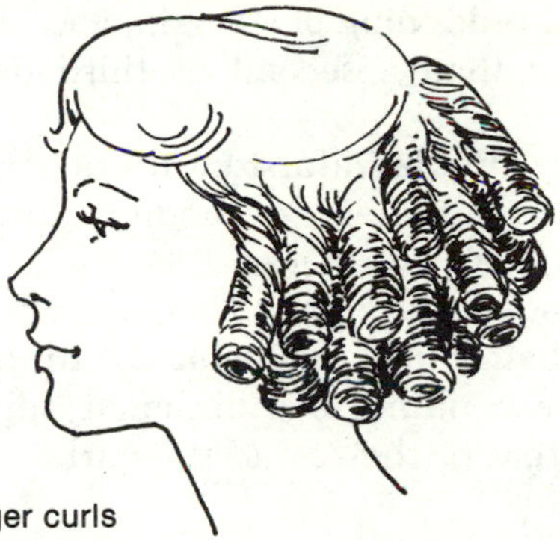

finger curls

finger dexterity (fĭn′gẽr dĕks-tẽr′ĭ-tē): skill and ease in using the fingers.

fingernail (fĭn′gẽr-nāl): the horny protective substance (hard keratin) on the upper surface of the fingers and thumb; the nail.

fingernail brush (fĭn′gẽr-nāl brŭsh): a small brush with semihard bristles, used to cleanse the fingers and nails during the manicure procedure.

fingernail buffer (fĭn′gẽr-nāl bŭf′ẽr): a padded implement used for polishing the nails without nail enamel; used to stimulate blood to the nail bed.

fingernail composition (fĭn′gẽr-nāl kŏm-pō-zĭ′shûn): the material which composes the nail, mainly keratin, a protein substance which forms the base of all horny tissue.

fingernail file (fĭn′gĕr-nāl fīl): a steel instrument with fine filing edges designed for filing and shaping the fingernails; an emery board with sandpaper surfaces is also used to smooth and shape the nails.

fingernail mender (fĭn′gẽr-nāl mĕn′dẽr): an adhesive product used to mend split or broken nails.

fingernail polish (fĭn′gẽr-nāl pŏl′ĭsh): a clear or colored enamel used to beautify and protect the nails.

fingernail polish remover (fĭn′gẽr-nāl pŏl′ĭsh rē-mo͞ov′ẽr): a product containing acetone, usually formulated with some water, lanolin fragrance and coloring agents; used to remove nail enamel.

fingernail reconstruction (fĭn′ger-nāl rē-kŏn-strŭk′shûn): a process in which a substance is applied to the natural nail, then shaped to form an artificial nail to replace the damaged natural nail or to add length to the nail.

fingernail repair (fĭn′gẽr-nāl rē-pâr′): the art of restoring and mending damaged nails by replacing the natural nail with an artificial nail or by sculpturing technique.

fingernail sculpturing (fĭn′gẽr-nāl skŭlp′-chẽr-ĭng): a technique using a product to build and form realistic artificial nails.

fingernail shapes (fĭn′gẽr-nāl shāps): the general classification of nail shapes, as square, rounded, oval and pointed.

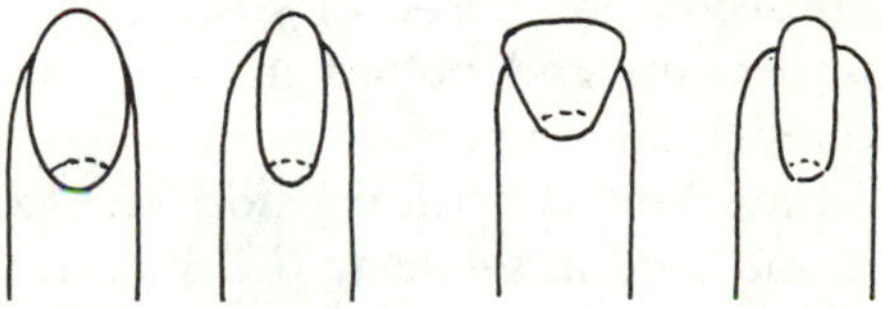

fingernail shapes

finger shield (fĭn′gẽr shēld): a small metal cap worn to protect the finger.

finger stall (fĭn′gẽr stôl): a finger shaped covering of plastic or rubber; used as a protector for sensitive or injured fingers.

finger test (fĭn′gẽr tĕst): a test given to determine the degree of porosity in the hair.

fingertip (fĭn′gẽr-tĭp): the extreme end of a finger.

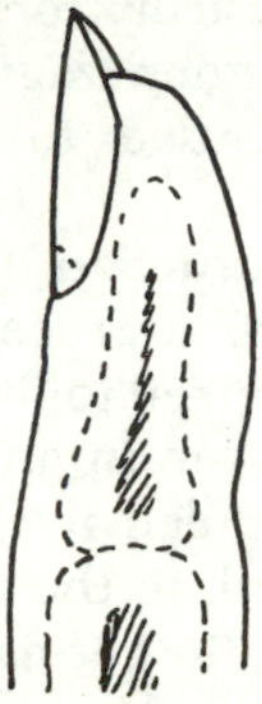

fingertip

finger wave (fĭng′ẽr wāv): the process of setting the hair in a pattern of waves through the use of the fingers, a comb and a setting solution.

finger wave comb (fĭn′gẽr wāv kōm): a small tapered comb used to sculpture finger waves in the hair.

finish (fĭn′ĭsh): the final phase of a combout; the final touches to achieve a desired effect or to correct imperfections.

finishing cream (fĭn′ĭsh-ĭng krēm): an emulsion composed of stearic acid in water, utilized before makeup is applied.

finishing knot (fĭn′ĭsh-ĭng nŏt): the technique used in securing the final strand of hair, on a wig or hairpiece, to make certain that the hair does not become loose.

finishing rinse (fĭn′ĭsh-ĭng rĭns): a conditioning rinse used as the final step of a shampoo or chemical service to close the cuticle and normalize the pH of the hair.

firelighting (fīr′ līt-ĭng): a coloring technique of tone on tone, red on red by single or double tinting process, depending on the desired results.

first degree burn (fûrst dă-grē′ bûrn): a mild burn characterized by some pain and reddening of the skin, and less severe than a second or third degree burn.

first quality hair (fûrst kwăl′ĭ-tē hâr): human hair in good condition used in wigs and hairpieces.

fishhook (fĭsh′ho͞ok): a flaw in the curling of hair which results in the tip of the hair bending in a direction opposite to that of the rest of the curl.

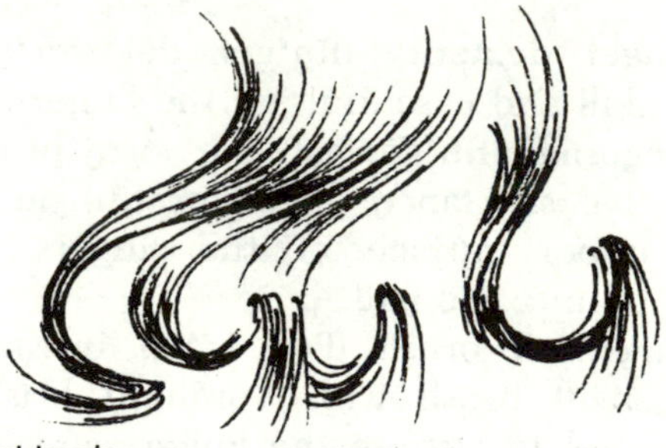

fishhook

fish oil (fĭsh oyl): a fatty oil from fish used in the manufacture of soaps; hydrogenated fish oil.

fish skin (fĭsh skĭn): a special material, used in wiggery, to cover the tips of springs or in some cases the entire spring, to prevent rust and discoloration.

fission (fĭsh′ûn): reproduction of bacteria by cellular division; the splitting of an atomic nucleus.

fissure (fĭsh′ûr): a narrow opening made by separation of parts; a furrow; a slit.

fitting (fĭt′ĭng): pertaining to the adjusting of a wig or hairpiece to the proper size.

E-F

fixative (fĭk′să-tĭv): a hairdressing used to keep hair in place; in cold waving, an agent that stops the chemical action of the cold waving solution and sets or hardens the hair; a chemical agent capable of stopping the processing of the chemical hair relaxer and hardening the hair in its new form; neutralizer; stabilizer.

flabby (flăb′ē): wanting firmness; flaccid.

flaccid (flăk′sĭd): flabby; relaxed; being without bone.

flagella (flă-jĕl′ă): slender whip-like processes which permit locomotion in certain bacteria.

flair (flâr): a sense of artistry; natural talent or ability.

flake (flāk): a small particle of a substance; to scale or chip as shedding of the skin in a dandruff condition; sloughing off of the epidermis due to dryness.

flammable (flăm′ă-b'l): capable of being easily ignited and burning with great rapidity.

flare (flâr): to spread outward; to add width.

flare curl (flâr kûrl): a pin curl that is rolled and placed so that it stands slightly away from the scalp; semi-stand-up curl.

flat (flăt): having a horizontal surface with no hollows or projections.

flatter (flăt′ĕr): to display to advantage; to enhance the individual's facial features through hairstyle or makeup.

flattop hairstyle (flăt′tŏp hâr′stīl): a hairstyle for men in which the hair is cut short on top so that the ends create a horizontal line.

flat weft (flăt wĕft): the most common type of weaving hair on silks; woven on three silks.

flat winding (flăt wīnd′ĭng): winding the hair on a rod without twisting.

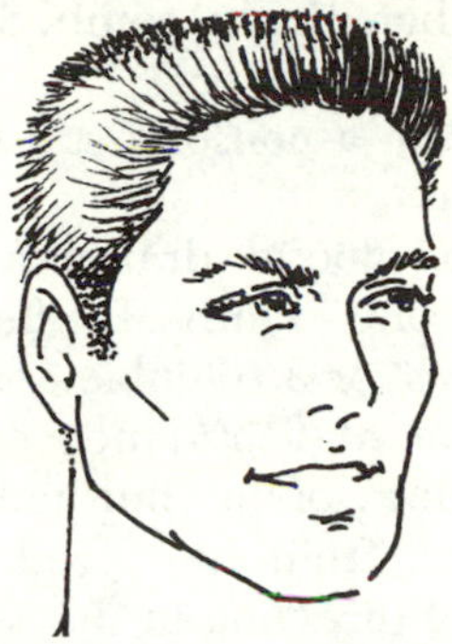

flattop hairstyle

flaxen (flăx′ĕn): a pale, straw color; a term used to describe light blonde hair.

fleshy (flĕsh′ē): pertaining to fullness, plumpness; as fleshy cheeks.

flex (flĕks): to bend, especially repeatedly; as to exercise a muscle.

flexible (flĕk′sĭ-b′l): capable of being bent; pliable; not stiff.

flexor (flĕk′sôr): a muscle that bends or flexes a part or a joint.

flexor carpiulnaris (flĕx′sâr kär′pĭ-ŭl-nâr′ĭs): the extensor muscles of the wrist, which are involved in bending the hand backward.

flick (flĭk): a quick, sharp movement.

flip (flĭp): to turn over or up; a hairstyle with the ends of the hair turned upward.

floral bouquet (flôr′âl bo͞o-kā′): a combination of flower fragrances.

floral fragrance (flôr′âl frā′grăntz): a fragrance characterized by the scent of one flower.

floral perfume (flôr′âl pûr′fūm): perfume made from flowers.

florid (flŏr′ĭd): flushed; tinged with red; ruddy.

flow (flō): smooth movement; free and graceful movement.

fluctuate (flŭk′tû-āt): to shift back and forth; to move like a wave.

fluff (flŭf): hair that is combed so that it has a soft, airy effect.

fluid (flo͞o′ĭd): a nonsolid substance; liquid or gas.

fluid dram (flo͞o′ĭd drăm): a measure equal to one eighth of a fluid ounce, 60 minims, or 3.70 cubic centimeters.

fluid movement (flo͞o′ĭd mo͞ov′ment): the appearance of a finished coiffure achieved from a predetermined change of direction in the setting pattern.

fluid ounce (flo͞o′ĭd aùns): one sixteenth of a pint (29.5737 cubic centimeters).

fluorescent (flo͞o′ôr-ĕs′n't): an ability to emit light after exposure to light; the wave length of the emitted light being longer than that of the light absorbed.

flush (flŭsh): to become red in the face due to emotion, fever or a skin condition which causes blood to rush to the under surface of the skin; to blush.

flyaway (flī′ă-wā): of or pertaining to an excessive electrostatic condition of hair which causes individual hair strands to repel one another and stand away from the head.

fly weft (flīwĕft): fine weaving used for the top row of postiche made of weft.

foam (fōm): a bubbly or frothy mass produced by products such as soap, detergents or bath beads.

foamer (fō′mĕr): a substance which creates an excessive amount of foam.

foil (foyl): a very thin sheet of metal once used in the construction of permanent wave pads; presently used in color technique of slicing or weaving out small strands of hair and placing in color covered foil for processing.

fold (fōld): to turn or bend back so that one part covers or lies alongside another; to close or wrap; wind; the space between two folded parts.

folic acid (fō′lĭk ăs′ĭd): vitamin B complex, found in green, leafy vegetables and some animal products.

follicle (fŏl′ĭ-k′l): a small secretary cavity or sac; the depression in the skin containing the hair root.

follicular (fŏ-lĭk′û-lăr): affecting or arising from the follicles.

folliculitis (fŏ-lĭk-û-lī′tĭs): an inflammation of any follicle.

folliculose (fŏ-lĭk′û-lōs): full of follicles.

folliculosis (fŏ-lĭk-û-lō′sĭs): a disease in which there is excessive development of the follicles.

Food and Drug Administration (F.D.A.) (fo͞od and drŭg ăd-mĭn-ĭs-strā′shûn): an agency of the United States Federal Government responsible for ensuring that cosmetics, drugs and foods are safe, correctly packaged and truthfully labeled.

foot (fo͞ot): the terminal section of the limb of a vertebrate animal upon which it stands, rests or moves.

footrest (fo͞ot′rĕst): a small stool or platform upon which to place the feet; the extension of the service chair used in a salon upon which the client may place his or her feet.

foramen (fô-rā′mĕn): a passage or opening through a bone or membrane.

forces (fôr′sĕz): the causes that produce change or stop the motion of a body; representation of curvature motion; clockwise or counterclockwise.

forearm (fôr′ärm): the part of the arm between the elbow and the wrist.

forehead (fôr′ĕd): the part of the face from the eyebrows to the hairline.

foreign matter (fôr′ĭn măt′ĕr): undesirable substance or particles from outside the body, found on or in the skin, hair, nails or body, occurring where they are not normally found.

forelock (fôr′lŏk): a small section of hair growing over the forehead.

foreside (fôr′sīd): the front part or front side.

form (fôrm): the outline of the overall hairstyle as seen from all angles.

formaldehyde (fôr-măl′dê-hīd): a pungent gas possessing powerful disinfectant and preservative.

formalin (fôr′mă-lĭn): a 37% to 40% solution of formaldehyde in water.

formation (fôr-mā′shûn): the manner in which a thing is formed or shaped.

formula (fôr′mû-lă): a prescribed method or rule; a recipe or prescription.

forward curls (fôr′wôrd kûrlz): curls directed toward the face; curls wound in a clockwise direction on the left side of the head; on the right side of the head such curls would be in a counterclockwise direction.

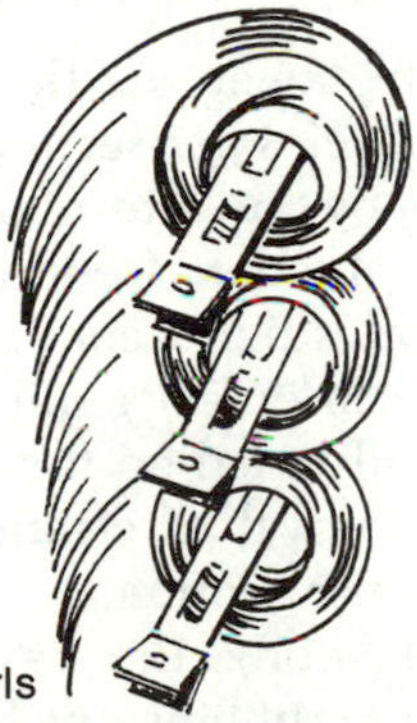

forward curls

forward wave (fôr′wôrd wāv): a wave shaped toward the face.

fossa (fŏs′ă); pl., **fossae** (-ē): a depression, furrow or sinus below the level of the surface of a part.

foul (foul): offensive to the senses; disagreeable or unpleasant.

foundation base (faun-dā′shûn bās): in wig making, the supporting base upon which the hair is fastened and secured; a cosmetic, usually tinted, in liquid, cream, or powdered form, used as a base for makeup applications.

foundation cream (faun-dā′shûn krēm): a cream sometimes used in place of a colored makeup base or as a protective film applied before the makeup base and/or powder.

foundation, net (faun-dā′shûn, nĕt): a fine, stiffened net used for most foundational hairpieces.

fraction (frăk′shûn): a quantity less than a unit; a part of something.

fracture (frăk′chẽr): the breaking or cracking of a bone or cartilage.

fragile hair (frăj′âl hâr): hair which is lacking in normal flexibility, tensile strength and resilience and is usually brittle and easily broken.

fragilitas (fră-jĭl′ĭ-tăs): brittleness.

fragilitas crinium (fră-jĭl′ĭ-tăs krī′nē-ûm): brittleness of the hair.

fragment (frăg′mênt): a small detached portion.

fragrance (frā′grans): a pleasant, agreeable odor; a product ingredient used to enhance cosmetic and other products; products used on the person such as perfume, toilet water, cologne, etc.

fragrant (frā′grănt): having an agreeable odor.

frail (frāl): easily broken or damaged; delicate.

frame (frām): in hairstyling, hair arranged to create a pleasing outline for the face.

franchise (frăn′chīz): authorization given by owner, corporation, group or founder to do business under their regulations.

fraudulent claim (frôd′û-lênt clām): a clain characterized by, founded on, or obtained by fraud.

frayed (frād): worn away, especially an edge of cloth, by friction or use.

freckle (frĕk′l): a yellow or brown spot on the skin; lentigo.

free edge (frē ĕj): part of the nail body extending over the fingertip.

free hand (frē hănd): a hand position and kind of stroke used when shaving the face.

free styling (frē stīl′ĭng): a technique using the fingers of one hand with a hand-held dryer in the other; to direct and style the hair.

French braiding (Frĕnch brād′ĭng): a technique of hair braiding using four strands of hair interlaced close to the head to form a pattern.

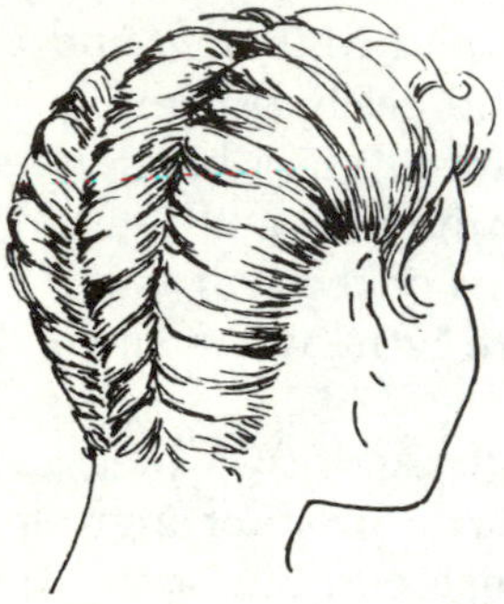

French braiding

French flow technique (Frĕnch flō tĕk-nēk′): a styling technique which employs double rollers or pin curls in an oblong design.

French fluff (Frĕnch flŭf): a combination of prepared tint and shampoo which is applied to the hair like a regular shampoo; adds some color and brightness to faded hair; see soap cap.

French knot (Frĕnch nŏt): in hairstyling, a hairstyle where the hair is smoothed off the face and gathered into a twisted roll at the nape of the neck; also called classic knot or chignon.

French lacing (Frĕnch lās′iňg): the technique of combing small sections of hair from the ends toward the scalp causing it to form a cushion upon which the hair is combed into the desired style; also called teasing.

French seam (Frĕnch sēm): a hairstyle created by combing the hair at the back of the head into a smooth, vertical, flat roll with the ends of the hair folded under.

French twist (Frĕnch twĭst): a vertical seamlike arrangement at the back of the head.

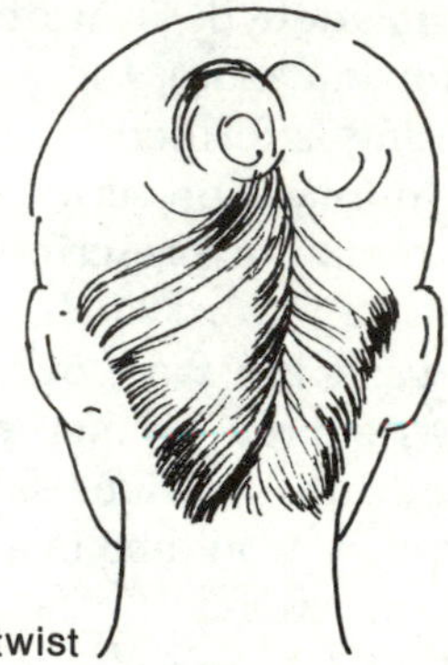

French twist

frequency (frē′kwĕn-sē): the number of complete cycles per second of current produced by an alternating current generator; standard frequencies are 25 and 60 cycles per second.

freshener (frĕsh′ĕn-ēr): a mild liquid cosmetic usually used on the skin following the removal of cleansing cream; skin freshening lotion.

friction (frik′shun): the resistance encountered in rubbing one body against another.

fringe (frĭnj): hair that partially or completely covers the facial area near the hairline; a small hairpiece.

frizzy (frĭz′ē): hair formed into small tight curls or narrow waves.

frontal (frŭn′tâl): in front; relating to the forehead; the bone of the forehead.

frontal artery (frŭn′tâl är′tĭr-ē): the supraorbital artery which supplies blood to the forehead and upper eyelids.

frontal bone (frŭn′tâl bōn): the bone

forming the forehead; the anterior part of the skull forming the forehead.

frontalis (frŭn-tăl′ĭs): anterior portion of the epicranium; muscle of the scalp.

frontal nerve (frŭn′tâl nûrv): a somatic sensory nerve which innervates the skin of the upper eyelids, the forehead and the scalp.

frontal vein (frŭn′tâl vān): the diploic vein of the frontal bones.

frostbite (frôst′bīt): injury to the skin and subcutaneous tissues caused by exposure to extreme cold.

frosting (frôst′ĭng): to lighten or darken (reverse frosting) small selected strands of hair over the entire head to blend with the rest of the hair.

frosting cap (frôst′ĭng kăp): a plastic cap-like head covering with small holes through which strands of hair are pulled to the surface to be tinted, lightened or darkened as desired.

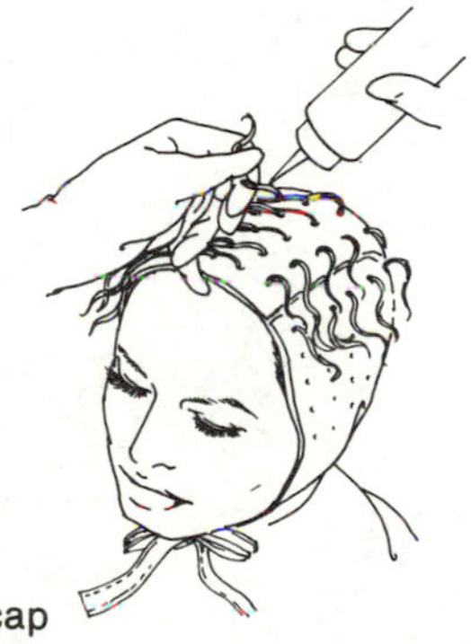

frosting cap

fruity blend (frōō′tē blĕnd): pertaining to fragrances based on the aromas of various fruits and combinations of fruits; as lemon, lime, peach, etc.; used in grooming products.

fuchsia (fyōō′shă): a bright bluish-red color.

full base (fŏŏl bās): placement of a roller or a curl directly and completely on its base.

full complement (fŏŏl kŏm′plê-mênt): complete; containing all of the essential or required substances.

fuller's earth (fŏŏl′erz ûrth): a soapy clay often used as a foundation for packs and masks.

fulling (fŏŏl′ĭng): a massage movement in which the limb is rolled back and forth between the hands.

full stem (fŏŏl stĕm): a curl or curling device such as a roller that is rolled up to the base part.

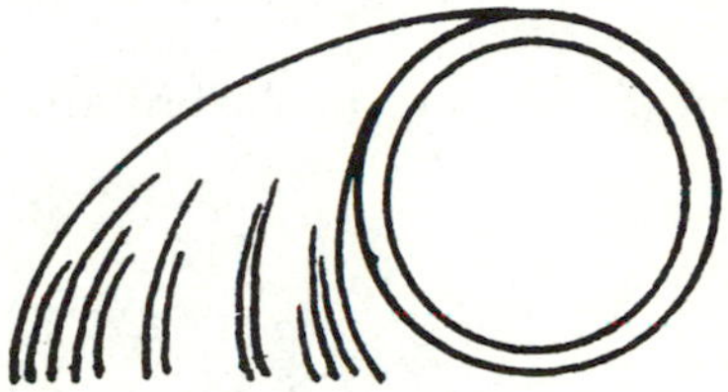

full stem

full stem curl (fŏŏl stĕm kûrl): a curl that is fastened completely off its base to give mobility to the curl; also called long stem curl.

full stem curl

full twist (fŏŏl twĭst): a rope-like winding of the hair on the rod in spiral permanent waving.

fume (fūm): a smoke, vapor or gas, especially one that is irritating.

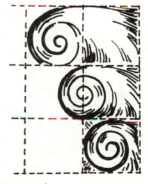

fumigant (fū′mĭ-gănt): a gaseous sub-

stance capable of destroying pathogenic bacteria.
fumigate (fū′mĭ-gāt): disinfect by the action of smoke or fumes.
function (fŭnk′shûn): the normal or special action for which a part is especially suited or used.
fundamental (fŭn-dă-mĕn′tâl): basic; essential; basic rule or principle.
fungicide (fŭn′jĭ-sīd): a substance formulated to destroy fungi.
fungus (fŭn′gûs): a vegetable parasite; a spongy growth of diseased tissue on or in the body.
furfurol (fûr′fū-rōl): a colorless aromatic fluid obtained in the distillation of bran with sulphuric acid.
furrow (fŭr′ō): a groove; wrinkle.
furuncle (fū′rŭn-k'l): a small skin abscess (boil).
fuscin (fŭs′ĭn): the black pigment of the retina.
fuscous (fŭs′kûs): grayish brown; dusky.
fuse (fūz): to liquify by heat; a special device which prevents excessive current from passing through a circuit.
fusion (fū′zhûn): the act of uniting, blending or melting together; something formed by fusing.
fuzz (fŭz): fine, lightweight hair.

G

galea aponeurotica (gā′lê-ă ă-pŏn-û-rŏt′ĭ-kă): the flat tendon joining the frontalis and occipitalis muscles in the scalp.

gallon (gâl′ĕn): a liquid measure equal to 4 quarts or 8 pints; in metric 3.78 liters.

galvanic current (găl-văn′ĭk kŭr′ênt): a direct, continued current having a positive and a negative pole; named for Galvani (1737–1798).

galvanic machine (găl-văn′ĭk mă-shēn′): an apparatus with attachments designed to produce galvanic current; used in the treatment of facial and scalp conditions.

galvanic multiple needle technique (găl-văn′ĭk mŭl′tĭ-p'l nē′d'l tĕk-nēk′): a technique used to remove superfluous hair permanently by use of galvanic current and several needles.

galvanic skin response (GSR) (găl′văn-ĭk skĭn rē-spŏns): the electrical reaction of the skin to stimulas by the galvanometer; used to measure the skin's responses to electrical current.

galvanism (găl′vă-nĭz′m): a constant current of electricity, the action of which is chemical.

galvanothermy (găl′vă-nō-thûr′mē): the production of heat by galvanism; used in therapeutic treatments.

gamma globulin (găm′ă glŏb′û-lĭn): a globulin in the blood plasma which contains antibodies effective against pathogenic microorganisms.

gamma rays (găm′ă rāz): a kind of powerful electromagnetic radiation having a frequency greater than X rays.

ganglion (găn′glē-ôn); pl., **ganglia** (-ă): subcutaneous tumors; bundles of nerve cells in the brain, in organs of special sense or forming units of the sympathetic nervous system.

gangrene (găn-grēn′): the dying of tissue due to interference with local nutrition.

gardenia (gär-dē′nē-ă): a tropical flower of yellow or white whose essence is used in perfumery.

garlic (gär′lĭk): a member of the onion family of vegetables; used in cookery, some cosmetics and medicines; nutritionally, it provides sulphur to hair follicles and skin, regulates oil glands and speeds removal of toxins from the system.

gastric (găs′trĭk): pertaining to the stomach.

gastric juice (găs′trĭk jo͞os): the digestive fluid secreted by the glands of the stomach.

gastrointestinal (găs′trô-ĭntĕs′tĭ-nâl): pertaining to both the stomach and intestines.

gaudy (gô′dē): showy; garish; flashy.

gauge (gāj): to estimate; appraise; judge.

gauze (gôz): a thin open-meshed cloth used for dressings and for facial masks in some types of facial treatments.

gauze grit (gôz grĭt): a wide meshed gauze generally used as the underneath layer of a hairpiece.

gauze mask (gôz măsk): a mask made by cutting a piece of thin open mesh cloth (cheesecloth) to fit over the client's face and neck; the material is moistened with warm water, applied to the face, then the mask ingredients such as fresh crushed fruit or other thin substance is applied over the cloth. The purpose of the gauze is to keep the mask from running or crumbling.

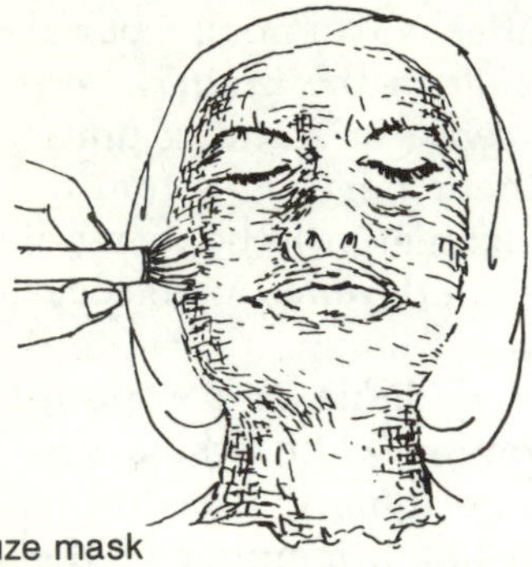

gauze mask

gauze, silk (gôz, sĭlk): a fine gauze silk material, having a flesh look, and used in the construction of wigs and hairpieces.

gel (jĕl): a substance comprised of a solid and a liquid which exists as a solid or semisolid mass.

gelatine (jĕl′ă-tĭn): the tasteless, odorless, brittle substance extracted by boiling bones, hoofs and animal tissues; used in various foods, medicines, etc.

gene (jēn): the ultimate unit in the transmission of hereditary characteristics.

general infection (jĕn′ĕr-âl ĭn-fĕk′shûn): an infection affecting large areas of the body.

generator (ǰen′ĕr-ā-tĕr): one who, or that which generates, causes or produces.

generic (jĕ-nĕr′ĭk): pertaining to a genus or class of related things.

generic product (jĕ-nĕr′ĭk prŏd′ŭkt): a product, especially a drug, not protected by a trademark and not registered.

genetics (ǰe-nĕt′ĭks): the science that deals with the heredity and variation of organisms.

gentian (ǰen′shên): an American herb used in astringents and cleansing products.

genuine (jĕn′yo͞o-ĭn): authentic; real.

geriatrics (jĕr′ē-ăt′rĭks): the branch of medicine which deals with the physical and psychological changes that affect humans during the aging process.

germ (jûrm): a microorganism that causes disease; a microbe; a bacillus.

germicidal (jûr-mĭ-sī′dôl): destructive to germs.

germicide (jûr′mĭ-sīd): any chemical that will destroy germs.

germination (jûr-mĭ-nā′shûn): the formation of an embryo from an impregnated ovum; the first act of growth in a germ, seed or bud.

germinative (jûr′mĭ-nā-tĭv): having power to grow or develop.

germinative layer (jûr′mĭ-nā-tĭv lā′ĕr): stratum germinativum; the deepest layer of the epidermis resting on the carium.

germ layer (jŭrm lā′ĕr): any of three primary layers of cells from which the various organs of most embryos develop by further differentiation.

gerontology (jĕr′ôn-tŏl′ô-jē): the scientific study of the processes and problems of aging.

gift spots (gĭft spŏts): leukonychia; spots of whiteness on the nails, often caused by a blow to the nail or by nutritional deficiency.

ginger (jĭn′jĕr): a product of a tropical plant used in medicinal preparations and in cookery.

ginseng (jĭn′sĕng): an herb native to China and North America; used as a stimulant and in some hair and skin preparations.

glabrous (glā′brûs): smooth; without hair.

glamor, glamour (glăm′ĕr): fascinating, alluring and often illusory glorification.

gland (glănd): a secretory organ of the body.

glandular (glăn′dû-lăr): pertaining to a gland.

glimmer (glĭm′ẽr): a rouge which imparts a glossy appearance.

glint (glĭnt): brightness; luster; shine.

globule (glŏb′ūl): a small, spherical droplet of fluid or semifluid material.

glomus tumor (glō′mŭs to͞om′ẽr): a tumor affecting the digits; usually painful, bluish and benign.

glossal (glôs′âl): pertaining to the tongue.

glossing (glôs′ĭng): a technique in hair tinting and conditioning which creates a highlight effect on the hair.

glossopharyngeal (glôs-ô-fă-rĭn′gē-âl): the ninth cranial nerve; pertaining to the pharynx and tongue.

glossy (glŏs′ē): smooth and shining; highly polished.

glucose (glo͞o′kōs): a monosaccharide (dextrose) found in fruit and other foods and in the blood; the chief source of energy for living organisms; used in the treatment of dehydration.

glued wig (glo͞od wĭg): a type of wig in which glue is placed on the base or netting, and the hair is attached to the glued surface.

glutamate (glo͞ot′ă-māt): a salt or ester of glutamic acid used to enhance the flavor of foods; used as an antioxidant in cosmetics to prevent spoilage.

glutamic acid (glo͞o-tăm′ĭk ăs′ĭd): an amino acid from vegetable or grain protein, used in cosmetics as an antioxidant and as a softener in permanent wave solutions.

gluteus muscle (glo͞o-tē′ûs mŭs′l): any of three muscles of the buttocks.

glutin (glū′tĭn): a protein obtained from gelatin.

glycerin (glĭs′ẽr-ĭn): a colorless, oily substance obtained by hydrolysis of fats and by synthesis; manufactured from the natural substance, glycerol; used as a solvent, emollient and humectant.

glycerol monostearate (glĭs′ẽr-ōl mŏn-ô-stē′-rāt): pure white or cream-colored, wax-like solid with faint odor; used as an emulsifying agent for oils, waxes and solvents; acts as a protective coating for various cosmetics.

G-H

glycine (glī′sēn): aminoacetic acid.

glycogelatin (glī′kō-jĕl′ă-tĭn): an ointment base containing gelatin and glycerin.

glycogen (glī′kô-jĕn): animal starch.

glycol (glī′kôl): any dihydric aliphatic alcohol; ethylene alcohol; useful as a solvent.

glycolic acid (glī-kŏl′ĭk ăs′ĭd): a possible intermediate in the metabolism of carbohydrates and proteins, found in cane sugar and some fruit.

goiter (goy′tẽr): enlargement of the thyroid gland.

gold (gōld): in hairdressing, a term used to indicate the presence of yellow tones; not ashy.

gold bands (gōld băndz): uneven effect and brassy areas, occurring in some hair lightening procedures.

golden (gōl′dên): bright, like the color of gold; golden blond; the color of gold tones.

golden seal (gōl′dên sēl): an herb having a yellow rootstock; a source of hydrosline (a crystalline alkaloid); used in astringents as a mild antiseptic; used for acne, dandruff and like conditions.

gonads (gō′nădz): primary sex glands; ovaries and testes.

gonorrhea (gŏn-ô-rē′ă): a contagious venereal disease caused by the presence of the gonococci bacteria in the genital tract.

G-H

gooseflesh (go͞os′flešh): skin marked by a raised appearance around the hair follicles caused by the contraction of the arrectore pilorum muscles; a condition caused by cold or emotional changes affecting the body.

grab (grăb): to react very rapidly to some stimulus; in haircoloring, pertaining to color that takes quickly.

graceful (grās′fûl): pleasing in form, line or movement.

graduate (grăd′û-āt): in hairstyling, to layer the hair.

graduated haircut (grăd′û-ā-tĕd hâr′kŭt): a haircut in which subsections of hair are cut in layers longer from the inner layer to the outer layer; a haircut displaying up-angle cutting.

gram (grăm): the basic unit of mass or weight in the metric system.

granular layer (grăn′û-lär lā′ĕr): the stratum granulosum of the skin.

granules (grăn′ū-lz): small grains or particles.

granulosum (grăn-û-lōs′ûm): grandular layer of the epidermis.

grapefruit oil (grāp-fro͞ot′ oyl): an oil obtained from the fresh peel of the grapefruit; used in fragrances and fruit flavorings.

grape-seed oil (grāp-sēd oyl): an oil expressed from grape seeds; used in hypoallergenic lubricating creams and lotions.

graphite (grăf′īt): a soft, black form of carbon used in pencils and as a pigment in some cosmetics.

G.R.A.S. (generally recognized as safe); a list established by Congress in 1958 to designate food additives that are not harmful when used as intended.

grattage (gră-tahzh′): the scrubbing, scrapping or brushing of a part during treatment.

gravity (grâv′ĭ-tē): the effect of the attraction of the earth upon matter; the quality of having weight.

gray (grā): any achromatic color mixture of black and white; gradation of black and white.

grayed (grād): in coloring, dulled or diluted by the addition of gray.

grease (grēs): oil; fat; oily matter.

great auricular (grāt ô-rĭk′û-lär): a nerve affecting the face, ears, neck and parotid gland.

greater multangular (grā′tĕr mŭl-tăn′gû-lär): trapezium; bone of the wrist.

greater occipital (grā′tĕr ŏk-sĭp′ĭ-tâl): sensory and motor nerve affecting the splenius complexus and scalp.

great saphenous vein (grāt să-fē′nûs vān): a large superficial vein in the leg.

great toe (grāt tō): the first inner digit of the foot.

green (grēn): the color between blue and yellow in the spectrum; the result of mixing equal parts of yellow and blue (primary colors) to achieve the secondary color, green.

green algae (grēn ăl′jē): a class of algae in which the cells containing chlorophyll are dominant; source of chlorophyll used in some grooming products.

green soap (grēn sōp): a soft soap made from hydroxides of potassium and sodium, and containing linseed oil; used as a cleanser for certain skin problems; also called tincture of green soap.

greige (grāj): a color between gray and beige as seen in some unfinished, unprocessed or raw fibers.

grip (grĭp): to hold firmly; to grasp.

gristle (grĭs′′l): cartilage, the tough, elastic connective tissue in the body.

grit gauze (grĭt gôz): a very firm, wide-meshed gauze; used in the manufacture of wigs underneath the silk gauze top layer; the grit gauze is the material into which the hair is knotted and anchored.

grizzled (grĭz′âld): streaked or flecked with gray; graying.

groom (grōōm): to make neat or tidy.

groove (grōōv): the hollow part of a curling iron into which the rod fits; a long narrow depression.

gross (grōs): in mathematics, a unit of quantity comprising 12 dozen.

ground (graủnd): in electricity, the connection of an electrical current with the earth through some form of conductor, such as a ground wire which connects an electrical apparatus with the ground object.

ground wire (graủnd wīr): a wire which connects an electric current to a ground.

growth (grōth): lengthening of hair, nails, etc.; the process of growing larger, longer; increase in size or maturity; abnormal formation of tissue such as a tumor.

growth direction (grōth dĭ-rĕk′shûn): the direction in which the hair grows from the scalp.

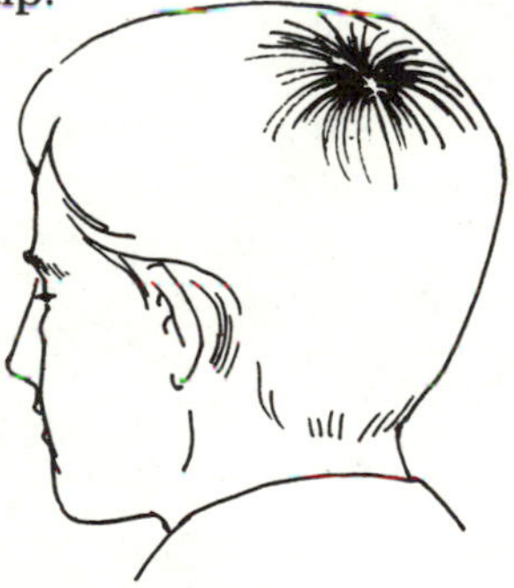

growth direction

growth pattern (grōth păt′ĕrn): the direction in which the hair grows.

guarantee (găr-ăn-tē′): a contract, pledge, promise to pay or act according to agreement.

guide (gīd): something that serves as a model to follow or provides information; a rule to follow.

guideline (gīd′līn): in hairdressing, a hair strand used for a general shaping pattern; hair usually at the hairline cut to a specific length to serve as a guide for determining the length of the rest of the section.

gum (gŭm): a water soluble, viscous vegetable secretion.

gum arabic (gŭm âr′ă-bĭk): acacia gum; a gum obtained from African acacia trees; used in facial masks, hair sprays, setting lotions and powders; a stabilizer, emulsifier and gelling substance.

gummy (gŭm′ē): a gum-like substance; sticky.

guttate (gŭt′āt): drop-like form, characterizing certain cutaneous lesions.

gynecology (gī′nă-kŏl′ă-jē): the science and branch of medicine dealing with the diseases of women, particularly those affecting the sexual organs.

H

H (āch): in chemistry, the symbol for hydrogen.

hack (hăk): in haircutting, to cut the hair in an irregular or unskilled fashion; in massage, to use short chopping movements with the side of the hand.

hacking (hăk′ĭng): a chopping stroke made with the edge of the hand in massage.

hackle (hă′k'l): an oblong board designed with metal upright teeth through which hair or other fiber is pulled in order to remove tangles; a disentangling device used in wig making.

hair (hâr): a slender filament of protein keratin found on most mammals; an appendage or outgrowth of the skin whose root is by the follicle in the corium and subcutaneous tissue.

hair analysis (hâr ă-năl′ĭ-sĭs): the examination of the hair to determine its condition: such as strength, elasticity, porosity, moisture content, etc.; the study of the mineral and chemical content of hair.

hair analyzer (hâr ăn′âl-ĭ-zer̃): an instrument designed to test the hair for chemical content and/or to determine its condition.

hairband (hâr′bănd): an elasticized band used to hold the hair in place during a facial treatment; a decorative ribbon or material worn to hold the hair back from the face.

hair bleaching (hâr blēch′ĭng): diffusing the natural pigment of the hair so it appears almost colorless; see hair lightening.

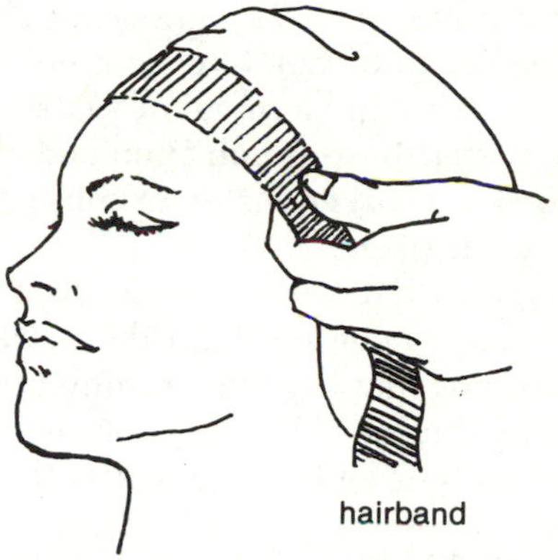

hairband

hair bobbing (hâr bŏb′ĭng): the term once used to describe the cutting of women's and children's hair.

hairbrush (hâr′brŭsh): an implement designed with bristles on one end and a handle on the other; used for grooming and styling the hair.

hair bulb (hâr bŭlb): the part of the hair which holds the root; the part which encloses the hair papilla; the lower extremity of the hair.

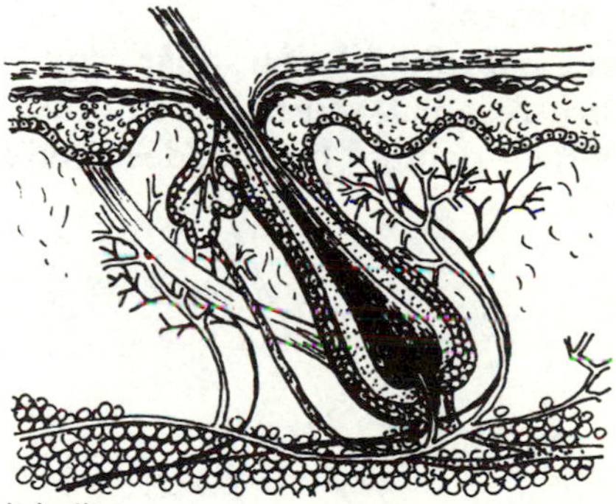

hair bulb

hair canal (hâr kă-nâl): the space in the hair follicle occupied by the hair root.

hair care products (hâr kâr prŏd′ŭkts):

products formulated especially for the hair to condition, cleanse and beautify the hair.

hair cell (hâr sĕl): an epithelial cell with hairlike out growths, especially those in the organ of Corti in the inner ear.

hair clip (hâr clĭp): a metal or plastic device with prongs which open and close to secure a curl or curler, or subsection of hair in place.

hair clipper (hâr klĭp′ĕr): an implement designed to cut and trim the hair.

hair clipping (hâr klĭp′ĭng): removing the hair by the use of hair clippers; removing split hair ends of the hair with scissors.

hair cloth (hâr klôth): a protective covering placed around the client's shoulders to protect clothing during haircutting or other hair care procedures.

hair, coarse (hâr, kôrs): hair which is extremely large in circumference.

hair color filler (hâr kŭl′ĕr fĭl′ĕr): a product used to fill porous spots in the hair and deposit base color during the lightening, tinting or perming process.

hair coloring (hâr kŭl′ĕr-ĭng): the procedures by which the hair color is changed.

hair coloring brush (hâr kŭl′ĕr-ĭng brŭsh): a flat, short-bristled brush with a long pointed handle, designed to be used in applying a coloring product to the hair.

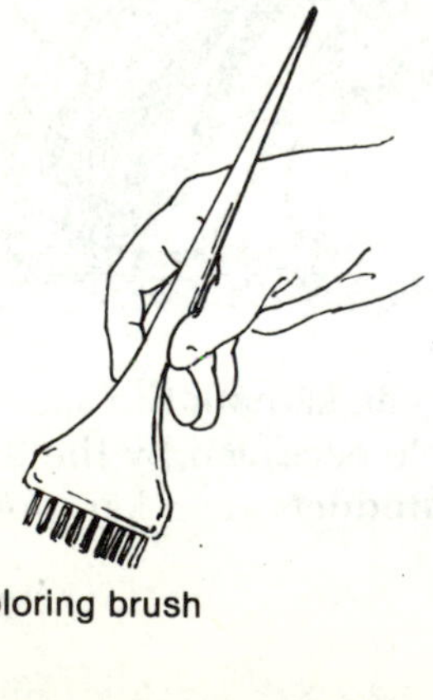

haircoloring brush

hair coloring classification (hâr kŭl′ĕr-ĭng klăs′ĭ-fĭ-kā′shûn): the three main categories of hair coloring; temporary, semipermanent and permanent.

hair coloring tint (hâr kŭl′ĕr-ĭng tĭnt): oxidative color; also called penetrating tint, synthetic tint, para tint and amino tint; used in permanent hair coloring.

hair color processing machine (hâr kŭl′ĕr prŏ′sĕs-ĭng mă-shēn′): a machine designed to increase the developing action of tints.

hair color remover (hâr kŭl′ĕr rē-mōōv′ĕr): a product formulated to remove tint from the hair.

hair color rinse (hâr kŭlĕr rĭns): a temporary rinse used to color and highlight the hair.

hair color spray (hâr kŭl′ĕr sprā): a spray, usually gold or silver, applied from an aerosol container, generally used for shows and special effects.

hair composition (hâr kŏm′pō-zĭ′shûn): hair is chiefly composed of protein keratin; the primary elements in average hair are: carbon, 50.65%; hydrogen, 6.36%; nitrogen, 17.14%; sulfur, 5.0%; and oxygen, 20.85%; hair also contains phosphorus in measurable amounts; the exact composition varies with the type of hair, depending to a large extent on age, race, sex and color.

hair condition (hâr kôn-dĭ′shûn): average condition; the state of health of a generally healthy, normal head of hair.

hair conditioner (hâr kôn-dĭ′shûn-ĕr): a product formulated to be used in the hair to improve its health and appearance.

hair cortex (hâr kôr′tĕks): the layer of hair between the cuticle and the medulla.

hair crayons (hâr krā′ŏns): sticks of coloring material compounded with soaps or synthetic waxes; used to retouch the hair growth between tintings.

haircut (hâr′kŭt): the act of cutting the hair; the result of cutting the hair.

haircut, blunt (hâr′kŭt, blŭnt): refers to a haircut in which there is no elevation; hair is cut off squarely, without taper, so all hairs are the same length.

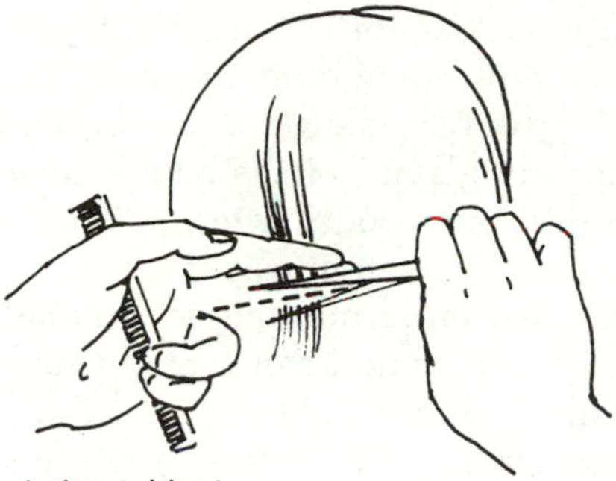

haircut, blunt

haircut circular (hâr′kŭt sûr′kū-lär): a haircut with medium to high elevation that blends when combed in any direction.

haircut, geometric (hâr′kŭt jē′ô-mĕt′rĭk): haircut using straight lines, zig-zag and unusual designs; the front perimeter and sides are cut into flattering designs.

hair cuticle (hâr kū′tĭ-k'l): the outside, horny layer of the hair composed of transparent, overlapping cells pointing away from the scalp toward the hair ends.

haircut, shag (hâr′kŭt, shăg): a haircut combining high and low elevation with fringed effect around the hairline.

haircut, reverse elevation (hâr′cŭt rē′-vẽrz ĕl′ē-vā′shŭn): the longest length of hair is at the lower hairline with the hair cut progressively shorter toward the crown and toward the front hairline.

haircut, tailored neckline (hâr′kŭt tāl′-ord nĕk′līn): a hairline length with low elevation in the nape section; haircut with fitted napeline.

haircut tapering (hâr′kŭt tā′pẽr′ĭng): cutting the hair at various lengths within the strands.

G-H

haircut thinning (hârkŭt thĭn′ĭng): cutting off small strands of hair at the scalp to reduce bulk.

haircutting (hâr′kŭt-ĭng): shortening and thinning of the hair, and molding the hair into a becoming style; hair shaping.

haircutting comb (hâr′kŭt-ĭng kōm): a comb specifically designed to be used in haircutting; usually it is narrow with short, fine teeth.

haircutting implements (hâr′kŭt-ĭng ĭm′-plă-mênts): the tools used to cut, trim and shape the hair: scissors, thinning shears, straight razor, combs, hair clippers, razors with safety guards.

haircutting kit (hâr′kŭt-ĭng kĭt): a case designed to hold the implements used in haircutting.

haircutting lotion (hâr′kŭt-ĭng lō′shŭn): a liquid applied to wet hair before cutting to aid the cutting process.

haircutting shears (hâr′kŭt-ĭng shērz): scissors designed to cut and shape the

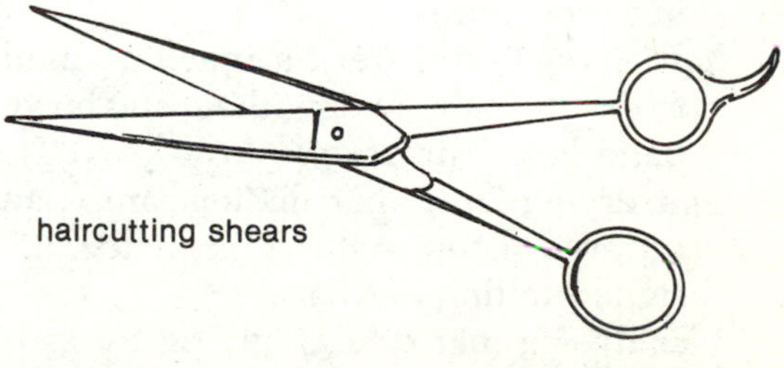

haircutting shears

G-H

hair; special thinning shears are used to remove excess bulk.

haircut under elevation (hâr′kŭt ŭn′dẽr ĕl-ĕ-vā′shûn): the shortest length of the hair is at the lower hairline; hair is cut progressively longer toward the top of the head, causing each layer to overlap to cover hair underneath; used in "page boy" styles.

hair density (hâr dĕn′sĭ-tē): the amount of hair strands per square inch on the scalp, generally broken into categories according to color; approximate number of hairs: blond hair, 140,000; brown hair, 110,000; black hair, 108,000; red hair, 90,000.

hair design (hâr dē-zīn′): the art of styling the hair; a specific style or trend.

hair, direction (hâr, dĭ-rĕk′shûn): the direction in which the hair flows in the final combout.

hair disease (hâr dĭ-zēz′): disease affecting the hair or scalp; see trichology.

hairdresser (hâr′drĕs-ẽr): a term for cosmetologist.

hairdressing (hâr′drĕs-ĭng): art of arranging the hair into various becoming shapes or styles.

hairdressing adhesive (hâr′drĕs-ĭng ăd-hē′sĭv): a substance used to hold small curls in place.

hairdresser's dermatitis (hâr′drĕs-ẽrz dûr-mă-tīt′tĭs): an inflammation of the skin caused by coming in contact with irritating substances used in hairdressing procedures.

hair dryer (hâr drī′ẽr): a machine used to dry the hair; chair with drying hood; hand held hair dryer.

hair drying lamp (hâr drī′ĭng lămp): an infrared lamp with a reflector designed to dry wet hair.

hair dyeing (hâr dī′ĭng): giving the hair new and permanent color by impregnating it with a coloring agent.

hair ends (hâr ĕndz): the last one to one half inch of hair growth furthest from the scalp.

hair filler (hâr fĭl′ẽr): a commercial product used to provide fill for porous spots in the hair during tinting, lightening and permanent waving.

hair, fine (hâr, fīn): hair which is extremely small in circumference.

hair follicle (hâr fŏl′ĭ-kl): the depression in the skin containing the hair root.

hair glands (hâr glănz): the sebaceous glands (oil glands) of the hair follicles.

hair goods (hâr gōōdz): wigs, hairpieces and decorative items for the hair.

hair lace (hâr lās): a net foundation made of stiffened human hair which is used in wig making.

hair lacquer (hâr lăk′ẽr): a product used to hold a hairstyle in place; usually used in spray form.

hairless (hâr′lĕs): without hair; bald.

hairlift (hârlĭft): an instrument employed to raise hair into proper balanced position while combing.

hair lightening (hâr lī′tĕn-ĭng): a chemical process involving the diffusion of the natural color pigment or artificial color from the hair.

hairline (hâr′līn): the line around the top of the head at which the hair ends, the edge of the growth of the hair around the face.

hairline tip (hâr′līn tĭp): the thin line at the tip of the nail where excess nail polish is removed during the manicure.

hair loss (hâr lôs): alopecia; unnatural loss of hair or premature baldness.

hair net (hâr nĕt): a cap-shaped, open mesh head covering made of nylon or rayon, used to hold the hair in place while drying; also made in a three-cornered scarf style which is tied over the head.

hair oil (hâr oyl): an oil used to lubricate dry hair and scalp.

hair ornament (hâr ôr′nă-mênt): a decorative object added to the finished hairstyle; comb, ribbon, feathers, bow, clasp, etc.

hair papilla (hâr pă-pĭl′ă): a small cone-shaped elevation at the bottom of the hair follicle.

hair parting (hâr pärt′ĭng): separating the hair by a line to comb or create a set, or as an aid in styling the hair; the sectioning of hair in order to apply tint or bleach to the scalp.

hairpiece (hâr′pēs): toupee; a small wig used to cover top or crown of the head; added piece of hair used in some women's hairstyles.

hairpin (hâr′pĭn): a slender, elongated "U" shaped pin of plastic or metal, used to secure the hair in place; a pin shaped like a clasp with ridges or plain sides.

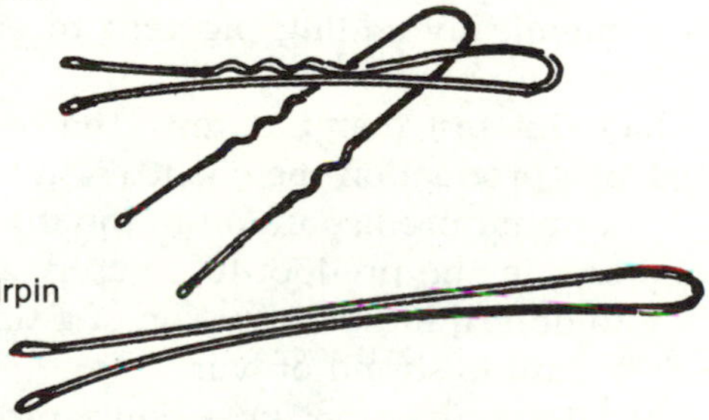
hairpin

hair pressing (hâr prĕs′ĭng): a method of temporarily straightening overcurly hair by means of a heated iron or comb.

hair pressing cream (hâr prĕs′ĭng krēm): a cream used in hair pressing as a protective lubricant for the hair.

hair pressing oil (hâr prĕs′ĭng oyl): an oily or waxy mixture used in hair pressing.

hair relaxer (hâr rē-lăks′ĕr): a chemical product used to soften or remove natural curl from the hair.

hair relaxing (hâr rê-lăk′sĭng): a method used to chemically straighten overcurly hair so that it can be styled in less curly arrangements.

hair restorer (hâr rê-stôr′ĕr): a haircoloring preparation containing metallic dye; not used professionally.

hair roll (hâr rōl): a sausage-like shape, in various lengths; used to fill under hair in order to create special effects.

hair roller (hâr rōl′ĕr): a tube-shaped device made of metal, plastic or other material of various lengths and diameters; used to set hair following a shampoo.

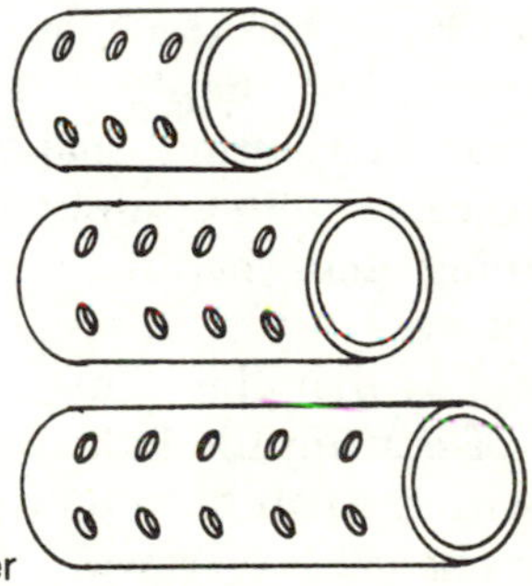
hair roller

hair roller pick (hâr rōl′ĕr pĭk): a toothpick-shaped plastic pick used to hold a hair roller in place.

hair roller pin (hâr rōl′ĕr pĭn): a flat, long, closed "U"-shaped pin, used to secure hair rollers.

hair root (hâr ro͞ot): that part of the hair contained within the follicle.

G-H

hair sample (hâr săm′p'l): a swatch of hair taken from a client's hair for purposes of testing or matching.

hair set (hâr sĕt): the technique of placing the hair into roller or pin curl patterns, finger waving or other manipulations, then combing and brushing into a finished style.

hair set tape (hâr sĕt tāp): a type of tape which is used to assist in the foundation of hairlines and curves when the hair is too short to set on rollers or in pin curls.

hair setting product (hâr sĕt′ĭng prŏd′ŭkt): a lotion, spray or gel used to make the hair easier to set and to hold the finished style in place.

hair shaft (hâr shăft): the portion of hair which projects beyond the skin, consisting of an outer layer, the cuticle; an inner layer, the cortex; and an innermost layer, the medulla.

hair shapers (hâr shāp′ẽrs): an implement for haircutting shaped like a straight razor with a safety guard.

hair shaping (hâr shāp′ĭng): the art of haircutting.

hair shingling (hâr shĭng′lĭng): the technique of cutting the hair close to the nape with the hair becoming gradually longer toward the crown.

hair slithering (hâr slĭth′ẽr′ĭng): the process used in thinning and tapering the hair at the same time, using scissors.

hair softener (hâr sof′ĕn-ẽr): a hair pomade, hair cream, cream rinse or similar substances that tend to remain on the hair for better texture and control.

hair spray (hâr sprā): a hair cosmetic applied in the form of a mist.

hair straightener (hâr strāt′ên-ẽr): a chemical agent or an iron used to straighten overcurly hair.

hair straightening (hâr strāt′nĭng): straightening overcurly hair by use of chemical agents or a heated mechanical device.

hair stream (hâr strēm): the natural direction in which the hair grows after leaving the follicle.

hairstyle (hâr stīl): a way of wearing the hair; a coiffure.

hairstyling (hâr′ stīl-ĭng): the art of dressing the hair.

hairstylist (hâr′stīl-ĭst): a specialist in the creation and design of hair fashions.

hair, superfluous (hâr, sōō-pẽr′flōō-ûs): unwanted or excess hair on the face or body.

hair test (hâr tĕst): a sampling of how the hair will react to a particular treatment.

hair texture (hâr tĕks′chŭr): the general quality of hair as to coarse, medium or fine; the feel of the hair.

hair thinning (hâr thĭn′ĭng): a procedure to reduce the bulk and density of hair.

hair tint (hâr tĭnt): a permanent hair coloring.

hair tinting (hâr tĭnt′ĭng): the act of chemically adding pigment to either virgin or tinted hair.

hair tint test (hâr tĭnt tĕst): the testing of a product on the client's skin to determine predisposition to the ingredients in the product to be used; a test to determine the reaction of a tint on a sample strand of hair.

hair tonic (hâr tŏn′ĭk): a liquid product for cleansing the hair and toning the scalp.

hair transplant (hâr trănz′plănt): a surgical procedure for transferring tufts of hair from one area of the scalp to a bald area.

hair treatment (hâr trēt′mênt): a procedure using appropriate products to improve the condition of the hair and scalp.

hair trim (hâr trĭm): trimming; cutting the hair slightly; following the existing lines.

hair weaving (hâr wēv′ĭng): the practice of sewing wefts of hair into a foundation, attached to the remaining hair on the head, in an effort to eliminate the appearance of baldness.

hair weft (hâr wĕft): a section of woven hair.

hairy (hâr′ē): having excessive hair growth; hirsute.

hairy nevus (hâr′ē nē′vŭs): a mole; a pigmented, brownish growth covered with hair.

half base (hăf bās): the placement of a roller or a curl one-half off the base.

half moon (hăf mōōn): in manicuring, a term pertaining to the light, crescent shape at the base of each nail which may be polished or left unpolished; lunula.

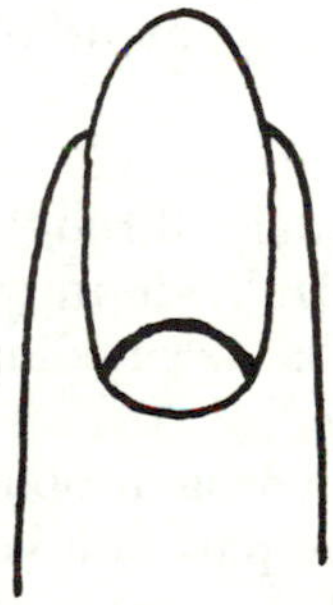
half moon

half stem (hăf stĕm): a technique by which a curl is rolled and placed one half off its base; pertains to rollers, pin curls, and perm wave rods.

half tone (hăf tōn): a semitone, halfway between a highlight and a shadow.

half twist (hăf twĭst): a term used in permanent waving to designate a type of winding, flat on one side of the rod and twisted on the other side in each revolution.

half wig (hăf wĭg): a hairpiece formed on one half of a wig base to blend with the natural hair on the head.

halitosis (hăl-ĭ-tō′sĭs): offensive odor from the mouth; foul breath.

hallux (hâl′ŭks): the first and innermost digit of the foot; the great toe.

halo (hā′lō): lengths of layered hair, on a ventilated or wefted foundation band, which is used over the top of the head or to encircle the head.

halo lightening (hā′lō līt′ĕn-ĭng): lightening the hairline area to create a halo effect.

halo wrap (hā′lō răp): a permanent wave created by wrapping vertical rods at the perimeter.

halve (hăv): to divide into two equal parts; to take half.

hamamelis (hăm-ă-mē′lĭs): a shrub of eastern North America having hazel-like leaves and small yellow flowers appearing after the leaves have fallen; witch hazel is an extract of this plant, and is used as an astringent.

hamate (hā′māt): hooked, unciform; a bone of the wrist.

hamstring (hăm′strĭng): in human anatomy, one of the tendons at the back of the knee; tendon of the biceps, flexor femoris.

hand (hănd): in human and primate anatomy, the part of the upper limb distal to the forearm and comprising the corpus, metacarpul and fingers (digits); the part attached to the wrist, top or back of the hand, palm, fingers and thumb.

G-H

hand care (hănd kâr): pertaining to beneficial exercises and grooming of the hands and nails.

hand care products (hănd kâr prŏd′ŭkts): any cream, lotion or other preparation used to soften and smooth the skin of the hands and to aid in care of the nails.

hand clippers (hănd klĭp′ĕrz): an implement used in haircutting; see clippers.

hand-held implement (hănd-hĕld ĕm′-plă-mênt): an item such as a blow-dryer, clippers, scissors, and facial apparatus, held in the hand and used to perform a service.

handmade (hănd′mād): made by hand, as differentiated from machine made.

hand massage (hănd mă-säzh′): a series of massage movements for the hands, included with a manicure.

hand mirror (hănd mĭr′ôr): a small mirror with a handle used in the salon to enable the client to view the back and sides of the finished hairstyle.

handtied (hănd tīd): a process in wig making whereby individual hairs are inserted in the mesh foundation and knotted individually with the aid of a needle; this type of wig is also referred to as a ventilated hairpiece.

hanging curls (hăng′ĭng kûrlz): curls hanging downward from the head.

hangnail (hăng′nāl): a tear in a strip of epidermis at the side of the nail; agnail.

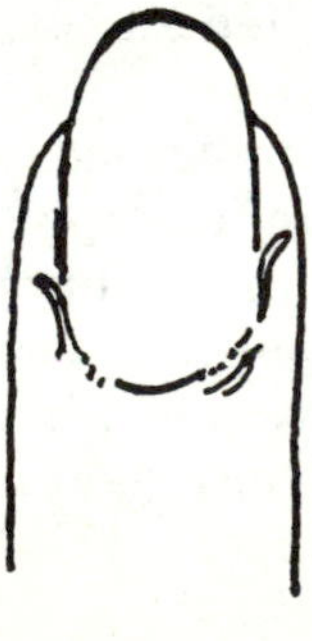

hangnail

hard (härd): firm; solid; difficult.

hardener (här′dĕn-ĕr): a substance used to strengthen the fingernails.

hard goods (härd go͞odz): pertaining to apparatus, machines, implements; also hardware.

hard press (härd prĕs): a technique in thermal hair straightening of repeating the procedure to remove all the curl.

hard rubber (härd rŭb′ĕr): a substance used in the manufacture of combs for the cosmetology and barbering industry.

hard soap (härd sōp): a soap made with sodium hydroxide; a white solid, bar-shaped soap, or a yellowish or white powdered soap.

hard sore (härd sôr): also called a chancre sore; a primary lesion which forms a hard crust.

hard water (härd wô′tĕr): water containing certain minerals; does not lather with soap.

harmony (här′mô-nē): an orderly or pleasing arrangement of shapes and lines.

haversian canals (hă-vûr′zhûn kă-nălz): small channels through which the blood vessels divide in the bone.

hazel (hā′zĕl): a medium yellowish brown color.

H-bond: see hydrogen bond.

head (hĕd): the part of a vertebrate animal at the top or front of a spinal column containing the sense organs: eyes, ears, nose and the mouth.

headband (hĕd′bănd): a band, usually of material, worn to hold the hair back from the face.

headdress (hĕd′drĕs): an ornamental addition to the hair; the style in which the hair has been arranged; a coiffure.

head lice (hĕd līs): small flat insects which may infect humans; an external parasite (pediculus capitis) found on the head.

heal (hēl): to cure.

health (hēlth): state of being whole or sound in body and mind.

heart (härt): a hollow muscular organ which by contracting rhythmically, keeps up the circulation of the blood.

heat (hēt): high temperature; to be or become warm or hot.

heat, electric (hēt, ê-lĕk′trĭk): the heat produced in a conductor by the passage of an electric current through it.

heater (hēt′ẽr): an apparatus used to warm products used in some grooming services; an example is the electric heater for warming wax used in facials and to remove superfluous hair.

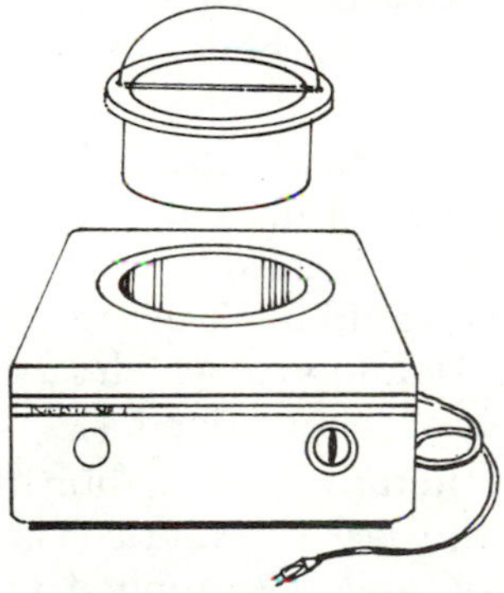

heater

heating cap (hēt′ĭng kăp): an insulated cap, containing interwoven electric wires, which is used for heating the hair and scalp in some corrective treatment.

heating coil (hēt′ĭng koyl): electric coil which heats the air in a hair dryer.

heat lamp (hēt lămp): a reddish brown, coated glass bulb which produces infrared light; used as an aid in heat treatments.

heat rash (hēt răsh): also called miliaria, an acute, inflammatory disease of the sweat glands characterized by lesions and itching papules; prickly heat.

heat regulation (hêt rĕg-û-lā′shûn): a system of permanent waving employing either machines or chemicals to generate heat; a means of controlling the amount of heat generated by chemical or mechanical means.

heat rollers (hēt rōl′ẽrs): electric or steam preheated rollers for setting the hair.

heat treatment (hēt trēt′mênt): a treatment given with the aid of a heat lamp which produces infrared light.

heat wave (hēt wāv): a permanent wave accomplished by changing the hair structure from an ordinary and natural straightness to one of curliness or waviness by using heat and mild chemicals.

heat waving (hēt wāv′ĭng): a method of permanent waving using machines or chemicals to produce heat.

heavy hair (hĕv′ē hâr): dense, thick hair having more than average weight and mass.

heavy side of the head (hĕ′vē sīd of the hĕd): the side of the head to which most of the hair is directed.

Heberden's disease (hē′bẽr-dĕnz dĭ-zēz′): arthritis; a degenerative joint disease affecting the fingers and hand; often deforming the bone structure.

heel (hēl): in human anatomy, the round, posterior part of the foot behind the arch and back of the ankle; also the heel of the hand, the part of the hand near the wrist and adjoining the thumb.

height (hīt): the distance from the base to the top.

helcoma (hĕl-kō′mă): an ulcer.

helical (hĕl′ĭ-kâl): shaped like a spiral.

helical winding (hĕl′ĭ-kâl wīnd′ing):

G-H

G-H

winding the hair from the scalp to the ends; see spiral waving.

heliotherapy (hē′lē-ô-thĕr′ă-pē): the therapeutic use of solar energy; use of the sun's rays as a beneficial treatment.

helix (hē′lĭks): spiral formation; the structural arrangement of polypeptide chains in the hair.

hem (hĕm): the bent-over edge of a piece of material which has been turned under to avoid fraying; in wig work, the netting and the binding.

hemal, haemel (hē′mâl): relating to the blood or blood vessels.

hematidrosis, hemidrosis (hĕm′ă-tĭ-drō′-sĭs, hĕm-ĭ-drō′sĭs): the excretion of sweat stained with blood or blood pigment.

hematocyst (hĕ-mă′tô-sĭst): a cyst containing blood.

hematocyte (hĕ-mă′tô-sīt): a blood corpuscle.

hematology (hē′mă-tŏl′ō-jē): the science of the blood, its functions, composition and diseases.

hemi (hĕm′ĭ): a prefix signifying half.

hemifacial (hĕm′ĭ-fā′shâl): pertaining to one side of the face.

hemoglobin; haemoglobin (hē′mă-glō-bĭn): the coloring matter of the blood; the oxygen-carrying pigment in the blood and iron-containing protein in red blood cells.

hemorrage (hĕm′ô-râj): heavy or uncontrollable bleeding.

hemostatic (hēm-ō-stăt′ĭk): a substance used to control bleeding; also referred to as a styptic.

henna (hĕn′ă): the leaves of an Asiatic thorny tree or shrub used as a dye, imparting a reddish tint; also used as a cosmetic.

henna, compound (hĕn′ă, kŏm′paund): Egyptian henna to which has been added one or more metallic preparations.

henna intensifier (hĕn′ă ĭn-tĕn′sĭ-fī-ĕr): an additive for henna that increases its color value.

henna leaves (hĕn′ă lēvs): leaves of the henna plant from which a red dye is extracted; the dye may be used on hair but is not used on eyebrows or eyelashes.

henna shampoo (hĕn′ă shăm-pōō′): a shampoo to which henna has been added to add color and luster to the hair.

henna, white (hĕn′ă, hwīt): magnesia plus peroxide and ammonia.

herb (ûrb, hûrb): a plant with leaves, stems or parts used in cookery and in medicinal and cosmetic preparations.

herbal (hûrb′âl): pertaining to herbs.

herbal extracts (hûrb′âl ĕks′trăkts): substances from herbs used in various products.

herbal shampoo (hûr′b'l shăm′pōō): shampoo containing substances extracted from bark, roots and herbs known to aid in cleansing the hair and scalp; shampoo to which saponin products have been added.

herbal therapy (ûr′bâl, hûr′bâl thĕr′ă-pē): the use of etheric oils of plants and natural oils, applied to the skin as a stimulant and to impart a sense of physical well being.

hereditary (hĕ-rĕd′ĭ-tĕ-rē): descending from ancestor to heir; genetically transmitted from parent to offspring.

heredity (hĕ-rĕd′ĭ-tē): the genetic capacity of the organism to develop ancestral characteristics; the transfer of qualities or disease from parents to offspring.

herpes (hûr′pēz): an inflammatory disease of the skin characterized by small vesicles in clusters.

herpes facialis (hûr′pēz fă-shē-ā′lĭs): a type of herpes simplex affecting the face, usually the lips and mouth; cold-sore.

herpes simplex (hûr′pēz sĭm′plĕks): fever blister; cold sore.

hexachlorophenol (hĕx-ă-klô-rô-fē′nôl): white, free-flowing powder, essentially odorless; used as a bactericidal agent in antiseptic soaps, deodorant products, including soaps, and various cosmetics.

hidroa (hī-drō′ă): a skin lesion associated with or caused by profuse sweating.

hidrosis (hi-drō′sĭs): abnormally profuse sweating.

high caloric diet (hī′ kăl-ôr′ĭk dī′ĕt): a diet containing 3,000 or more calories per day.

high colored (hī kŭl′ẽrd): deep or brilliant rosy color; exaggerated color.

high elevation (hī ĕl′ă-vā′shûn): haircutting term indicating that hair is held 90 degrees or more from the head form and then cut, causing it to fall in a layered effect.

high fashion (hī fă′shûn): a current fashion trend in clothing, hairstyling or hair coloring.

high fashion blonding (hī fă′shûn blŏnd′-ĭng): the special process of coloring in which the hair is lightened and then toned.

high frequency machine (hī frē′qwĕn-sē mă-shēn′): a machine which produces violet rays, used for facial and scalp treatments.

high frequency, tesla (hī frē′kwĕn-sē, tĕs′lă): violet ray; an electric current of medium voltage and medium amperage.

highlight (hī′līt): brightness or luster added to hair by some artificial means; a lighter cosmetic applied to a facial feature to improve its contours.

highlighting (hī′līt-ĭng): coloring some of the hair strands lighter than the natural color to add the illusion of sheen; applying a lighter cosmetic to a facial feature to improve its contours.

G-H

highlighting shampoo tint (hī′līt-ĭng shăm-pōō′ tĭnt): a permanent hair tint mixed with peroxide and shampoo; used when a very slight change in hair shade is desired.

high molecular weight (hī mô-lĕk′ū-lăr wāt): large size and density of a specific molecular construction.

high style (hī stīl): the newest hair fashion; an up-to-the-minute design.

hip (hĭp): in human anatomy, the part of the body below the waist on either side of the pelvis.

hip bone (hĭp bōn): the innominate bone.

hirsute (hûr′sūt, hẽr-sūt′): hairy; having coarse, long hair; shaggy.

hirsuties (hûr-sū′shĭ-ēz): hypertrichosis; growth of an unusual amount of hair in unusual locations, as on the faces of women or the backs of men; hairy; superfluous hair.

hirsutism (hûr′sû-tĭzm): pertaining to an excessive growth or cover of hair, especially in areas not normally covered with excessive hair.

histologists (hĭs-tŏl′ô-jĭsts): those who apply themselves to the science of histology.

histology (hĭs-tŏl′ô-jē): the science of the minute structure of organic tissues; microscopic anatomy.

hives (hīvz): urticaria; a skin eruption.

hoary (hôr′ē): gray or white with age.

Hodgkin's disease (hŏj′kĭnz dĭs-ēz′): a disease characterized by enlargement of the lymph nodes, lymphoid tissue and the spleen; a progressive and sometimes fatal condition, named after Dr. Thomas Hodgkin (1798–1866).

hold (hōld): pertaining to the ability of a hair spray to keep a hairstyle in place.

holding angle (hōld′ĭng ăng′'l): angle at which the hand is held while cutting hair from the headform.

G-H

homogenizer (hō-mŏj′ĕ-nīz-ẽr): a substance that produces a uniform suspension of emulsions from two or more normally immiscible substances.

homogenous (hō-mŏj′ê-nûs): having the same nature or quality; a uniform character in all parts.

hone (hōn): a fine grit stone used to sharpen a cutting tool, such as a razor; used for haircutting or for shaving the beard.

honey (hŭn′ē): mel; the product of the honey bee; considered to be a health-giving food and sometimes used in facial and other cosmetic products.

honeycomb base (hŭn′ē-kōm bās): a lightweight, openly woven base on a wig through which a person's own hair can be pulled through the openings and blended with the artificial wig hair.

honeysuckle (hŭn′ē-sŭk′'l): a large climbing shrub with white or crimson flowers, valued for its pleasing fragrance; used in perfumery.

hops (hŏps): a climbing herb with scaly fruit; produces an astringent and moisturizing substance; provides amino acids for cell renewal.

horizontal (hŏr-ĭ-zŏn′tâl): parallel to the horizon; level; opposed to vertical.

hormone (hôr′mōn): a secretion produced in and by one of the endocrine glands, such as the pituitary, thyroid, adrenals, etc.; and carried by the blood stream or body fluid to another part of the body or body organ to stimulate functional activity.

hormone cream (hôr′mōn krēm): a cosmetic containing hormones.

horny (hôr′nē): composed of or resembling horns; a keratoid substance; having the hard texture of horns.

horse chestnut (hôrs chĕs′nŭt): a tree bearing chestnut-like fruit, digitate leaves and clusters of flowers; used in preparations for facial treatments; said to tighten pores, stimulate and speed healing of the skin.

horsetail (hôrs′tāl): an herb with hollow, jointed stems used in products for the skin and hair; contains vitamin C and acts as an astringent and healing substance.

hot brush (hŏt brŭsh): an electric curling iron with metal body and firm bristles, shaped like a round brush; used to style the hair when it is dry.

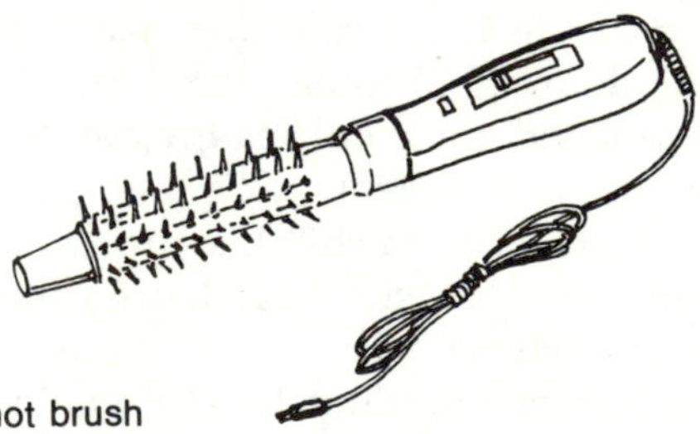

hot brush

hot comb (hŏt kōm): a thermal iron used in hair pressing; also an electric appliance designed to dry the hair as it is being styled.

hot iron (hŏt ī′ûrn): another term for curling iron.

hot oil (hŏt oyl): a warmed oil used in facial and manicure treatments.

hot rollers (hŏt rōl′ẽrs): rollers that are

preheated before being placed in the hair.

hue (hū): pertaining to a particular color, tint or shade; gradation of color.

human hair (hū′mân hâr): hair that grows on a human being; the facial, head or body hair of a person.

human hair wig (hū′mân hâr wĭg): a wig made with Asiatic or European hair, considered to be of excellent quality.

humectant (hū-mĕk′tânt): a substance which absorbs moisture or promotes retention of moisture; a substance having affinity for water, with the stabilizing action on water content of a material.

humeral (hū′mĕr-âl): pertaining to the humerus; the shoulder or shoulders.

humerus (hū′mĕr-ûs): the bone of the upper part of the arm.

humid (hū′mĭd): containing moisture, vapor or water; damp.

humidity (hū-mĭd′ĭ-tē): dampness; a moderate amount of wetness especially of the atmosphere.

hyacinth (hī′ă-sĭnth): a fragrant bell-shaped flower cultivated for use in perfumery; the color purple-blue.

hydrate (hī′drāt): a compound formed by the union of water with some other substance; to combine a substance with water; to add moisture to the skin.

hydrating agent (hī′drāt-ĭng ā′jĕnt): a substance used in facial treatments to restore moisture to a dry (dehydrated) skin.

hydration (hī-drā′shûn): the chemical union of a substance with water.

hydro (hī′drô): a prefix denoting water; hydrogen.

hydrocarbon (hī′drô-kär′bôn): charcoal; any compound consisting only of hydrogen and carbon.

hydrochloric acid (hī′drô-klô′rĭk ăs′ĭd): a compound of hydrogen and chlorine.

hydrocyst (hī′drō-sĭst): a cyst containing a watery fluid.

hydrocystoma (hĭd-rô-sĭs-tō′mă): a variety of sudamina appearing on the face, especially of women in middle and advanced life.

hydrogen (hī′drô-jên): in chemistry, the symbol H; the lightest element; it is an odorless, tasteless, colorless gas found in water and all organic compounds; hydrogen acceptor: a substance which, on reduction, accepts hydrogen atoms from another substance called a hydrogen donor.

hydrogenate (hī′drô-jên-āt): to combine or treat with hydrogen.

hydrogenated lanolin (hī′-drô-jên-āt′ĕd lăn′ô-lĭn): lanolin treated with hydrogen so that it retains its emollient qualities while losing unwanted odor, color and tackiness; used in cosmetic preparations such as creams, lotions, powders, sprays, suntan products, hair and nail preparations and perfumes.

hydrogen bond in hair (hī′drô-jĕn bŏnd in hâr): in hair chemistry; the molecular association between an atom of hydrogen and an atom of oxygen in the hair forming an electromagnetic bond; gives strength and elasticity to hair and form to the hair when it is dry.

hydrogen bond (physical bond) (hī′drō-jĕn bŏnd): in chemistry, the bond formed between two molecules when the nucleus of a hydrogen atom, originally attached to a fluorine, nitrogen or oxygen atom of a second molecule of the same or different substance.

hydrogen ion concentration (hī′drô-jĕn ī′ôn kŏn-sĕn-trā′shûn): also called pH, a measure of the degree of acidity or alkalinity of an aqueous solution and expressed on a scale of 0–14, where

7 is neutral, 0.0–6.9 indicates degreasing acidity, and 7.1 to 14.0 indicates increasing alkalinity.

hydrogen peroxide (hī′drô-jĕn pĕr-ŏk′-sīd): a powerful oxidizing agent; in liquid form it is used as an antiseptic, as a neutralizer and for the activation of lightness and hair tints; the most common strength for cosmetology use is 6% (20 volume).

hydrolysis (hī-drŏ′lĭ-sĭs): chemical process of decomposition involving splitting of a bond with the addition of the elements of water (hydrogen and oxygen).

hydrolyze (hī′drō-līz): to decompose as a result of the incorporation and splitting of water; the two resulting products divide the water: the hydroxyl group being attached to one and the hydrogen atom to the other.

hydrolyzed elastin (hī′drô-līz′d ĭ-lăs′tĭn): the product (hydrolysate) of animal ligaments and other connective tissue used in creams formulated to help retain the skin's elasticity.

hydromassage (hī′drō-mă-säzh′): massage by means of moving water.

hydrometer (hī-drŏm′ĕ-tĕr): an instrument used to measure the strength (volume) of peroxide and other liquids.

hydrophilic (hī-drō-fĭl′ĭk): capable of combining with or attracting water.

hydrophobia (hī-drô-fō′bē-ă): rabies in humans; morbid fear of water.

hydroquinone (hī-drō-kwĭ-nōn′): a chemical compound used as an antioxidant and bleaching agent in some cosmetic preparations.

hydrosis (hī-drō′sĭs): excretion of perspiration.

hydrosoluble (hī-drō-sŏl′ū-b'l): soluble in water.

hydrotherapy (hī′drô-thĕr′ă-pē): the scientific use of water in the treatment of injuries, diseases or for mental well-being; physical therapy using water.

hydroxic cellulose (hī-drŏk′sĭk sĕl′û-lōs): a chemical employed as a thickening agent; a chemical used to make a watery liquid thick.

hydroxide (hī-drŏks′īd): any compound formed by the union of OH (one oxygen atom joined with one hydrogen atom) with a group of atoms known as a radical.

hygiene (hī′jēn): the science of preserving health.

hygienic (hī-jĭ-ĕn′ĭk): having to do with preserving health.

hygroscopic (hī-grô-skŏp′ĭk): readily absorbing and retaining moisture.

hyoid (hī′oyd): pertaining to the "U" shaped bone situated at the base of the tongue that supports the tongue and its muscles.

hyper (hī′pĕr): a prefix denoting excessive; above normal; above; beyond.

hyperacidity (hī-pĕr-ă-sĭd′ĭ-tē): an excess of acidity.

hyperemia (hī′pĕr-ē′mē-ă): the presence of an excessive quantity of blood in a part of the body.

hyperhidrosis, hyperidrosis (hī′pĕr-hĭ-drō′sĭs, hī′pĕr-ĭ-drō′sĭs): excessive sweating.

hyperkeratinization (hī′pĕr-kĕr-ă-tĭn-ĭ-zā-shûn): see hyperkeratosis.

hyperkeratosis (hī-pĕr-kĕr-ă-tō′sĭs): hypertrophy (excessive growth) of the corneous (horny) layer of the skin and associated with hypertrophy of the prickle cell layer, and the granular layer of the skin.

hyperkeratosis subungualis (hī′pĕr-kĕr-ă-tō′sĭs sŭb-ŭn-gwā′lĭs): hypertrophy affecting the nail bed.

hyperostosis (hī-pĕr-ŏs-tō′sĭs): excessive

growth or thickening of bone tissue.

hyperpigmentation (hī′pĕr-pĭg-mĕn′-tāshûn): a condition characterized by the production of more melanin in some areas of the skin than in others.

hyperplasia (hī′pĕr-plā′zē-ă): excessive formation of tissue; an increase in the size of a tissue or organ because of an increase in the number of cells.

hypersecretion (hī-pĕr-sê-krē′shûn): excessive secretion.

hypersensitivity (hī-pĕr-sĕn-sĭ-tĭv′ĭ-tē): unusually affected by external agencies or influences to which a normal individual does not react.

hypertrichosis, hypertricosis (hī′pĕr-trĭ-kō′sĭs): a condition of excessive development or abnormal growth of the hair; superfluous hair.

hypertrophica, acne (hī′pĕr-trŏf′ĭ-kă): vulgaris in which the lesions leave conspicuous pits and scars upon healing.

hypertrophy (hī-pĕr′trō-fē): abnormal increase in the size of a part or an organ; overgrowth; abnormal growth.

hypo (hī′pô): a prefix denoting under; beneath; lower state of oxidation.

hypoallergenic (hī-pô-ăl-ĕr-jĕn′ĭk): having a lower than usual tendency to cause allergic reactions.

hypodermal (hī′pô-dûr′mâl): lying beneath the epidermis.

hypodermic (hī′pô-dûr′mĭk): of or relating to parts beneath the skin; placed or introduced beneath the skin.

hypodermis (hī′pô-dûr′mĭs): in human anatomy, the subcutaneous tissue.

hypoglossal (hī′pô-glŏ′sâl): under the tongue; the twelfth cranial nerve.

hyponychium (hī′pô-nĭk′ē-ûm): the thickened stratum corneum of the epidermis that lies underneath the free edge of the nail.

hypothalamus (hī′pô-thăl′ă-mûs): the part of the brain that regulates many metabolic body processes.

hypothenar (hī-pŏth′ĕ-när, hī-pō-thēn′-ăr): the fleshy eminence on the palm of the hand over the metacarpal bone of the little finger; also the prominences on the palm at the base of the fingers.

hypothermia (hī′pô-thûr′mē-ă): a condition of abnormally low body temperature.

hypothesis (hī-pŏth′ĕ-sĭs): an assumption or theory proposed to account for facts.

hypoxia (hī-pŏk′sē-ă): inadequate supply of oxygen in the tissues.

hyssop (hĭs′ŭp): an herb of the mint family; used in medicine and cosmetic preparations; valued as an astringent and for its healing properties.

I

ice (īs): frozen water.

ice bag (īs băg): also called ice pack; a flexible, waterproof container used to hold ice; it is wrapped in a towel and applied to the part of the face or body to be treated.

ice cube (īs kūb): frozen water in the shape of a small block; used in ice bags and in some facial procedures to contract the pores.

ice pick scars (īs-pĭk skärz): large visible open pores that look as if the skin has been punctured with an icepick or similar object; this scar is caused by a deep pimple or cyst that has destroyed the follicle as infection worked its way to the surface of the skin.

icing (īs′ĭng): in haircoloring, a term for frosting only half of the head, either the front or back of the head.

ichthyosis (ĭk-thê-ō′sĭs): a skin disease in which the skin becomes rough with diminished sweat and sebaceous secretion; fishskin disease.

ichthyotic (ĭk-thê-ŏt′ĭk): characterized by a skin disease accompanied by scaling.

ide (īd): a word termination denoting certain types of compounds.

identical (ī-dĕn′tĭ-kâl): exactly alike or equal.

illumination (ĭl-lū′mĭ-nā′shûn): the action or state of making light, luminous or shining; in hair coloring, a process whereby one area of the head is lightened two or three shades.

imagery (ĭm′ÿ-rē): the forming of a mental image; creative thinking.

imbalance (ĭm-băl′êns): the state of being out of balance.

imbibition (ĭm-bĭ-bĭsh′ûn): the act of sucking up moisture.

imbricated (ĭm′brĭ-kāt′ĕd): overlapped, as scales in skin disease.

imbrications (ĭm-brĭ-kā′shûnz): cells arranged in layers overlapping one another; tiny overlapping of scales found in the hair cuticle; overlapping of layers of tissue in the closure of wounds or repair of defects.

immerse (ĭ-mûrs′): to plunge into; dip; submerge in a liquid.

immersion (ĭ-mûr′shûn): plunging or dipping into a liquid especially so as to cover completely.

immiscible (ĭ-mĭs′ĭ-b′l): not capable of being mixed, as oil and water.

immobile (ĭ-mō′b′l): incapable of being moved; motionless.

immune (ĭ-mūn′): safe from attack; protected from disease by vaccination or natural defenses.

immunity (ĭ-mūn′ĭ-tē): freedom from or resistance to disease.

immunodermatology (ĭm-ū-nō-dûr-mă-tŏl′ō-jē): the study of the immune system as related to skin disorders and their treatment.

immunology (ĭm-ū-nŏl′ō-jē): the branch of medical science that deals with immunity to diseases.

impair (ĭm-pâr′): to make worse; to render less than perfect; to cause to lose quality.

impearl (ĭm-pûrl′): to make pearly; to pearlize a cosmetic product to give a sheen.

impedance (ĭm-pēd′ns): the resistance in an electric current to an alternating current.

impenetrable (ĭm-pĕn′ă-tră-b'l): incapable of being penetrated.

imperfect (ĭm-pûr′fĭkt): falling short of perfection; defective; unfinished.

impermeable (ĭm-pûr′mē-ă-b'l): impenetrable; not capable of being penetrated; impervious to moisture.

impervious (im-pur′vē-us): impenetrable; incapable of being passed through.

impetigo (ĭm-pĕ-tī′gō): an eruption of pustules, caused by staphylococci or streptococci, which rupture or become crusted; occurring chiefly on the face around the mouth and nostrils.

implant (ĭm-plănt′): to imbed; to insert and fix firmly.

implement (ĭm′plĕ-mĕnt): an instrument or tool.

impregnated (ĭm-prĕg′nāt-ĕd): fertilized; saturated.

impure (ĭm-pyŏŏr′): containing some form of contamination; lacking purity; adulterated.

in (ĭn): a prefix denoting not; negative; within; inside.

inappropriate (ĭn-ă-prō′prē-ĭt): unsuitable, not fitting; as a hairstyle unsuitable for facial structure.

incandescent (ĭn-kăn-dĕs′ĕnt): giving forth light and heat.

inch (ĭnch): a measure of length equal to the twelfth part of a foot; 2.54 centimeters.

incision (ĭn-sĭzh′ûn): a cut; a cut of soft body tissue made with a knife or similar instrument.

inclined (ĭn-klīnd′): forming an angle with a line or plane; bent or bowed.

include (ĭn klōōd′): to make a part of something; add to a category; comprise.

incombustible (ĭn-kŏm-bŭs′tĭ-b'l): fireproof; not flammable.

increase layering (ĭn-krēs′lā-ĕr′ĭng): cutting to produce a layered effect with progressivelylongerlengths.

increasing graduation (ĭn-krēs′ĭng grăj'-ōō-wā′shûn): graduation within two non-parallel lines; it increases as it moves back from the face.

incretion (ĭn-krē′shûn): the secreting of a substance, such as oil, from the sebaceous glands.

incrust (ĭn-krŭst′): also encrust; to form a crust or a coating.

incrustation (ĭn-krŭs-tā′shûn): the state of having crusts or scales; the formation of a crust or hard coating.

incubation (ĭn-kû-bā′shûn): the act or process of hatching or developing; the period of time between infection of an individual with an infectious disease and the appearance of symptoms.

incurable (ĭn-kyŏŏr′ă-b'l): not capable of being cured.

incurvate (ĭn-kûr′vāt): to cause to curve inward.

indelible (ĭn-dĕl′ĭ-b'l): cannot be removed, erased, blotted out or eliminated; permanent; lasting.

indemnity (ĭn-dĕm′nĭ-tē): compensation for loss.

indent (ĭn′dĕnt): an inward depression or hollow.

indentation (ĭn-dĕn-tā′shûn): the curved depth, valley or hollowness created by the formation of curls or waves in the hair.

indentation curl (ĭn-dĕn-tā′shûn kûrl): pin curl technique in which the stem is combed flat against the scalp and the curl is rolled up to stand up away from the head; used to create a hollow or valley in the finished style.

indentation roller (ĭn-dĕn-tā′shûn rōl′ĕr):

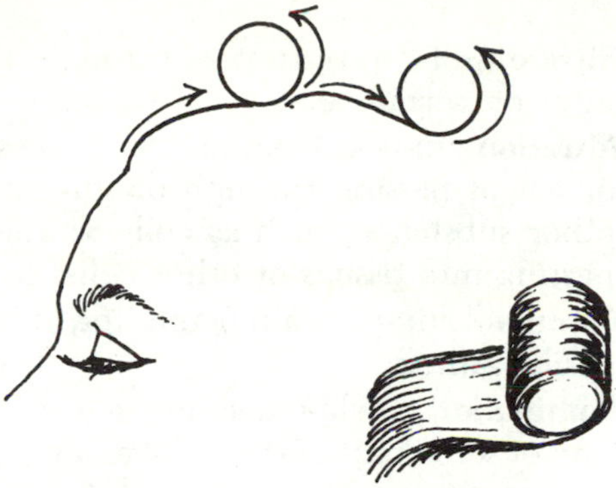

indentation roller and indentation curl

setting technique in which the stem is combed flat against the scalp and the roller is rolled upward, away from the head; used to create a hollow or valley in the finished style.

index (ĭn′dĕks): an alphabetical list of items from a printed work; the first finger next to the thumb.

Indian cress (ĭn′dē-ăn krĕs): an herb used in some skin care products and as a dandruff control agent; contains amino acids, sulphur and antibiotics.

indicator (ĭn′dĭ-kā-tẽr): an apparatus or instrument used to show changes in conditions such as color or the degree of acidity or alkalinity.

indigo (ĭn′dĭ-gō): a blue dye.

indirect point (ĭn′dĭ-rekt poynt): partings of an oval shape using curved or straight lines; the first parting is out of the circumference, then intersections all form one point.

indispensable (ĭn-dĭs-pĕn′să-b'l): absolutely necessary.

individual (ĭn-dĭ-vĭj′o͞o-âl): separate; distinguished from others of the same kind.

individual eyelashes (ĭn-dĭ-vĭj′o͞o-âl ī′lăsh′ĕz): separate, artificial eyelashes that are applied to the eyelids one at a time.

individualize (ĭn-dĭ.vĭj′o͞o-ă-līz): to distinguish from others; to give a client a particular hairstyle or haircut.

induction (ĭn-dŭk′shûn): the process by which an electrified or magnetic state is produced through nearness with a charged body or presence in a magnetic field.

inductor (ĭn-dŭk′tẽr): an electrical apparatus or part that acts inductively upon another.

indurata, acne (ĭn-dû-rā′tă, ăk′nē): deeply seated papular eruptions with hard tubercular lesions.

indurate (ĭn′dû-rāt): to make hard or firm.

induration (ĭn-dû-rā′shûn): the process or act of hardening; a spot or area of hardened tissue.

inefficiency (ĭn′ĕ-fĭsh′ên-sē): quality, state or fact of being wasteful of time or energy or not producing the effect intended or desired within a given expenditure of time or energy.

inelasticity (ĭn-ê-lăs-tĭs′ĭ-tē): in cosmetology, the ability to stretch but not return to its former shape, as overbleached or limp hair; aging skin or muscles.

inert (ĭn-ûrt′): inactive; lacking the power to move.

infect (ĭn-fĕkt′): to cause infection; to contaminate.

infection (ĭn-fĕk′shûn): the invasion of body tissues by disease germs.

infection, general (ĭn-fĕk′shûn, jĕn′ẽr-âl): the result of disease germs gaining entrance into the bloodstream and circulating throughout the entire body.

infection, local (ĭn-fĕk′shûn, lō′kâl): infection confined to only certain portions of the body such as an abscess.

infectious (ĭn-fĕk′shûs): capable of spreading infection.

infectious allergy (ĭn-fĕk′shûs ăl′ẽr-je):

delayed hypersensitivity induced by an infectious agent.

infectious dermatitis (ĭn-fĕk′shûs dûr-mă-tī′tĭs): an inflamed irritation of the skin resulting from the irritating effect of a substance.

infectious mononucleosis (ĭn-fĕk′shûs mŏn-ô-nū-klē-ō′sĭs): a contagious disease characterized by a swelling of the lymph nodes, fever, and sore throat; also called glandular fever.

inferior (ĭn-fĭr′ē-ẽr): situated lower down, or nearer the bottom or base; of lesser quality.

inferioris (ĭn-fĭr-ē-ŏr′ĭs): below; lower.

inferior labial artery (ĭn-fĭr′ē-ẽr lā′bē-âl är′tĭr-ē): artery that supplies blood to the lower lip.

inferior labial nerve (ĭn-fĭr′ē-ẽr lā′bē-âl nûrv): in the skin of the lower lip.

inferior labial vein (ĭn-fĭr′ē-ẽr lā′bē-âl vān): a vein that drains the region of the lower lip into the facial vein.

inferior maxilla (ĭn-fĭr′ē-ẽr măk-sĭl′ă): the lower jawbone or mandible.

inferior ophthalmic vein (ĭn-fĭr′ē-ẽr ŏf-thăl′mĭk vān): a vein that supplies blood to the eye, orbit and adjacent facial structures.

inferior palpebral nerve (ĭn-fĭr′ē-ẽr păl′pĕ-brâl nûrv): a nerve that receives stimuli for the lower eyelid.

inferior palpebral vein (ĭn-fĭr′ē-ẽr păl′pĕ-brâl vān): a vein that drains blood from the lower eyelids to the facial veins.

inferior terbinate (ĭn-fĭr′ē-ẽr tûr′bĭ-nāt): the nasal concha; an irregular scroll-shaped bone situated on the lateral wall of the nasal cavity.

inferior vena cava (ĭn-fĭr′ē-ẽr vēn′ă kāv′ă): the large vein that carries blood to the heart from the abdomen, feet and legs; located in front of the vertebral column to the right of the aorta.

infiltrate (ĭn-fĭl′trāt): to pass through; to filter or permeate.

infiltration (ĭn-fĭl-trā′shûn): the process or act of passing through or into another substance, such as cells or fluid passing into tissues or other cells.

inflammable (ĭn-flăm′ă-b'l): tending to be easily ignited.

inflammation (ĭn-flă-mā′shûn): a condition of some part of the body as a reaction to injury, irritation or infection characterized by redness, heat, pain and swelling.

inflate (ĭn-flāt′): to swell or distend by filling with air or gas.

influenza (ĭn-flū-ĕn′ză): an acute, highly contagious viral disease characterized by sudden onset, fever, prostration, and severe aches and pains; grippe.

informal (ĭn-fôrm′âl): not in the usual or prescribed form; relaxed; casual.

infra (ĭn′-fră): a prefix denoting below; lower.

inframandibular (ĭn′fră-măn-dĭb′û-lâr): below the lower jaw.

infraorbital (ĭn′fră-ôr′bĭ-tâl): below the orbit, in the floor of the orbit; a sensory and motor nerve affecting the cheek muscles, nose, and upper lip.

infrared (ĭn′fră-rĕd′): pertaining to that part of the spectrum lying outside the visible spectrum and below the red rays.

infratrochlear (ĭn′fră-trŏk′lē-âr): sensory nerve affecting the lacrimal sac, the skin of the nose and the inner muscle of the eye.

ingestion (ĭn-jĕs′chûn): the act of taking substances, especially food, into the body.

ingredient (ĭn-grē′dē-ênt): any part of a compound; that which enters into the composition of a mixture.

ingrown (ĭn′grōn): growing inward; an ingrown hair or nail.
ingrown hair (ĭn′grōn hâr): a hair that has grown so that the normally free end is embedded in or underneath the skin, sometimes causing an infection.
ingrown nail (ĭn′grōn nāl): a nail that has grown into the flesh instead of toward the tip of the finger or toe, sometimes causing an infection.
inhalation (ĭn-hă-lā′shûn): the breathing in of air and other vapors.
inhale (ĭn-hāl′): to draw in the breath; to inspire.
inhibit (ĭn-hĭb′ĭt): to check or restrain; prohibit.
inhibition (ĭn-hĭ-bĭsh′ûn): the diminution or arrest of the function in an organ.
inject (ĭn-jĕkt′): to force into; to force fluid through a syringe or needle; to force fluid into an injector rod.
injector rod (ĭn-jĕk′tẽr rŏd): a permanent wave rod designed with openings into which wave lotion and neutralizer may be injected after the hair is wound on the rod.
injury (ĭn′jo͝or-ē): damage or hurt.
inner (ĭn′nẽr): interior; internal; inward.
inner and outer circle (ĭn′ẽr and out′ẽr sûr′k'l): terms employed in hair sectioning to indicate an inner section with a preshaped base and an outer section with a slanted or oblique base.
inner and outer technique (ĭn′ẽr and aù-t′ẽr tĕk′nēk): in hairdressing, the technique of expanding a circle.
inner circle (ĭn′ẽr sûr′k'l): in hair sectioning; a pieshaped base; the outer circle is on a slanted base.
innermost (ĭn′ẽr mōst): the inmost part; the farthest inward from the outermost part.
inner perimeter (ĭn′ẽr pă-rĭm′ĭ-tẽr): in hairstyling, the hair length and density in the inner area excluding the hairline.
innervation (ĭn-ẽr-vā′shûn): distribution of nerves in a part of the body.
innominate (ĭ-näm′ĭ-nĭt): having no specific name or names; anonymous; generally applied to certain anatomical structures.
innominate artery (ĭ-näm′ĭ-nĭt är′tĭr-ē): an artery that distributes blood to the right side of the head and to the right arm.
innominate bone (ĭ-näm′ĭ-nĭt bōn): one of two large irregular bones that form the pelvis; hipbone.
innominate veins (ĭ-näm′ĭ-nĭt vānz): veins of the neck.
innovate (ĭn′ô-vāt): to create or introduce something new and original, such as a new hairstyle.
innovation (ĭn-ô-vā′shûn): to introduce new methods or ideas.
inoculation (ĭn-ŏk-û-lā′shûn): the injection of a disease agent to cause a mild form of the disease to build immunity to that disease.
inorganic (ĭn-ôr-găn′ĭk): composed of matter not arising from natural growth or living organisms.
inorganic chemistry (ĭn-ôr-găn′ĭk kĕm′ĭs-trē): the branch of chemistry dealing with compounds lacking carbon, or containing carbon only in the form of cyanides, carbides or carbonates.
inorganic hair dye (ĭn-ôr-găn′ĭk hâr dī): a nonvegetable, nonanimal hair coloring material.
inorganic nutrients (ĭn-ôr-găn′ĭk no͞o′trē-ênts): minerals needed in the daily diet.
insanitary, unsanitary (ĭn-săn′ĭ-tĕ-rē, ŭn-): not sanitary or healthful; unclean enough to be injurious to health.

I-J

inseparable (ĭn-sĕp′är-ă-b'l): incapable of being separated.
insert (ĭn-sûrt′): to put or thrust in; to set, so as to be within.
insertion (ĭn-sûr′shûn): act of inserting; that which is set in; portion of muscle at more movable attachment.
inside (ĭn′sīd): an inner side or surface.
inside curve (ĭn′sīd kûrv): a concave (inward) curve cut in the hair.
inside movement (ĭn′sīd mo͞ov′mĕnt): pertaining to an indentation, a curve or movement keeping the hair close to the head.
insolation (ĭn-sô-lā′shûn): exposure to the rays of the sun; sunstroke.
insoluble (ĭn-sŏl′û-b'l): incapable of being dissolved or very difficult to dissolve.
inspiration (ĭn-spĭr-ā′shûn): the feeling or impulse leading to a creative idea; the act of inhaling.
inspire (ĭn-spīr′): to influence or motivate a person; to inhale.
instantaneous (ĭn-stên-tā′nē-ûs): done, occurring or acting immediately.
instant hair roller (ĭn′stênt hâr rō′lẽr): an electronically heated hair roller used to style the hair while it is dry.

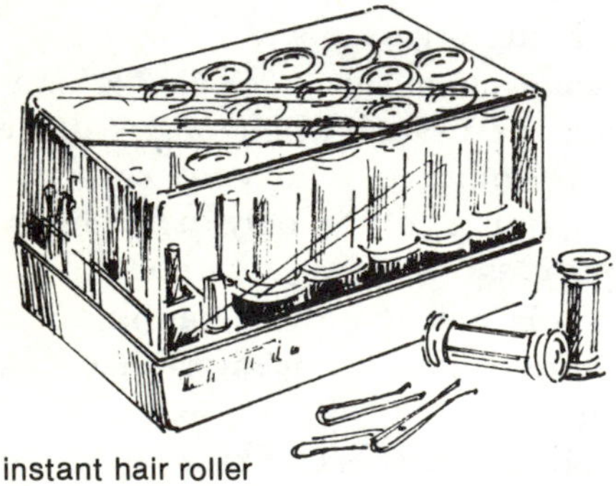
instant hair roller

instep (ĭn′stĕp): the dorsal part of the human foot on the medial side; the arched upper part of the foot.
instructor (ĭn-strŭk′tẽr): one who instructs; a teacher; a licensed cosmetologist with teaching credentials; a person with the required licenses and experience to teach a subject or subjects.
instrument (ĭn′stro͞o-mênt): device or tool for performing cosmetology work.
insulate (ĭn′sû-lāt): to separate by nonconductors to prevent transfer of electricity or heat.
insulation (ĭn′sû-lā′shûn): nonconducting substance.
insulator (ĭn′sû-lā-tẽr): a nonconducting material or substance used to cover electric wires.
insulin (ĭn′-sû-lĭn): a hormone secreted by the pancreas that regulates carbohydrate and fat metabolism.
insurance (ĭn-sho͝or′êns): protection against loss or injury.
insure (ĭn-sho͝or′): to make sure or secure.
integument (ĭn-tĕg′û-mênt): a covering, especially the skin.
integumentary system (ĭn-tĕg′û-mên′tär-ē): pertaining to the skin and its functions.
intensify (ĭn-tĕn′sĭ-fī): to increase; to make stronger or more intense.
intensity (ĭn-tĕn′sĭ-tē): the amount of force per unit area, as of heat, light or current; the quality of being intense.
inter-(ĭn′tẽr): a prefix denoting amid; between; among.
intercellular (ĭn-tẽr-sĕl′û-lẽr): between or among cells.
intercostal (ĭn-tẽr-kŏs′tâl): between the ribs.
intercostal muscles (ĭn-tẽr-kŏs′tâl mŭs'ls): muscles lying between adjacent ribs.
intercostal nerves (ĭn-tẽr-kŏs′tâl nûrvz): the branches of the thoracic nerves in the intercostal spaces (spaces between the ribs).

interior (ĭn-tĭr′ē-ẽr): inner or internal part of anything; situated within; occurring or functioning on the inside.

interlace (ĭn-tẽr-lās′): to weave strands of hair.

interlocking (ĭn′tẽr-lŏk′ĭng): a type of back combing which does not pack or mat the hair at the scalp; this technique causes the strands of hair to cling to each other and gives better control.

intermediate (ĭn-tẽr-mē′dē-ât): between two extremes; being or occurring at the middle place or degree.

intermediate supraclavicular nerve (ĭn-tẽr-mē′dē-ât so͞o′pră-klă-vĭk′yo͞o-lẽr nûrv): nerve that receives stimuli from the skin of the anterior part of the neck and chest wall.

intermittent heat (ĭn-tẽr-mĭt′ênt hēt): interrupted heating period; electric current turned on and off during a steaming procedure.

intermuscular (ĭn-tẽr-mŭs′kū-lẽr): situated between the muscles.

internal (ĭn-tûr′nâl): pertaining to the inside; inner part.

internal absorption (ĭn-tẽr′nâl ăb-sôrp′-shûn): the normal digestive assimilation of foods and liquids.

internal carotid artery (ĭn-tẽr′nâl kă-rŏt′ĭd är′tĭr-ē): the artery that distributes blood to the cerebrum, the eye, the forehead, nose and internal ear.

internal carotid nerve (ĭn-tẽr′nâl kă-rŏt′ĭd nûrv): a sympathetic nerve serving the internal carotid artery and its branches.

internal jugular vein (ĭn-tẽr′nâl jŭg′yo͞o-lăr vān): the vein located at the side of the neck to collect blood from the brain and parts of the face and neck; see jugular vein.

internal respiration (ĭn-tẽr′nâl rĕs-pĭ-rā′shûn): an exchange of gases between the blood and the capillaries and tissues of the body.

international color ring (ĭn-tẽr-nă′shûn-âl kŭl′ẽr rĭng): also called J and L color ring; a ring of color samples used to match hair colors, originated by Jacques Leclebort and accepted by the industry as standardization of colors for manufacturers of hair goods.

international unit (I.U.) (ĭn′tẽr-năsh′ŭn-âl ū′nĭt): the amount of a substance, such as a vitamin or antibiotic that produces a biological effect and has had established an accepted measure of the activity or potency of the substance.

interosseous (ĭn-tẽr-ŏs′ê-ûs): lying between or connecting bones.

interosseous artery, anterior (ĭn-tẽr-ŏs′ê-ûs är′tĭr-ē, ăn-tĭr′ē-ẽr): artery that supplies blood to the muscles of the deep anterior part of the forearm.

interosseous artery, posterior (ĭn-tẽr-ŏs′ê-ûs är′tĭr-ē, pŏs-tĭr′ē-ẽr): artery that supplies blood to the posterior forearm.

interosseous membrane of the forearm (ĭn-tẽr-ŏs′ê-ûs mĕm′brān): pertaining to the strong, fibrous membrane between the radius and the ulna; forearm.

interosseous membrane of the leg (ĭn-tẽr-ŏs′ê-ûs mĕm′brān): the strong, fibrous sheet between the margins of the tibia and the fibula.

interosseous nerve (ĭn-tẽr-ŏs′ê-ûs nûrv): a somatic, sensory nerve distributed in the ankle joint.

interparietal (ĭn-tẽr-pă-rī′ĕ-tâl): between walls; between parietal bones.

interpenetrate (ĭn-tẽr-pĕn′ă-trāt): to pervade; permeate; penetrate thoroughly.

interpose (ĭn-tẽr-pōz′): to place or put between the parts.

interstice (ĭn-tĕr′stĭs): a narrow opening between adjoining parts.

intertwist (ĭn-tĕr-twĭst′): to join strands by twining or twisting together.

intervascular (ĭn-tĕr-văs′kyo͞o-lăr): situated between vessels.

interweave (ĭn-tĕr-wēv′): to blend small strands of hair into a pattern.

intestinal (ĭn-tĕs′tĭn-âl): pertaining to the intestines.

intestine (ĭn-tĕs′tĭn): the digestive tube from the stomach to the anus.

intra- (ĭn′tră-): a prefix meaning inside of; within.

intraarterial (ĭn′tră-är-tĭr′ē-âl): within or directly into an artery.

intraarticular (ĭn-tră-är-tĭk′yo͞o-lăr): within a joint.

intracardiac (ĭn′tră-kär′dē-ăk): occurring within or situated in the heart.

intracellular (ĭn-tră-sĕl′ū-lăr): occurring or within a cell or cells.

intracorneal (ĭn-tră-kor′nē-âl): within the horny layer of the skin; also, within the cornea of the eye.

intracranial (ĭn-tră-krā′nē-âl): occurring within the cranium.

intracuticular (ĭn′tră-kyo͞o-tĭk′ū-lăr): within the epidermis.

intradermal (ĭn-tră-dûr′mâl): within the dermis.

intradermal nevus (ĭn-tră-dûr′mâl nē′-vûs): a skin lesion containing melanocytes located in the dermis.

intraepidermal (ĭn-tră-ĕp-ĭ-dûr′mâl): within the epidermis.

intramuscular (ĭn′tră-mŭs′kyo͞o-lăr): affecting the inside of the muscle.

intraneural (ĭn-tră-nyo͞o′râl): within a nerve.

intumesce (ĭn′tyo͞o-mēs′): to swell, expand or enlarge.

invasion (ĭn-vā′zhûn): the process in which bacteria or other microorganisms enter the body.

inventory (ĭn′vĕn-tôr-ē): a list of stock items; an accounting of products on hand; a record of supplies used and to be reordered.

inversion (ĭn-vûr′shûn): the act of turning inward.

inverted triangle (ĭn-vûr′tĕd trī′ăng'l): a face shape having a narrow chin, broad cheeks and broad forehead.

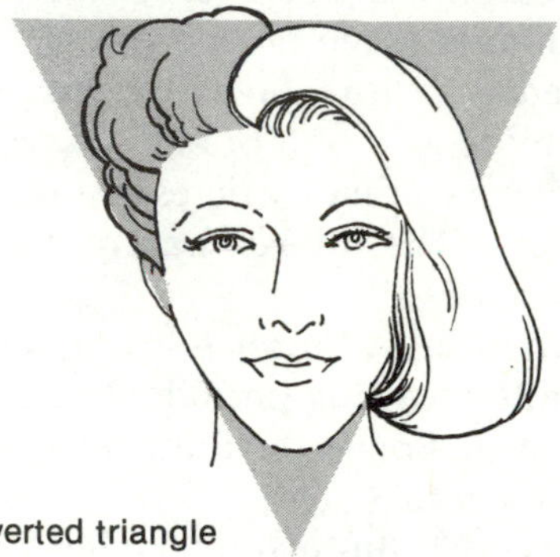

inverted triangle

inverter (ĭn-vûr′tĕr): a device for converting direct current into alternating current.

invisible (ĭn-vĭz′ĭ-b'l): not capable of being seen.

invisible light (ĭn-vĭz′ĭ-b'l līt): light that cannot be seen with the naked eye, but can be felt; examples are infrared and ultraviolet light.

involuntary (ĭn-vŏl′ûn-tĭr′ē): functioning or acting independently of the will or conscious control.

involuntary muscle (ĭn-vŏl′ûn-tĭr′ē mŭs'l): a muscle that functions automatically without the action of the will.

involute (ĭn′vô-lyo͞ot): in hairdressing, having ends rolling upward; curving; spiraling.

inward (ĭn′wărd): toward the inside.

iodine tincture (ī′ô-dīn tĭnk′chûr): a solution of iodine and sodium iodide in diluted alcohol; used as a local antiinfective.

iododerma (ī-ō-dô-dûr′mă): a skin condition caused by the injection of iodine compounds.

iodoform (ī-ō′dô-fôrm): a yellow crystalline compound formed by the action of iodine on alcohol and potash, used as an antiseptic for wounds and sores.

ion (ī′ŏn): an atom or group of atoms carrying an electric charge; when negatively charged, called "anions"; when positively charged, called "cations."

ionic bond (ī-on′ĭk bŏnd): the chemical bond between charged atoms or ions.

ionization (ī-ŏn-ĭ-zā′shûn): the separating of a substance into ions.

ionto mask (ī-ŏn′tō măsk): a mask of spongy material which covers the face, and is used with a galvanic machine during the process of the ionization or disincrustation facial treatment.

iontophoresis (ī-ŏn′tō-fôr-ē′sĭs): the process of introducing water soluble products into the skin with the use of electric current, such as the use of the positive and negative poles of a galvanic machine.

ionto rollers (ī-ŏn′tō rōl′ĕrz): metal rollers attached to a galvanic machine used to aid the penetration of creams or lotions into the skin during a facial treatment.

iridescence (ĭr-ĭ-dĕs′êns): the quality of being iridescent; a varied play of colors creating a sheen as in a soap bubble or mother of pearl.

iris (ī′rĭs): the colored muscular disk-like diaphragm of the eye which regulates the size of the pupil.

iron (ī′ûrn): a metallic element with the symbol Fe, required in the human diet; recommended amount is approximately 10 milligrams daily.

iron heater (ī′ûrn hē′tĕr): a small, compact electric heater used to heat thermal curling irons.

iron holder (ī′ûrn hōl′dĕr): an apparatus designed to hold a thermal curling iron.

irons (ī′ûrnz): heated implements designed to wave or curl the hair while it is dry.

I-J

irregular (ĭ-rĕg′û-lăr): lacking symmetry; unevenly shaped or arranged.

irreparable (ĭ-rĕp′ă-ră-b'l): damaged beyond repair.

irreversible (ĭr-ê-vĕr′sĭ-b'l): not capable of being reversed.

irrigate (ĭr′ĭ-gāt): to flush with water; to spray; to refresh with water.

irritability (ĭr-ĭ-tă-bĭl′ĭ-tē): the quality or state of being readily excited or stimulated to annoyance.

irritant (ĭr′ĭ-tênt): something that irritates, excites or stimulates.

irritate (ĭr′ĭ-tāt): to make inflamed or sore.

irritation (ĭr-ĭ-tā′shûn): the reaction of tissues or nerves to overstimulation.

isochromatic (ī′sō-krō-măt′ĭk): having the same color throughout; matched in color.

isometric (ī-sō-mĕ′trĭk): having equal measurements in several dimensions.

isometric exercise (ī-sō-mĕ′trĭk ĕks′ĕr-sīz): an exercise for the muscles in which contractions are counteracted by equal force exerted by the opposing muscles.

isopropyl alcohol (ī-sō-prō′pĭl ăl′kô-hôl): a homologue of ethyl alcohol; used as a solvent and rubefacient.

isopropylamine (ī-sō-prō′pĭl-lă′mĭn): a substance produced from acetone; an emulsifier used in many hair grooming creams and lotions.

isothermal (ī-sō-thûr′mâl): of equal temperature; without change in temperature.

itch (ĭch): an irritating sensation on the skin causing a desire to rub or scratch the affected area; any of various skin conditions such as scabies.

ithylordosis (ith-ĭ-lôr-dō′sĭs): lordosis unaccompanied by lateral curvature of the spine.

itis (ī′tĭs): suffix meaning inflammation of a specific part; e.g., arthritis, dermatitis, inflammation of the skin or joint; such terms are often preceded by the word infectious, as in infectious dermatitis.

ive (ĭv): a word termination signifying relating or belonging to, such as active.

ivory (ī′vă-rē): the smooth, yellowish white dentine substance of tusks; the creamy, white color of ivory; a light skintone resembling ivory.

ize (īz): a word termination forming transitive verbs, such as sterilize.

J

jack (jăk): in electricity a plug in device used to make electrical contact.

jagged (jăg′ĭd): having rough, uneven edges.

jasmine (jăs′mĭn): a fragrant flowering plant of the olive family used in fragrances.

jaundice (jôn′dĭs): yellowness of the skin, tissues and body fluids caused by deposits of bile pigments.

jaw (jô): either of two bony structures forming the framework of the mouth, the upper jaw (maxilla) and the lower jaw (mandible).

jawbone (jô′bōn): one of the bones forming the jaw, particularly the bone of the lower jaw of humans or animals.

jet (jĕt): a sudden spurt or gush of liquid or gas emitted from a narrow orifice, such as a shower head or shampoo bowl attachment.

jet black (jĕt blăk): deep black resembling hard, black jet stone or marble.

joint (joynt): a connection between two or more bones.

joint movement (joynt mo͞ov′mênt): the manipulating of a joint during massage.

jojoba (hŏ-hō′bă): an evergreen shrub which produces a bean from which oil is extracted for use in some cosmetic products.

jowl (jaŭl): the fleshy part of the lower jaw; a double chin.

jugal (jo͞o′gâl): pertaining to the cheek.

jugular (jo͞og′û-lâr, jŭg′û-lâr): pertaining to the neck or throat or the large veins in the neck.

jugular bulb (jo͞og′û-lâr bŭlb): superior bulb of the internal jugular vein.

jugular fossa (jo͞og′û-lâr fŏs′ă): the depression or cavity between the carotid canal and the stylomastoid opening containing the superior bulb of the internal jugular vein.

jugular nerves (jo͞og′û-lâr nûrvz): pertaining to nerves in the jugular area.

jugular trunk (jo͞og′û-lâr trŭnk): one of two connecting lymph trunks on the right and left sides of the head and neck; the right drains into the right lympathic duct; the left drains into the thoracic duct.

jugular vein (jo͞og′û-lâr vān): one of the largest veins on either side of the neck that returns blood from the brain, neck and parts of the face back to the heart.

jugular vein, anterior (jo͞og′û-lâr vān, ăn-tĭr′ē-ẽr): vein located in the middle of the neck that drains the anterior part of the neck.

jugular vein, external (jo͞og′û-lâr vān, ĕx-tûr′nâl): vein located parallel to arteries on the sides of the neck that returns blood to the heart from the face, head and neck.

jugular vein, internal (jo͞og′û-lâr vān, ĭn-tûr′nâl): vein that returns blood to the heart from the brain, face and neck.

jugular vein, posterior (jo͞og′û-lâr vān, pŏs-tĭr′ē-ẽr): vein situated in the occipital region and serves the skin and muscles in the upper back area of the neck.

junction nevus (jŭnk′shûn nē′vûs): a benign skin lesion containing nerve cells and located at the junction of the epidermis and dermis.

I-J

K

kaleidoscope (kă-lī′dô-skōp): a tube shaped object used to show constantly changing colors and patterns; used to study color.

kaolin, kaoline (kā′ô-lĭn): fuller's earth; porcelain clay; used in some cosmetics, but chiefly in facial packs; mud pack.

karaya gum (kă-ră′yă gŭm): Indian gum; a gum obtained in India and Africa from the trees of the genus Sterculia; used to make mucilages and wave set preparations.

keloid (kē′loyd): a thick scar resulting from excessive growth of fibrous tissue.

keloid acne (kē′loyd ăk′nē): a follicular infection with pustules which causes keloidal scarring; frequently affects black skin.

keratic (kĕ-răt′ĭk): pertaining to the cornea of the eye.

keratin (kĕr′ă-tĭn): a fiber protein characteristic of horny tissues: hair, nails, feathers, etc.; it is insoluble in protein solvents and has a high sulfur content; the principal constituent of hair and nails.

keratinization (kĕr′ă-tĭn-ī-zā′shûn): the process of being keratinized; development of a horny quality in a tissue.

keratitis (kĕr-ă-tī′tĭs): inflammation of the cornea of the eye.

keratoacanthoma (kĕr-ă-tō-ăk′ăn-thō′-mă): a skin nodule which usually occurs on hairy parts of the body and resembles squamous cell cancer of the skin.

keratoderma (kĕr-â-tô-dûr′mă): a horny condition of the skin, especially of the palms of the hands and soles of the feet.

keratoid (kĕr′ă-toyd): hornlike; horny tissue.

keratolytic (kĕr-ă-tô-lĭt′ĭk): an agent that causes exfoliation of the epidermis, as in skin peeling processes.

keratoma (kĕr-ă-tō′mă): a callosity; a horny tumor; an acquired thickened patch of the epidermis.

keratonosis (kĕr′ă-tō′no′sis): an anomaly in the horny structure of the epidermis.

keratoprotein (kĕr′â-tō-prō′tē ĭn): the protein of the horny tissues of the body which make up such structures as the hair, nails and epidermis.

keratosa, acne (kĕr-ă-tō′să ăk′nē): a rare form of acne consisting of horny plugs projecting from the hair follicles, accompanied by inflammation, usually at the angles of the mouth.

keratosis (kĕr-ă-tō′sĭs): any disease of the epidermis that is marked by the presence of circumscribed overgrowths of the horny layer.

ketone body (kē′tōn bod′ē): one of three related substances (acetone, methyl, ethyl).

ketones (kē′tōnz): acetone, methyl or ethyl; substances obtained by the oxidation of secondary alcohols; used as solvents in nail polish and polish removers.

khaki (kă′kē): a color between medium brown and tan.

kidney (kĭd′nē): one of a pair of glandular organs which excretes urine.

kil (kĭl): a clay from the Black Sea region widely used as an ointment in the treatment of skin diseases.

kilo (kē′lō): a prefix meaning thousand.

kilocalorie (kē′lō-kăl′ŏ-rē): the quantity of heat required to raise the temperature of one kilogram of water one degree centigrade.

kimono (kĭ-mō′nō): a loose, Japanese style robe or gown; used in salons to protect the client's clothing.

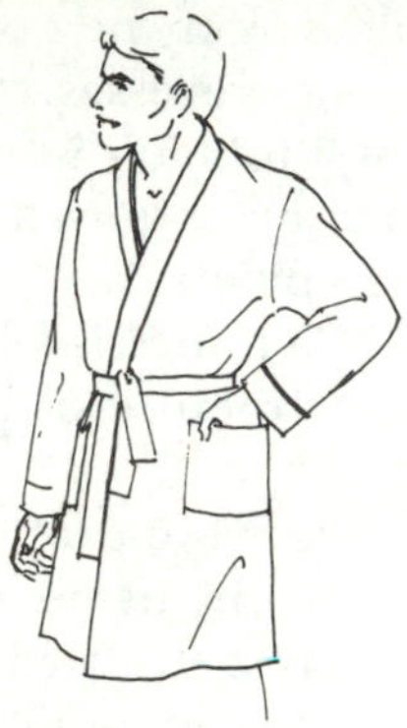

kimono

kinesics (kĭ-nē′sĭks): the study of body movements.

kinetics (kĭ-nĕt′ĭks): the branch of physics dealing with the effect of forces on the motion of physical objects or with changes on physical or chemical systems.

kinky (kĭnk′ē): very curly or closely twisted.

kit (kĭt): in cosmetology, a case containing the implements the cosmetologist needs to perform services.

kit

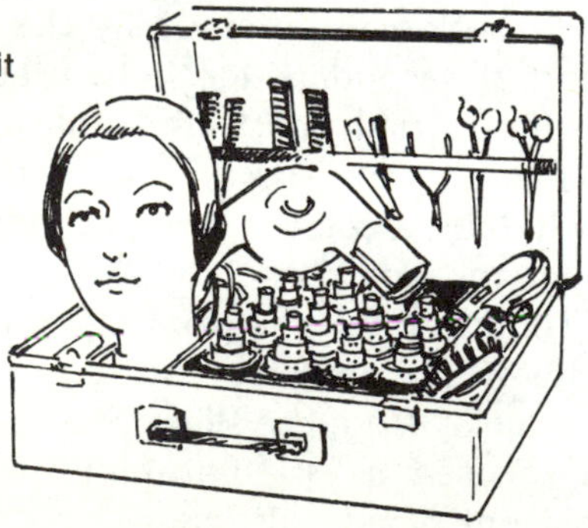

knead (nēd): to work and press with the hands as in massage.

knee (nē): the joint of the human leg that articulates the tibia, fibula and patella (knee cap).

knit (nĭt): to cause to draw together, as in the healing of bone.

knot (nŏt): to intertwine and loop strands of hair, fabric, rope, etc., to form a flat or oval mass.

knotted hair (nŏt′ĭd hâr): hair that has tangled, snarled lumps; see trichonodrosis.

knotting (ventilating) (nŏt′ĭng): the process by which hair is attached to the foundation in the creation of a wig or hairpiece; the actual knotting is also referred to as ventilating; there are two types of knotting generally used, single and double.

knotting gauze (nŏt′ĭng gôz): a very light type of silk net which has not been stiffened; it is used for men's hairpieces and for knotted partings.

knotting hook holder (nŏt′ĭng ho͝ok hōld′ĕr): a steel, pencil-shaped holder with an adjustable top, used to hold the knotting or parting hooks used in wig making.

knuckle (nŭk′′l): one of the joints of the fingers; the joints connecting the fingers to the hands.

knuckling (nŭk′lĭng): a massage movement made by using the knuckles of the four fingers of the hand to lightly tap the skin.

kohl (kōl): a preparation used to darken the edges of the eyelids.

koilonychia (koy-lō-nĭk′ē-ă): a dystrophy of the fingernails associated with nutritional deficiencies, such as of iron and calcium; the nails become thin and concave in shape; also called "spoon nails."

K-L

kosmetikos (kŏz-mĕt′ĭ-kōs): a Greek word meaning skilled in use of cosmetics and from which the word cosmetology is derived.

kyphoscoliosis (kī′fō-skō-lē-ō′sĭs): backward and lateral curvature of the spinal column.

kyphosis (kī-fō′sĭs): backward curvature of the spine; humpback.

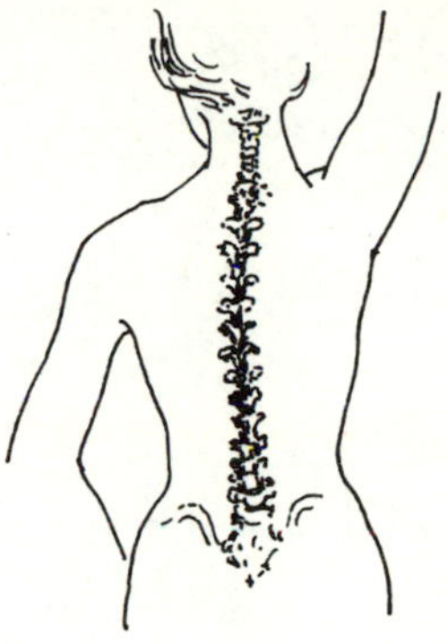
kyphosis

L

labdanum (lăb′dă-nŭm): a resin derived from the rockrose plant; used in some medicines, cosmetics and perfumery.

labia (lā′bē-ă); pl., **labium** (-ûm): pertaining to the lips.

labial artery, inferior (lā′bē-âl är′tĭr-ē, ĭn-fĭr′ē-ẽr): artery that supplies blood to the lower lip.

labial artery, superior (lā′bē-âl är′tĭr-ē, so͞o-pĭr′ē-ẽr): artery that supplies blood to the upper lip, septum and wing of the nose.

labial nerve, inferior (lā′bē-âl nûrv, ĭn-fĭr′ē-ẽr): nerve that distributes stimuli to the lower lip.

labial nerve, superior (lā′bē-âl nûrv, so͞o-pĕr′ē-ẽr): nerve that distributes stimuli to the skin of the upper lip.

labium (lā′bē-ûm); pl., **labia** (-ă): lip; a fleshy border or edge.

laboratory (lăb′ô-ră-tô-rē): a room containing apparatus for conducting experiments.

lac (lăk): milk or a milk-like substance.

lace (lās): a very fine flesh-colored mesh which is used to blend hairlines where they meet the skin; this type of lace, which is used primarily in men's hairpieces, gives a natural effect to the hairline.

lacerate (lăs′ẽr-āt): to tear the skin or tissue.

laceration (lăs-ẽr-ā′shûn): a tear of the skin or tissue.

lacing (lās′ĭng): a delicate, even backcombing along an entire strand of hair, giving the hair a lacy quality.

lacing, French (lās′ĭng, Frĕnch): a style of braiding; see French braid.

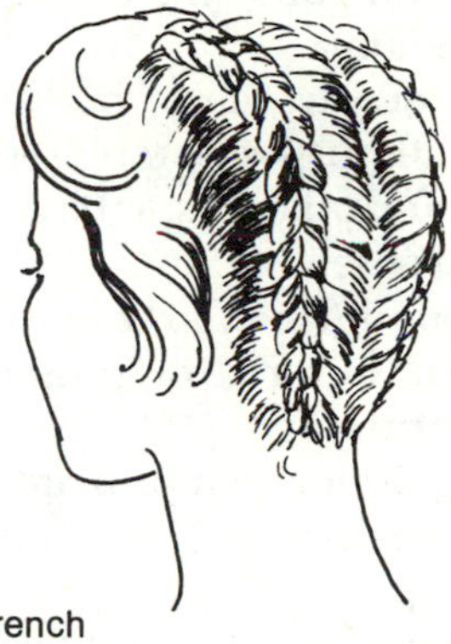

lacing, French

lacquer (lă′kẽr): a liquid cosmetic used on the hair or nails.

lacrimal (lăk′rĭ-mâl): pertaining to tears or weeping and the organs that secrete tears.

lacrimal artery (lăk′rĭ-mâl är′tĭr′ē): artery supplying blood to the eye and eyelid area.

lacrimal bone (lăk′rĭ-mâl bōn): small, thin bone resembling a fingernail; located in the anterior medial wall of the orbits (eye sockets).

lacrimal duct (lăk′rĭ-mâl dŭkt): either of the two tear ducts of the eyes.

lacrimal glands (lăk′rĭ-mâl glăndz): glands situated in the orbit of the eye in the depression of the frontal bone that secrete tears.

lacrimal nerves (lăk′rĭ-mâl nûrvz): nerves distributed in the area of the upper eye and eyelid and affecting the tear glands.

lacteals (lăk′tê-âlz): any one of the lymphatics of the intestines that take up chyle.

lactic acid (lăk′tĭk ăs′ĭd): a clear, syrupy

K-L

organic acid; used in skin freshening lotions.

lamina (lăm′ĭ-nă): a thin layer or scale.

lamp dry (lămp drī): to style the hair and dry it at the same time under an infrared heat lamp.

lamp, hot quartz (lămp, hŏt kwärtz): a general all purpose lamp used for skin tanning and other cosmetic and germicidal purposes.

lamp, infrared (lămp, ĭn′fră-rĕd): a lamp producing infrared rays; used in skin care treatments.

lamp, magnifying (lămp, măg′nĭ-fī′ĭng): a lamp used to analyze the skin or scalp.

K-L

lamp, ultraviolet (lămp, ŭl′tră-vī′ō-lĕt): pertaining to the three types of lamps used in cosmetology practice: glass bulb, hot quartz and cold quartz.

lamp, Wood's (lămp, wo͝odz): a lamp developed by Robert W. Wood, an American physicist, to help diagnose skin and scalp conditions.

lancet (lăn′cĕt): a small, sharp pointed instrument; used by dermatologists to pierce a papule.

lank (lănk): in cosmetology, describes hair that is long, lifeless; not curly.

lanolin (lăn′ô-lĭn): purified wool fat; used in some cosmetic preparations.

lanosterol (lăn-ô-stĭr′ôl): the fatty alcohol derived from lanolin (oil from sheep wool); used as a softening agent in hand creams and lotions.

lanthionine (lăn-thē′ô-nīn): a nonessential form of amino acid; bonding structure in the cortex resulting from processing with sodium hydroxide relaxer.

lanugo (lă-nū′gō): the fine hair which covers most of the body.

large intestine (lärj ĭn-tĕs′tĭn): the distal portion of the intestine which extends from the ileum to the anus, and consists of the cecum, colon and rectum.

larynx (lăr′ĭnks): the upper part of the trachea or windpipe; the organ of voice production.

laser (lāy′zer): an instrument that emits radiation as a beam of great power; used in surgical procedures and in research.

lash (lăsh): the short, fine hair of the upper and lower eyelids.

lateral (lăt′ĕr-âl): on or to the side.

lateral cutaneous nerve (lăt′ĕr-âl kyo͞otā′nē-ûs nûrv): nerve that receives stimuli from the skin of the lateral side of the forearm.

lateral nasal cartilage (lăt′ĕr-âl nāz′âl kär′tĭ-lĭj): the upper lateral cartilage of the nose.

lateral palpebral artery (lăt′ĕr-âl pâl′pă-brâl är′tĭr-ē): artery which supplies blood to the eyelids and surrounding area.

lateral vibration (lăt′ĕr-âl vī-brā′shûn): a massage movement using the palms of the hands to press firmly on the muscles while moving them from side to side in a vibrating motion; primarily for shoulder and back massage.

lather (lăth′ĕr): froth made by mixing soap and water.

lathering machine (lăth′ĕr-ĭng mă-shēn′): a machine used to produce lather or foam from soap and water that is used for shaving the face.

latissimus dorsi (lȧ-tĭs′ĭ-mŭs dôr′sī): a broad, flat superficial muscle of the back.

lattice hair braid (lăt′ĭs hâr brād): a technique of crossing and interlacing strands of hair to resemble a lattice.

laurel (lär′ĕl): an evergreen tree or shrub of the genus laurus; including cinnamon, sassafras and bay; used in some cosmetic and medicinal preparations.

lauric acid (lôr′ĭk ăs′ĭd): a fatty acid derived from laural oil and coconut oil; used in the manufacture of some soaps and cosmetic products.

lauryl alcohol (lôr′ĭl ăl′kô-hŏl): an alcohol derived from laurel oil and used in detergent products.

lavender (lăv′ĕn-dẽr): a plant of the mint family producing pale violet flowers; the oils and dried flowers are used in perfumery.

layer (lā′ẽr): a single thickness, fold or stratum.

layer, skin

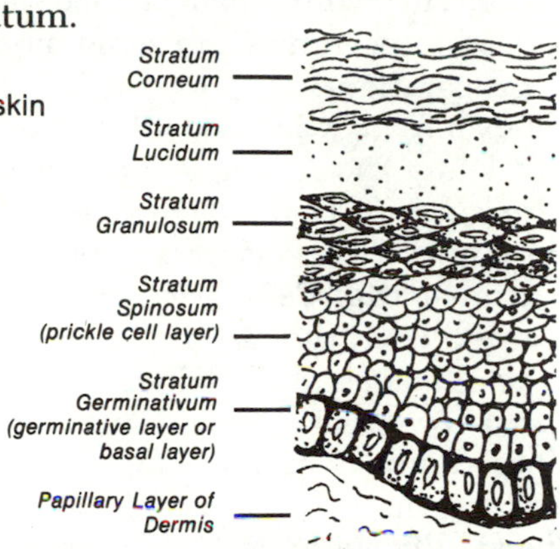

layer cutting (lā′ẽr kŭt′ĭng): cutting the hair into many thin layers by holding the hair at various angles from the head before cutting.

lecithin (lĕs′ĭ-thĭn): a colorless, crystalline compound soluble in alcohol; found in animal tissue and yolk of egg; used as an emulsifier, natural antioxidant and emollient in cosmetics.

lemongrass (lĕm′ôn-grăs): a tropical grass yielding a fragrant oil which is used in some cosmetic preparations.

lemon rinse (lĕm′ăn rĭns): a product containing lemon juice or citric acid; formerly used to eliminate soap curd from hair; used as a bleach to slightly lighten hair.

lentigines (lĕn-tĭdj′ĭ-nēz); pl., of **lentigo** (-tī′gō): the technical term for freckles.

lentigo (lĕn-tī′gō): a freckle; circumscribed spot or pigmentation in the skin.

lepid, lepido (lĕp′ĭd, lĕp ĭ-dō): a word part meaning pertaining to scaly skin conditions.

lesion (lē′zhûn): injury or damage which changes the structure of tissues or organs.

lesser multangular (lĕs′ẽr mŭl-tăn′gû-lâr): trapezoid; bone of the wrist.

lesser occipital (lĕs′ẽr ŏk-sĭp′ĭ-tâl): the nerve supplying muscles at the back of the ear.

lesson plan (lĕs′ôn plăn): a detailed set of directions in logical sequence, for teaching a subject or a skill.

leuc, leuk, leuco, leuko (lūk, lūk′ô): a combining form meaning white, colorless, weakly colored.

leucine (lo͞o′sēn): an essential amino acid produced by the breakdown of proteins.

leucocyte (lū′kō-sīt): white blood corpuscle, which performs the function of destroying disease causing germs.

leuconychia (lū-kô-nĭk′ē-ă): a whitish discoloration of nails; white spots.

leukoderma (lo͞o′kô-dûr′mă): a skin disorder characterized by light and dark areas, caused by a burn or disease which destroys the pigment producing cells.

leukotrichia (lū′kô-trĭk′ē-ă): whiteness of the hair; canities.

levator (lĕ-vā′tẽr): a muscle that elevates a part.

levator anguli oris (lĕ-vā′tẽr ăng′û-lī ŏr′ĭs): caninus; muscle that raises the angle of the mouth and draws it inward.

levator labii superioris (lĕ-vā′tẽr lā′bē-ī sû-pĭr-ē-ŏr′ĭs): quadratus labii superioris; muscle that elevates the upper lip and dilates the nostrils.

K-L

K-L

levator palpebrae (lĕ-vā′tĕr păl′pĕ-brē): muscle that raises the upper eyelid.
liability (lī′ă-bĭl′ĭ-tē): the state of being liable for one's products or services; the state of being obligated according to law; responsibility.
liability insurance (lī-ă-bĭl′ĭ-tē ĭn-shōōr′-ăns): the act or system of insuring against personal damage.
lice (līs): plural of louse; see pediculosis capitis.
license (līs′'ns): an official document granting permission to engage in a specified activity or to perform certain services.
lichen (lī′kĭn): a type of skin lesion with solid papules.
lichenification (lī-kĕn-ĭ-fĭ-kā′shŭn): the process by which the skin becomes hard and leathery.
lichenoid eczema (lĭk′ĕ-noyd ĕk′zĕ-mă): eczema characterized by papules on a reddened base, accompanied by a tingling and itching sensation.
lift (lĭft): a term used in hair coloring to indicate a lightening of the hair; to raise or cause to raise to a higher plane or position.
lift, face (lĭft, fās): a technique used by a surgeon to lift the skin of the face to create a more youthful appearance; see face lift and rhytidectomy.
lift, hair (lĭft, hâr): a fork-like comb employed in hair styling to raise the hair into a balanced position while combing.
ligament (lĭg′ă-mênt): a tough band of fibrous tissue, serving to connect bones, or to hold an organ in place.
light (līt): radiant energy that can be seen and felt; less than usual in weight, amount or force; not heavy.
lighten (līt′n): in hairstyling; to make the hair color lighter.
lightener (bleach): the chemical employed to remove color from the hair.
lightening retouch (līt′n-′ĭng rē′tŭch): the application of a lightening agent to the hair that has grown out since the first lightening application.
light therapy (līt thĕr′ă-pē): the application of light rays for treatment of disorders.
lilac (lī′lăk): the purple-pink flower used in perfumery; a purple-pink color.
lily of the valley (lĭl′ē of the vâl′ē): a perennial herb with oblong leaves and fragrant white, bell shaped flowers; used in perfumes and some medicinal preparations.
lime (līm): a white powder containing calcium dioxide; a small oval shaped green fruit of the citrus family.
limewater (līm-wôt′ĕr): a solution of calcium hydroxide that absorbs carbon dioxide from the air; used to neutralize acids and as an alkali in face masks and hair preparations.
limp (lĭmp): weak; lacking firmness or strength.
lineal albicantes (lĭn′ē-ă âl-bĭ-kăn′tēz): shiny white lines in the skin due to rupture of elastic fibers; often due to rapid weight loss or seen as stretchmarks following pregnancy.
linear (lĭn′ē-är): pertaining to or resembling a line or lines; straight.
line, linea (līn, lĭn′ē-ă): a thin, continuous mark used as a guide; a thin crease on the face or body.
linen (lĭn′ĕn): a fiber made from flax; used in pure form or combined with other textiles.
line of demarcation (līn ŏf dē-mär-kā′-shŭn): a visible line of separation; line separating colored hair from regrowth; line created where makeup is not blended evenly; line separating healthy from diseased tissue.
liniment (lĭn′ĭ-mênt): a medicated liquid

applied to the skin to relieve sore or inflamed conditions.

linoleic acid (lĭn-ô-lē′ĭk ăs′ĭd): an unsaturated fatty acid prepared from fats and oils; used as an emulsifier.

linseed (lĭn′sēd): the dried seeds of flax; contains a mucilage which is used as an emollient in some cosmetic preparations.

liodermia (lī′ō dûr′mē-ă): a condition of abnormal smoothness and glossiness of the skin.

liparotrichia (lĭp′ă-rō-trĭk′ē-ă): abnormal oiliness of the hair.

lip color (lĭp kŭl′ĕr): also called lipstick; a cosmetic in paste form, usually in a metal or plastic tube, manufactured in a variety of colors and used to color the lips.

lip color sealer (lĭp kŭl′er sēl′ĕr): a product resembling fingernail base coat; used to keep lip color from seeping into fine lines around the lips.

lipectomy (lī-pĕk′tô-mē): a surgical procedure to excise excessive fatty tissue.

lip gloss (lĭp glôs): a product formulated to add lubricating oil to the lips. Contains many of the same ingredients as lipsticks and is packaged in a small jar or lipstick tube.

lipid (lĭ′pĭd): any of a large class of organic substances insoluble in water, including fats, sterols and waxes.

lip liner (lĭp līn′ĕr): a colored pencil or brush used to outline the lips.

lipophilic (lĭp-ô-fĭl′ĭk): having an affinity or attraction to fat and oils.

liquefy (lĭk′wă-fī): to reduce to a liquid state, said of both solids and gases.

liquefying cream (lĭk′wă-fī′ĭng krēm): a cream that becomes liquid-like upon contact with the warmth of the skin.

liquid (lĭk′wĭd): a substance that flows and is capable of being poured, as water or oil.

liquid dry cleaner (lĭk′wĭd drī-klēn′ĕr): a product used to clean wigs and hairpieces.

liquid dry shampoo (lĭk′wĭd drī shăm-po͞o′): a dry cleansing fluid used to clean the hair without the use of shampoo and water.

liquid measure (lĭk′wĭd mĕzh′ĕr): a unit or system of units used to measure liquids.

liter (lē′tĕr): in the metric system, a measure of capacity equal to the volume of one kilogram of water at 4°C, or 1,056 liquid quarts.

litmus paper (lĭt′mûs pāp′ĕr): strips of paper containing coloring matter used in testing acidity or alkalinity of a product; red turns blue to indicate alkalinity and blue turns red to indicate acidity.

livedo (lĭ-vē′dō): a bluish, mottled discoloration of the skin.

liver (lĭv′ĕr): an internal organ which secretes bile for digestion.

liver spots (lĭv′ĕr spŏts): see choloasma.

lobe (lōb): a curved or rounded projection of a bodily organ or part; ear lobe.

localize (lō′kâl′īz): to confine to a specific area.

lock (lŏk): in hairstyling, a strand or ringlet of hair.

logarithm (lôg′ă-rĭth-ûm): the power to which a fixed number, the base, is raised in order to produce a given number; used as a measure of pH, indicating each change by one full digit equals a ten-fold change of acidity.

long face (lông fās): a face that is longer in proportion than an oval shape; a long oval or rectangular shaped face.

long stem roller (lông stĕm rōl′ĕr): in hairsetting, a roller that is placed completely off the base to create maximum movement and minimum volume.

loofah (lo͞o′fă): also luffa; a fibrous fruit of the gourd family; used as a sponge when bathing to stimulate circulation and to remove dead surface cells from the skin.

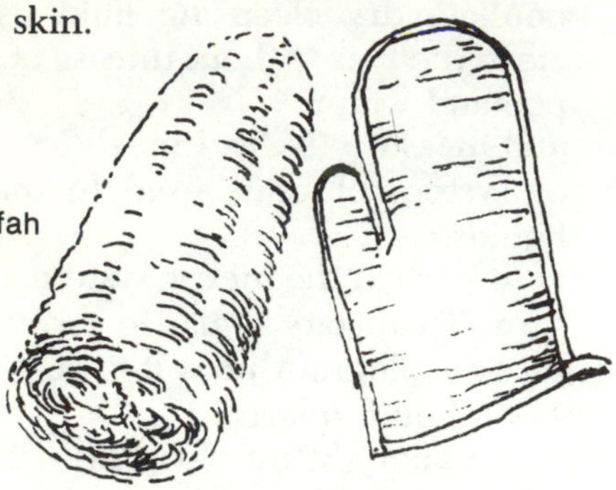
loofah

loose (lo͞os): free; not confined or restrained; not tight.

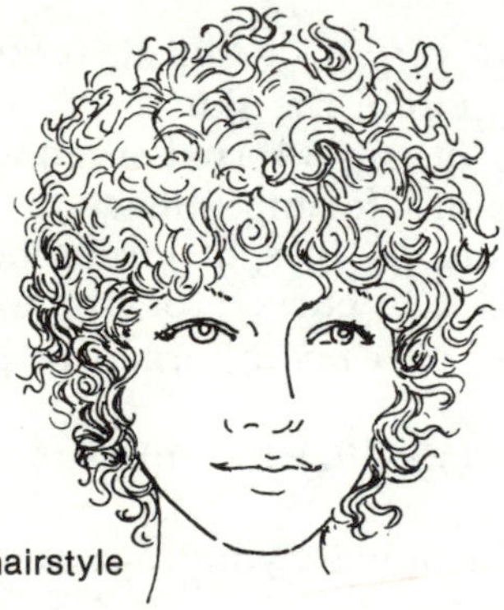
loose hairstyle

lordosis (lôr-dō′sĭs): a forward curvature of the lumbar spine; swayback.

lotion (lō′shûn): a liquid solution generally a cosmetic preparation for the hands, face and body.

louse (laůs); pl. **lice** (līs): an insect of the genus pediculus; an animal parasite infesting the hairs of the head.

low calorie (lō kăl′ô-rē): having a low caloric value; having fewer than usual number of calories.

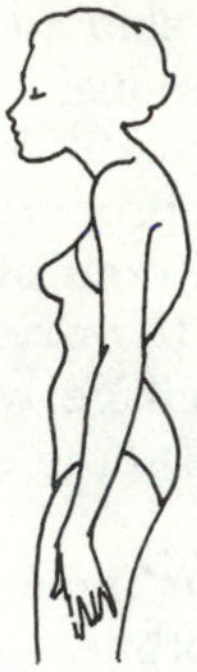
lordosis

low elevation (lō ĕl-ă-vā′shûn): hair cutting technique using slight layering.

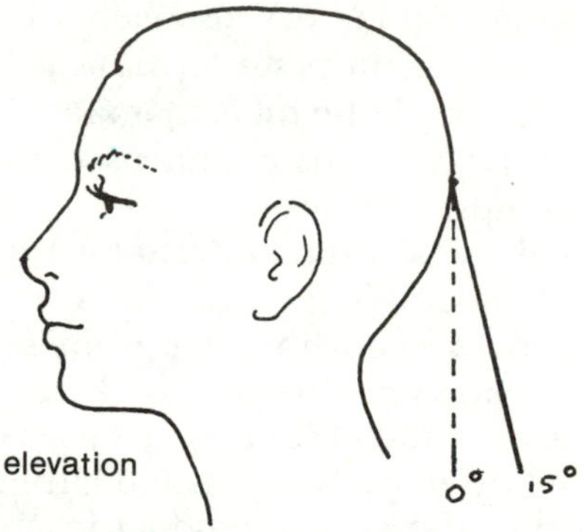

low elevation

low frequency (lō frē′kwĕn-sē): in electricity, pertaining to current characterized by a low rate of oscillation.

low lighting (lō′ līt′ĭng): the technique of coloring strands of hair darker than the natural color.

low molecular weight (lō mô-lĕk′û-lâr wāt): term used in cosmetology to indicate the ability of a substance to penetrate hair or skin tissue.

lubricant (lū′brĭ-kănt): an oily or slippery, smooth substance used to lubricate a part.

lucid (lū′sĭd): clear; transparent.

lucid layer (lū′sĭd lā′ĕr): the clear layer of the skin; the stratum lucidum; located below the stratum corneum and above the stratum granulosum.

lucidum (lū′sĭ-dŭm): the clear layer of the epidermis.

lukewarm (lo͝ok′wôrm): tepid; not hot; approximately body temperature: 98.6°F (Fahrenheit) or 37°C (Celsius).

lumbar region (lŭm′bär rē′jŭn): the area of the back lying lateral to the lumbar vertebrae.

lumbar vertebrae (lŭm′bär vûr′tĕ-brē): the bones which make up the vertebral column located in the lower part of the back; the five vertebrae associated with the lower part of the back.

luminous (lo͞o′mă-nûs): emitting or reflecting light; shiny.

lump (lŭmp): a small mass; a swelling or tumor.

lunate (lū′nāt): crescent-shaped.

lunate bone (lū′nāt bōn): semilunar; a bone of the wrist.

lung (lŭng): one of a pair of organs of respiration.

lunula (lū′nû-lă): the whitish, half-moon shape at the root of a fingernail.

lupus (lū′pŭs): any chronic and progressive ulcerative skin lesion.

lupus vulgaris (lū′pŭs vŭl-gâr′ĭs): tuberculosis of the skin.

luster (lŭs′tĕr): radiance; glossiness.

lye (lī): a solution of sodium or potassium hydroxide; a strong alkali substance used in making soap and other cleansing products.

lymph (lĭmf): a clear, yellowish fluid which circulates in the lymph spaces (lymphatics) of the body.

lymphagogue (lĭm′fŭ-gŏg): a substance that stimulates the flow of lymph.

lymphatic (lĭm-făt′ĭk): pertaining to, containing or conveying lymph.

lymphatic blockage (lĭm-făt′ĭk blŏk′ĭj): obstruction of lymphatic drainage.

lymphatic glands (lĭm-făt′ĭk glăndz): lymph nodes; the glands which produce white corpuscles and filter the lymph as it passes through them.

lymphatic system (lĭm-făt′ĭk sĭs′tĕm): consists of lymph flowing through the lymph spaces, lymph vessels, lacteals, and lymph nodes or glands.

lymph channels (lĭmf chăn′ĕlz): the lymph sinuses around lymphatic glands and vessels; a lymph channel that surrounds a nerve trunk.

lymph drainage massage (lĭmf drān′ĭg mă-säzh′): a method of massage which works upon lymph vessels and glands to eliminate watery stagnation of tissues (edemas) and to stimulate the flow of body fluids.

lymph node (lĭmf nōd): any of the gland-like bodies found in lymphatic vessels; also lymph glands.

lymphoderma (lĭm-fō-dûr′mē-ă): a disease of the lymphatics of the skin.

lysine (lī′sēn): an amino acid essential in nutrition to assure growth; used to improve protein content.

lysis (lī′sĭs): a combining form meaning to dissolve or loosen; the gradual disappearance of the symptoms of a disease, especially an infectious disease or fever.

M

macassor oil (mă-kăs′ẽr oyl): an oil obtained from Indonesia; used in some hairdressing preparations.

macerate (măs′ă-rāt): to reduce a solid to a soft mass by soaking in liquid.

maceration (măs-ă-rā′shûn): a process used in perfumery in which the petals and parts of flowers are plunged into hot oil, which absorbs essential oils, from which fragrances are made.

machineless (mă-shēn′lĕs): work performed without the use of machines; in cosmetology, pertaining to methods of permanent waving and facial treatments that require no machines.

machine made (mă-shēn′mād): a term used to indicate that a wig or hairpiece was made by machine and not by hand.

macro (măk′rō): large in size or duration.

macrofollicular (măk′rō-fŏl-ĭk′ū-lẽr): pertaining to or having large follicles.

macronychia (măk′rō-nĭk′ē-ă): excessive size of the nails.

macroscopic (măk-rō-skŏp′ĭk): visible to the naked eye.

macula (măk′ū-lă); pl., **maculae** (-lē): a spot or discoloration on the skin; a freckle; macule.

madarosis (măd-ă-rō′sĭs): loss of the eyelashes or eyebrows.

magenta (mă-jĕn′tă): the purplish-rose color produced from a fuchsin dye compound; fuchsia color.

magnesia (măg-nē′zē-ă): a skin freshener and an ingredient used in dusting powder; also used in some medicinal preparations such as laxatives and as an antacid.

magnesium carbonate (măg-nē′zē-ŭm kär′bô-nāt): perfume carrier and coloring material used in powders, shampoos and in some medicinal preparations.

magnesium sulfate (măg-nē′zē-ŭm sŭl′fāt): an ingredient used in medicinal preparations and in some shampoos formulated for oily hair.

magnetic (măg-nĕt′ĭk): pertaining to or having the properties of a magnet.

magnetic hair roller (măg-nĕt′ĭk hâr rō′lẽr): a plastic roller, either cylindrical or cone-shaped, used to shape and hold wet hair until it has been dried into the desired set.

magnetize (măg′nĕ-tīz): convert into a magnet; to communicate magnetic properties to.

magnify (măg′nĭ-fī): increase in fact or in appearance as by placement under a microscope; increase in size by use of a mirror or lens.

magnifying lamp (măg′nĭ-fī-ĭng lămp): an apparatus with a magnifying glass and source of light; used to examine the skin or scalp.

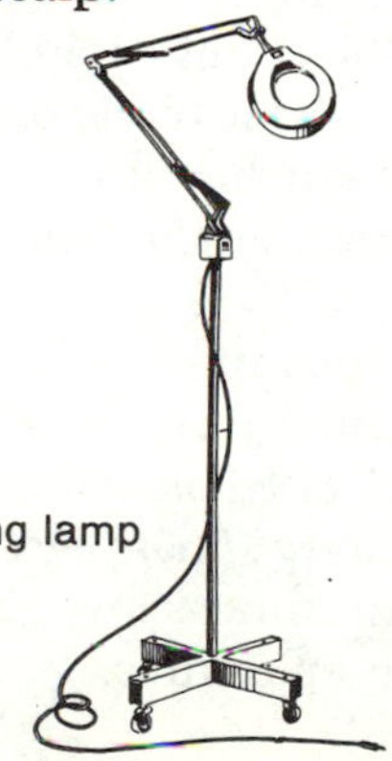

magnifying lamp

magnum (măg′nŭm): the largest bone in the distal row of the carpus, located at the center of the wrist.

mahogany (mă-hŏg′ă-nē): a reddish hard wood; a deep reddish-brown color.

maize (māz): in color, the deep shade of ripe yellow corn.

makeup (māk′ŭp): cosmetic products used to groom, color or beautify the face.

makeup base (māk′ŭp bās): a clear or colored cosmetic in liquid or cream form, applied to the face as a foundation before the application of powder, and cheek color.

makeup cape (māk′ŭp kāp): a garment made of cloth or plastic designed to be draped across the chest and shoulders of a client to protect clothing during a makeup application or other salon service.

M-N

malady (măl′ă-dē): a disease, illness or disturbed condition.

malar (mā′lăr): of or pertaining to the cheek; the cheekbone.

malformation (măl-fôr-mā′shûn): an abnormal or badly formed shape or structure, especially of the face or body.

malignant (mă-lĭg′nênt): a growth or condition endangering health; not benign.

malleable (mal′ê-ă-b'l): capable of being shaped or molded.

malleable block (măl′ê-ă-b'l blŏk): a head-shaped form, made of canvas and stuffed with sawdust, used for dressing-out and knotting the underside of a hairpiece.

malnutrition (măl-nû-trĭsh′ûn): poor nutrition resulting from inadequate consumption of nutrients.

malpighian layer (măl-pĭg′ē-ŭn lā′ẽr): the stratum mucosum; the deepest layer of the epidermis.

malpractice (măl-prăk′tĭs): in cosmetology, the negligent or improper treatment of a client while performing a service.

mandible (măn′dĭ-b'l): the lower jaw bone.

mandibular (măn-dĭb′û-lăr): pertaining to the lower jaw.

mandibular nerve (măn-dĭb′û-lăr nûrv): the fifth cranial nerve which supplies the muscles and skin of the lower part of the face.

manicure (măn′ĭ-kūr): the artful treatment and care of the hands and nails.

manicure bowl (măn′ĭ-kūr bōl): a vessel shaped to fit the hand and fingers; warm sudsy water is placed in the bowl and the fingers allowed to soak so that cuticles are softened before treatment.

manicure chair (măn′ĭ-kūr chấr): a chair designed to allow the manicurist to sit comfortably during the manicure service.

manicure implements (măn′ĭ-kūr ĭm′plê-mĕnts): the tools or equipment used for the manicuring procedure: nail file, cuticle pusher, cuticle scissor, cuticle nipper, emery board, buffer, etc.

manicure kit (măn′ĭ-kūr kĭt): a case or kit designed to carry the implements, equipment and supplies used for the manicure service.

manicure lamp (măn′ĭ-kūr lămp): a flexible light fixture attached to the manicure table to provide adequate light during the manicure.

manicure machine (măn′ĭ-kūr mă-shēn′): a small electrically powered machine designed to aid in giving a manicure; the machine has attachments for various implements.

manicure oil heater (măn′ĭ-kūr oyl hē′tẽr): a thermostatically controlled electric heating cup used to heat the oil or cream used on the hands and nails during the manicure service.

manicure supplies (măn′ĭ-kūr sŭ-plīz′): products and materials that are used for the manicure service: cotton, cosmetics, etc.

manicure table (măn′ĭ-kūr tā′b′l): a small table especially designed for the manicure service.

manicurist (măn′ĭ kūr-ĭst): one who professionally attends to the care of the hands and nails.

manikin: see mannequin.

manipulate (mă-nĭp′ū-lāt): to control; to handle skillfully.

manipulation (mă-nĭp-û-lā′shûn): act or process of treating, working or operating with the hands or by mechanical means, especially with skill.

mannequin; manikin (măn′ĭ kĭn): in cosmetology, a model of the human head manufactured with hair, to be used for practice work; in fashion, a model of a human figure used for display purposes.

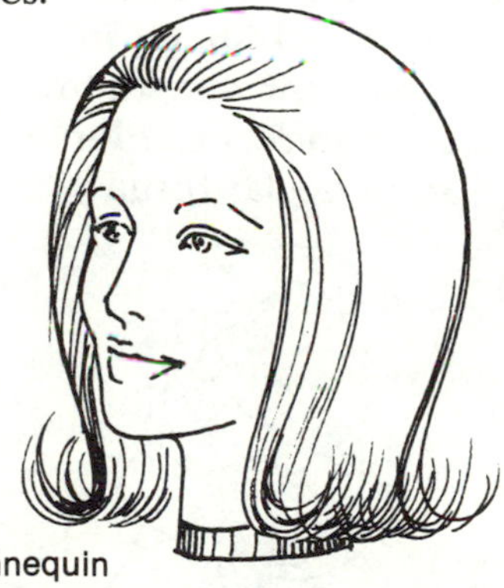

mannequin

mannequin case (măn′ĭ-kĭn kās): a box-like carrying case designed to hold the mannequin head and holder.

mannequin holder (măn′ĭ-kĭn hōl′dẽr): a clamp-like implement designed to be used to secure a mannequin head to a table top while it is in use.

mannequin slip-on (măn′ĭ-kĭn slĭp′ŏn): a glove-like mannequin form which can be slipped over another mannequin head to allow more varied practice routines.

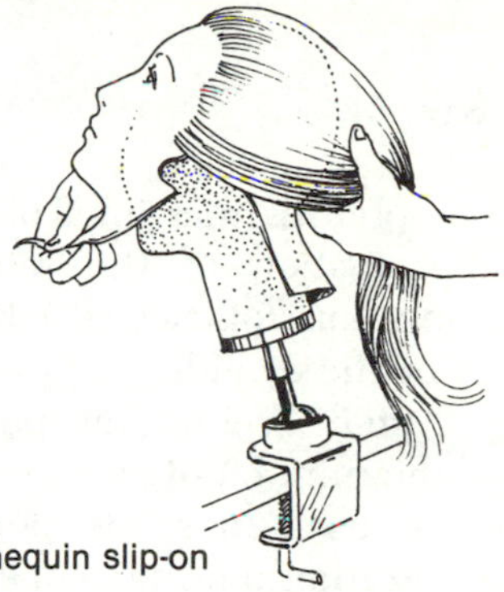

mannequin slip-on

M-N

mannitol (man′ă-tōl): a colorless, crystalline alcohol occurring in plants and animals; used as a humectant in creams and lotions.

mantle (măn′t′l): nail mantle, the fold of the skin into which the nail root is lodged.

manual (măn′ū-âl): done by hand or used by hand rather than by machines.

manus (mă′nûs); pl., **mani** (-nī): the hand.

marbleizing (mär′b′l-īz-ĭng): intertwining sections of light and dark shades of hair on one head.

marcel irons (mär-sĕl′ ī′ûrn): a curling (thermal) iron with a rod and groove attached to a handle that opens and closes; the iron is heated and strands of hair placed between the rod and groove to create curls or waves.

marcel wave (mär-sĕl′ wāv): a wave resembling a natural hair wave, produced by a thermal iron; originated by Francois Marcel, a French hairdresser.

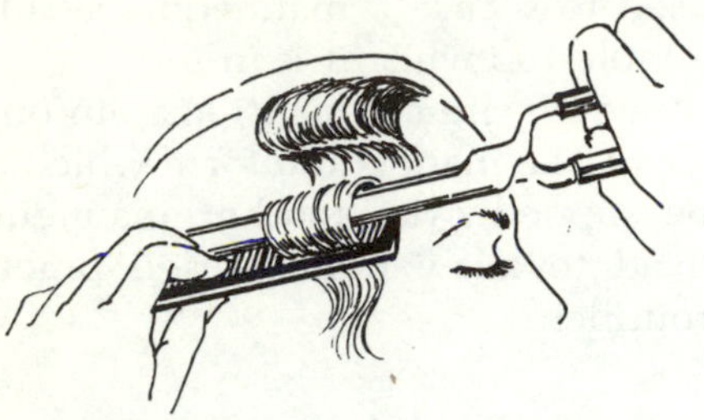

marcel wave

marginal blepharitis (mär′jĭn-âl blĕf-ă-rī′-tĭs): inflammation of the sebaceous glands and hair follicles that line the margins of the eyelids.

marjoram (mär′jĕr-ăm): a perennial plant of the mint family with aromatic properties; used in soaps, perfumes, hair preparations and in cooking.

M-N

maroon (mă-rōōn): a deep, dark red color.

marrow (măr′ō): a soft fatty substance filling the cavities of bone.

mascara (măs-kă′ră): a preparation used to darken the eyelashes.

mask; masque (măsk): to hide or conceal; to apply a substance to the face as part of a facial treatment; a special cosmetic formula applied to the face to benefit and beautify the skin.

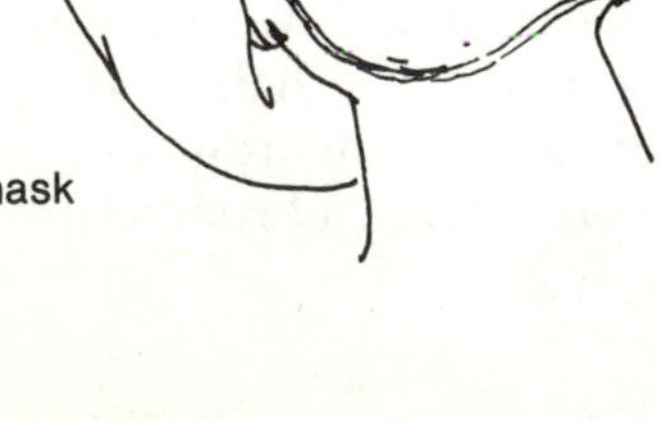

mask

masotherapy (măs′ō-thĕr′ă-pē): the treatment of the body by massage.

masque; mask (măsk): a preparation such as clay, paraffin wax, vegetables, fruits, gels or other beneficial substances, applied to the face as part of a facial treatment.

mass (măs): a quantity of matter in any given body, relatively large in size with no particular shape.

massage (mă-säzh′): manipulation of the body by rubbing, pinching, kneading, tapping, etc. to increase metabolism, promote absorption, relieve pain, etc.

massage compression (mă-säzh′ kŏm-prĕsh′ûn): pressure used in massage movements.

massage cream (mă-säzh′krēm): an emollient cream employed in skin treatment; designed to lubricate the skin; also referred to as tissue cream or nourishing cream.

massage equipment (mă-säzh′ ĭ-kwĭp′-mênt): implements used in massage manipulations.

massage movement direction (mă-säzh′ mōōv-mênt dī′rĕk′shûn): in massage, the direction of movement toward the origin of a muscle in order to avoid damage to muscular tissue.

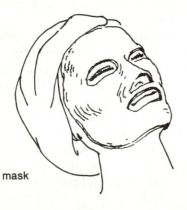

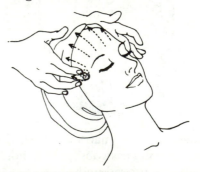

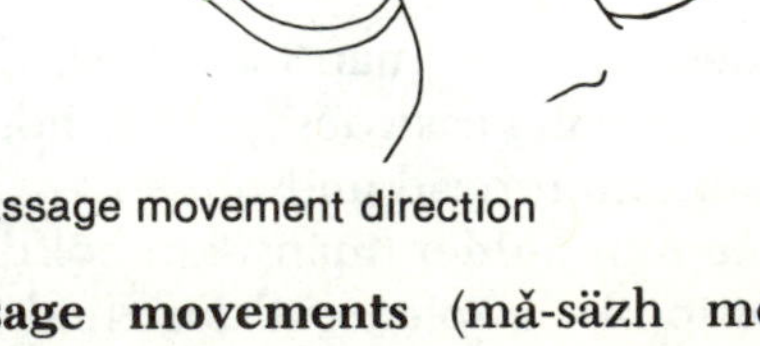

massage movement direction

massage movements (mă-säzh mōōv′-

mênts): specific movements used in facial and body massage; basic movements include: friction, joint, percussion, petrissage, stroking and vibration.

masseter (mă-sē′tĕr): one of the muscles of the jaw used in mastication.

masseteric artery (măs-ē-tĕr′ĭk är′tĭr-ē): the artery supplying blood to the muscles of the jaw (masseter).

masseteric nerve (măs-ē-tĕr′ĭk nûrv): a nerve in the face supplying the masseter muscle.

masseur (mă-sûr′); fem., **masseuse** (mă-sooz): man or woman who practices or gives massage.

masticate (măs′tĭkāt): to chew or to grind food with the teeth.

mastoid (măs′toyd): relating to the mastoid process; of or designating the projection of the temporal bone behind the ear.

mastoid process (măs′toyd prŏs′ĕs): a conical projection of the temporal bone.

materia medica (mă-tē′rē-ă mĕd′ĭ-kă): a compilation of drugs and substances used in medicine; the branch of medical science that deals with the sources, properties and preparation of drugs, and like substances.

matrix (mā′trĭks): the formative portion of a nail or a tooth; the intercellular substance of a tissue.

matte (măt): in makeup, a dull, nonshiny finish achieved by use of a special base or by applying face powder over foundation.

matter (măt′ĕr): a substance that occupies space and has weight.

matting (măt′ĭng): tangling the hair into a thick mass; another term for back combing.

maturation (măch′o͝o-rā′shûn): in skin care, the ripening or coming to a head of a pimple or other blemish.

mauve (mōv): a coal tar dye of a purple-rose shade; a moderate purple, violet or lilac color.

maxilla (măk-sĭl′ă): bone of the upper jaw.

maxillary (măk′sĭ-lĕr-ē): pertaining to the jaws.

maxillary artery (măk′sĭ-lĕr-ē är′tĭr-ē): artery that supplies blood to the lower regions of the face.

maxillary nerves (măk′sĭ-lĕr-ē nûrvz): the nerves of the upper part of the face.

mayonnaise (mā′ô-nāz′): a creamy salad dressing made of egg yolks, olive or other vegetable oils, lemon juice or vinegar; used as a hair conditioner.

M-N

measure (mĕzh′ĕr): a standard or unit of measurement, as a foot, yard, gallon, pound, ounce, etc.

mechanical (mĕ-kăn′ĭ-kâl): relating to a machine; performed by means of some apparatus; not manual.

mechanism (mĕk′ă-nĭz′m): mechanical construction; parts of a machine.

medial; median (mē′dē-ăl; -ûn): pertaining to the middle.

median nerve (mē′dē′ûn nûrv): the nerve located in the center of the arm that supplies blood to the arm and hand.

medicamentosus (mĕd-ĭ-kă-mĕn-tō′sûs): a skin eruption caused by a drug.

medicate (mĕd′ĭ-kāt): to treat a condition by use of drugs or other medications.

medicated ingredient (mĕd′ĭ-kāt′ĕd ĭn-grē′dē-ênt): a substance added to cosmetics to promote healing.

medicine (mĕd′ĭ-sĭn): a drug or other healing substance; the science of preventing, treating or curing diseases.

medium elevation (mē′dē-ûm ĕl-ĕ-vā′shûn): a term used in hairdressing to indicate that hair is held at approximately a 45 degree angle to the head while it is being cut.

medium hair (mē′dē-ûm hâr): a hair fiber neither especially large nor small in circumference, but of a thickness about halfway between fine and coarse.

medius (mē′dē-ûs): the middle finger.

medulla (mĕ-dŭl′ă): the pith of the hair; the marrow in the various bone cavities; soft inner portion of an organ.

medulla oblongata (mĕ-dŭl′ă ŏb-lŏn-gā′tă): the lowest or posterior part of the brain, continuous with the spinal cord.

medullary (mĕd′ū-lĕr-ē): pertaining to marrow or medulla.

medullary space (mĕd′ū-lĕr-ē spās): the cavity through the shaft of the long bones.

megalonychosis (mĕg′ă-lŏn-ĭ-kō′sĭs): noninflammatory hypertrophy of the nails.

melanin (mĕl′ă-nĭn): the dark pigment in the epidermis and hair, and in the choroid or coat of the eye.

melanism (mĕl′ă-nĭz′m): excessive pigmentation of the hair, skin, eyes, tissues or organs.

melanochroi (mĕl-ă-nŏk′rō-ē): a term used to describe very fair skin and very dark hair of Caucasians.

melanocyte (mĕ-lăn′ō-sīt): a melanin-forming cell.

melanocytic nevi (mĕl′ă-nō-sĭt′ĭk nē′vī): commonly called moles; brown spots sometimes having hair growing from them.

melanocytoma (mĕl′ă-nō-sī-tō′mă): a benign, heavily pigmented tumor.

melanoderma (mĕl′ă-nō-dûr′mă): abnormal darkening of the skin, usually in patches caused by accumulation or deposits of melanin.

melanodermatitis (mĕl′ă-nō-dûr-mă tī′-tĭs): an inflamed skin condition characterized by increased skin pigmentation.

melanogenesis (mĕl′ă-nō-jĕn′ĕ-sĭs): the formation of melanin.

melanoid (mĕl′ă-noyd): having dark pigment.

melanoma (mĕl-ă-nō′mă): a black or dark brown pigmented tumor.

melanonychia (mĕl-ă-no-nĭk′ē-ă): darkening of the fingernails or toenails.

melanophore (mĕl-ăn′ô-fôr): a pigment cell containing melanin.

melanosis (mĕl-ă-nō′sĭs): a condition in which dark pigment is deposited in the skin or other tissues.

melanotic sarcoma (mĕl-ă-nŏt′ĭk sär-kō′mă): a malignant melanoma.

membrane (mĕm′brān): a thin sheet or layer of pliable tissue surrounding a part, separating adjacent cavities, lining a cavity, or connecting adjacent structures.

mental artery (mĕn′tâl är′tĭr-ē): artery which supplies blood to the lower lip and the chin.

mentalis (mĕn-tā′lĭs): the muscle that elevates the lower lip and raises and wrinkles the skin of the chin.

mental nerve (mĕn′tâl nûrv): a nerve which supplies the skin of the lower lip and chin.

menthol (mĕn′thōl): an alcohol obtained from peppermint or other mint oils, often employed for its marked cooling effect.

menthyl salicylate (mĕn′thĭl să-lĭs′ĭ-lāt): an organic compound which is used as a filtering agent in sunburn preventives; produces an even tan by removing the majority of the ultraviolet rays.

mentum (mĕn′tûm); pl., **menti** (-ī): of or pertaining to the chin.

mercurochrome (mẽr-kū′rô-krōm): a germicide.

mercury bichloride (mûr′kû-rē bī-klō′-rīd): a powerful germicide; very poisonous.

mercury compound (mûr′kyoo-rē käm-pound′): quicksilver; used in face masks, bleaching creams, hair tonics and other cosmetics.

mesh (mĕsh): an open weave foundation used to attach hair in a hairpiece; a wig foundation or base made of a net material.

mesh hair roller (mĕsh hâr rō′lẽr): a roller covered with a woven mesh fabric, usually of nylon.

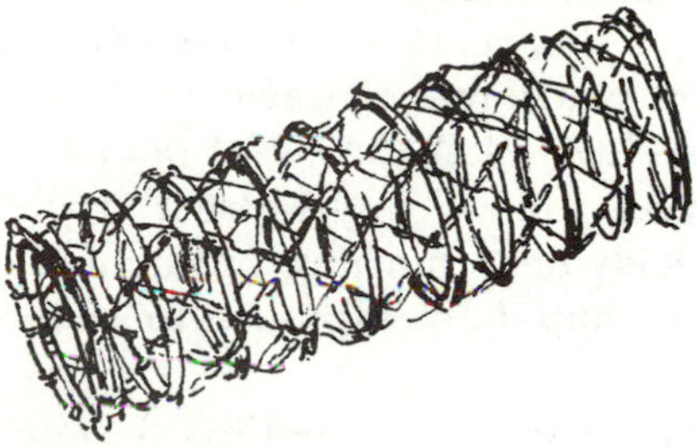

mesh hair roller

meso (mĕs′ô): a prefix denoting in the middle; intermediate.

mesomorph (mĕs′ô môrf): a body type characterized by a sturdy body structure and great strength.

mesorrhine (mĕs′ô-rīn): pertaining to a broad, high-bridged nose.

meta (mĕt′ă): a prefix signifying over; beyond; among; between change or transformation.

metabolism (mĕ-tăb′ô-lĭz'm): the constructive and destructive life process of the cell.

metacarpal (mĕt-ă-kär′pâl): pertaining to the bones of the palm of the hand.

metacarpal, dorsal (mĕt-ă-kär-pâl, dôr′-sâl): the vein that draws blood from the back of the hand.

metacarpal, palmar (mĕt-ă-kär′pâl, păl′mẽr): the main vein that draws blood from the palm of the hand.

metacarpus (mĕt-ă-kär′pûs): the bones of the palm of the hand; the part of the hand containing five bones between the carpus and phalanges.

metallic (mē-tâl′ĭk): relating to, or resembling metal.

metallic hair dye (mĕ-tâl′ĭk hâr dī): a solution containing metal, such as copper to change hair color gradually.

metaphase (met′ă-fāz): in biology, in meiotic cell division, the middle stage of mitosis when the cell chromosomes lie nearly in a single plane at the equator of the spindle forming the

metastasis (mĕ-tăs′tă-sĭs): the migration or transference of a disease from one site in the body to another by the conveyence of cells in blood vessels or lymph channels.

metatarsus (mĕt-ă-tär′sûs): the bones which make up the instep of the foot; the part of the foot between the phalanges and the tarsus, containing five bones.

metatoluene-diamine (mĕt-ă-tŏl′ū-ēn-dī-ăm ĭn): an oxidation dye used to provide lighter shades of red and blond; an aniline derivative type dye.

meter (mē′tẽr): an instrument for measuring the strength of an electric current in amperes; the basic metric unit of length, equal to 39.37 inches.

methodology (mĕth-ă-dŏl′ô-jē): principles, practices and particular procedures applied to a field of learning.

methyl alcohol (mĕth′ĭl ăl′kă-hŏl): meth-

M-N

anol, a solvent, flammable and toxic; used in the manufacture of formaldehyde and some disinfectants.

methyl salicylate (mĕth′ĭl să-lĭs′ĭ-lāt): the chief constituent of oil of wintergreen, used as a counter irritant, anesthetic and disinfectant.

metric (mĕt′rĭk): base on the meter as a unit of measurement; pertaining to the metric system; see metric conversion chart.

metric system (mĕt′rĭk sĭs′tăm): a decimal system of weights and measures based on the gram, from which measures of weights and mass are derived, and the meter, from which measures of area, length and volume are derived.

M-N

mica (mī′kă): a mineral occurring in the form of thin, shining, transparent plates.

micro (mī′krô): a prefix denoting very small; slight; millionth part of.

microbicide (mī-krō′bĭ-sīd): an agent that destroys microbes.

microcirculation (mī′krō-sẽr-kū-la′shûn): pertaining to the microvasculature; circulation of blood in the body's system of fine vessels (100 microns or less in diameter).

microfollicular (mī′krō-fŏl-ĭk′ū-lăr): characterized by very small follicles.

micron; mikron (mī′krŏn): a measurement equal to one thousandth of a millimeter or one millionth of a meter.

micronychia (mī′krō-nĭk′ē-ă): the presence of an abnormally small fingernail or toenail.

microorganism (mī′krô-ôr′gă-nĭz′m): microscopic plant or animal cell; bacterium.

microscope (mī′krô-skōp): an instrument for making enlarged views of minute objects.

microscopic (mī-krô-skŏp′ĭk): extremely small; visible only with the aid of a microscope; not visible to the naked eye.

mid (mĭd): a prefix denoting the middle part.

middle ear (mĭd′′l ēr): the portion of the ear between the tympanic membrane and the opening of the eustachian tube.

middle temporal artery (mĭd′′l tĕm′pôr-âl är′tĭr-ē): the artery that supplies blood to the temporal muscles.

midfrontal (mĭd-frŭn′tâl): pertaining to the middle of the forehead.

milia (mĭl′ē-ă): see milium.

miliaria (mĭl-ē-âr′ē-ă): an eruption of minute vesicles due to retention of fluid at the mouths of the sweat follicles.

miliaria profunda (mĭl-ē-ă′rē-ă prō-fŭn′-dă): a skin reaction in the sweat retention syndrome, characterized by papules located at the sweat pores.

miliaria rubra (mĭl-ē-ă′rē-ă rōōb′ră): prickly heat; burning and itching usually caused by exposure to excessive heat.

miliary fever (mĭl′ē-ă-rē fē′vẽr): sweating sickness; an infectious disease characterized by fever, profuse sweating, and the production of papular vesicular and other eruptions.

milium (mĭl′e-ûm); pl., **milia** (-ă): a small, whitish pearl-like mass in the epidermis due to retention of sebum; a whitehead.

milli (mĭl-ē): thousand; a combining form meaning one thousandth part of.

milliameter (mĭl-ē-ăm′ĕ-tẽr): an instrument which registers electric current in milliamperes; used to measure the amount of current required for a given treatment.

milliampere (mĭl′ē-ăm′pēr): one thousandth of an ampere.

milligram (mĭl′ĭ-grăm): a unit of weight in the metric system equal to one thousandth of a gram.

milliliter (mĭl′ĭ-lē-tĕr): a unit of capacity in the metric system equal to one thousandth of a liter; equivalent to a cubic centimeter.

millimeter (mĭl′ĭ-mē-tĕr): one thousandth of an meter.

mineral (mĭn′er-âl): any inorganic material found in the earth's crust.

mineral oil (mĭn′ĕr-âl oyl): white oil; oil found in the rock strata of the earth; a colorless, tasteless oil derived from petroleum and used in creams, lotions, moisturizing products, powders, lip and eye makeup, hairdressings and many other cosmetics; it is a widely used cosmetic lubricant and binder.

mini (mĭ′nē): combination form meaning miniature or of small dimensions; smaller than average.

minibraid (mĭ′nē-brād): thin strands of hair woven to form small braids.

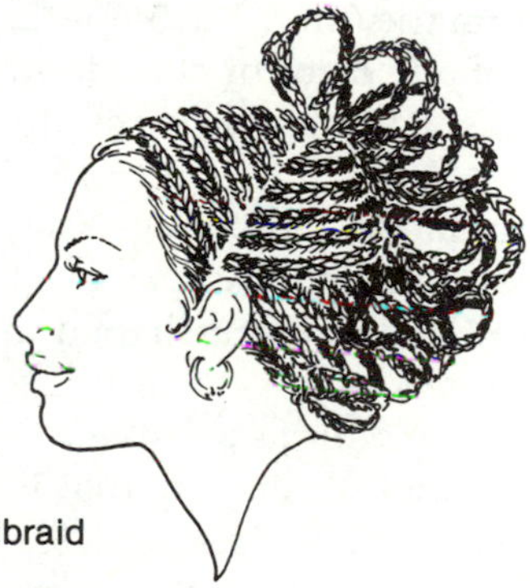

minibraid

minifall (mĭ′nē-fôl): a loose-hanging hairpiece (shorter than a regular fall) which is attached at the crown.

minishears (mĭ′nē-shērz): small scissors used to cut and layer hair in small graduations.

miniwig (mĭ′nē-wĭg): a very short wig or hairpiece.

minimize (mĭn′ĭ-mīz): to reduce to the smallest possible degree.

mink oil (mĭnk oyl): an oil produced by the small mammal (genus mustela); used in some cosmetics for its softening properties.

mint (mĭnt): any of several aromatic herbs used as a flavoring and in some cosmetic preparations.

minute (mī-nūt′): very small; tiny.

miscible (mĭs′ĭ-b'l): the property of certain liquids to mix with each other in equal proportions.

mitosis (mĭ-tō′sĭs): indirect nuclear division, the usual process of cell reproduction of human tissues.

M-N

mixing (mĭks′ĭng): the intermingling of hair of various shades and/or lengths.

mixture (mĭks′tyōōr): a preparation made by incorporating an insoluble ingredient in a liquid vehicle; sometimes used to identify an aqueous solution containing two or more solutes; a combination of two or more substances which are not chemically united.

mobility (mô-bĭl′ĭ-tē): the quality of being movable.

mode (mōd): a current style or fashion; a manner or method of doing something.

model (mŏd′'l): an object used as an example of something to be made or already existing; one who is hired to display clothes, hairstyles or merchandise.

moderate porosity (mŏd′ĕr-ât pôr-ŏs′ĭ-tē): category of normal hair in which the cuticle is close to the hair shaft.

modern blend (mäd′ûrn blĕnd): descriptive of a basic perfume type which contains aldehydes (a class of organic chemical compounds) and has its own distinctive fragrance.

modifier (mŏd′ĭ-fī-ẽr): anything that will change the form or characteristics of an object or substance.

moist (moyst): slightly wet; damp.

moisture (moyst′ûr): water or other liquid spread in very small drops in the air or on a surface.

moisture gradient (moyst′ûr grā′dē-ênt): the amount of moisture in the skin or hair.

moisturizer (moyst′ûr-īz-ẽr): a product formulated to add moisture to dry skin or hair.

mold (mōld): a fungus growth usually growing in dark, damp places; to form into a particular shape.

molded curl (mōld′ĕd kûrl): see carved curl.

molding (mōld′ĭng): the act of forming or directing hair into a desired pattern.

mole (mōl): a small brownish spot on the skin; pigmented nevis.

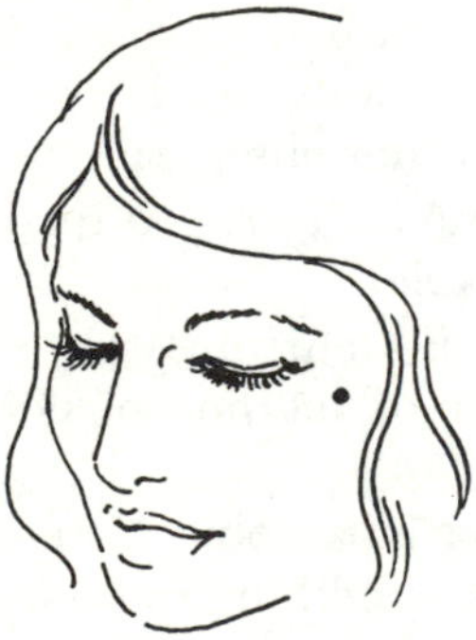

mole

molecular attraction (mô-lĕk′û-lăr ă-trăk′-shûn): the force which is exerted between two unlike molecules tending to draw them together and to resist separation.

molecular breakdown (mô-lĕk′û-lăr brāk′daún): the disrupting or disuniting of a molecular unit.

molecular weight (mô-lĕk′û-lăr wāt): the sum of the weights of the atoms of a molecule.

molecule (mŏl′ĕ-kūl): the smallest possible unit of any substance that still retains its characteristics.

molluscum (mŏ-lŭs′kûm): pertaining to a skin disease having waxy, dome-shaped nodules.

molluscum contagiosum (mŏ-lŭs′kûm kôn-tā-jē-ō′sûm): a viral disease of the skin, characterized by waxy, dome-shaped nodules.

molluscum fibrosum (mŏ-lŭs′kûm fī-brō′-sûm): a cutaneous tumor of the dermis, characterized by fibrous papules.

mongolism (mŏn′gō-lĭzm): a congenital disease characterized by yellowness of the skin and slightly slanting eyes; Down's syndrome.

monilethrix (mô-nĭl′ĕ-thrĭks): beaded hair; a condition in which the hairs show a series of constrictions, giving the appearance of fusiform beads.

mono (mŏn′ô): a prefix denoting one; single.

monochromatic (mŏn′ô-krō-măt′ĭk): consisting of one color or color family; displaying shades and tints of the same color.

monochromatism (mŏn-ô-krō′mă-tĭzm): total color blindness.

moons (mo͞onz): cresent-shaped areas at the base of the fingernails.

mordant (môr′dênt): a substance, such as alum, phenol, aniline oil, that fixes the dye used in coloring.

morphology (môr-fŏl′ă-jē): the branch of biology which deals with structure and form; it includes histology and cytology of the organism at any stage of its life history.

motile (mō′tĭl): having the power of movement, as certain bacteria.

motor (mō′tĕr): of or relating to muscular movement.

motor nerves (mō′tĕr nêrvz): nerves that carry impulses from nerve centers to muscles.

motor oculi (mō′tĕr ŏk′û-lī): third cranial nerve; the nerve controlling most of the eye muscles.

motor point (mō′tĕr poynt): a point on the skin over a muscle where pressure or stimulation will cause contraction of that muscle.

motor units (mō′tĕr ū′nĭts): muscle fibers which are controlled by nerve fibers.

mount (maůnt): that part of a wig (excluding the crown) or any hairpiece made of foundation net, hair lace, or gauze, on which hair is knotted.

mousse (mo͞os): a light, airy, whipped hair setting and sculpturing product resembling shaving foam; the whipped dessert called mousse.

mousy (maů′sē): hair color that is similar to the drab, grey-brown color of a mouse.

movement (mo͞ov′mênt): the change of place or position of hair; the rhythmic quality or motion of hair.

muco (mû′kō): a combining form meaning mucus or mucous membrane.

mucosa (mû-kō′să): mucous membrane.

mucosum, stratum (mû-kō′sûm strā′-tûm): mucous or malpighian layer of the epidermis; a deeper portion of the skin located in the germinative zone.

mucous membrane (mū′kûs mĕm′brān): a membrane secreting mucus which lines passages and cavities communicating with the air.

mucus (mū′kûs): a thick, slippery secretion produced by the mucous membranes to lubricate and cleanse the part.

mudpack (mŭd′păk): a thick, spreadable product, usually containing clay; used for facial and body treatments.

multi (mŭl′tĭ): many; more than one.

multicellular (mŭl′tĭ-sĕl′ū-lăr): having many cells.

multicolor (mŭl′tĭ-kŭl′ĕr): having many colors.

multidimensional (mŭl′tĭ-dī-mĕn′shûn-âl): having several dimensions.

multidirectional (mŭl′tĭ-dī-rĕk′shûn-âl): extending in many directions.

multilayered (mŭl′tĭ-lā′ĕrd): having several layers.

multiple (mŭl′tĭ-p’l): consisting of more than one.

murky (mûr′kē): thick, hazy in color; not clear.

muscle (mŭs′’l): the contractile tissue of the body by which movement is accomplished.

muscle-bound (mŭs′’l-boůnd): having tight, inflexible muscles.

muscle insertion (mŭs′’l ĭn-sûr′shûn): the distal point of muscle attachment.

muscle oil (mŭs′’l oyl): a vegetable oil in which either lecithin or cholestrin is dissolved; used in conjunction with massage to soften the skin and to help prevent fine lines.

muscle origin (mŭs′’l ôr′ĭ-jĭn): the proximal point of muscle attachment.

muscle strapping (mŭs′’l străp′ĭng): a heavy massage treatment used to reduce fatty deposits.

muscle tone (mŭs′’l tōn): the normal degree of tension in a healthy muscle.

muscular (mŭs′kû-lăr): relating to a muscle or the muscles.

musculi colli (mŭs′kū-lī kŏl′ī): the anterior muscles of the neck.

musculi dorsi (mŭs′kū-lī dôr′sī): the muscles of the back.

musk (mŭsk): a secretion with a penetrating odor, obtained from the male musk deer, and used in the making of some perfumes and medicines.

muslin (mŭz′lĭn): any of several plain-weave cotton fabrics of varying fineness.

mustache (mŭs′tăsh): the growth of hair on the upper lip.

mustache brush (mŭs′tăsh brŭsh): a small brush designed to groom the mustache.

mustache comb (mŭs′tăsh kōm): a small comb with fine teeth designed to groom the mustache.

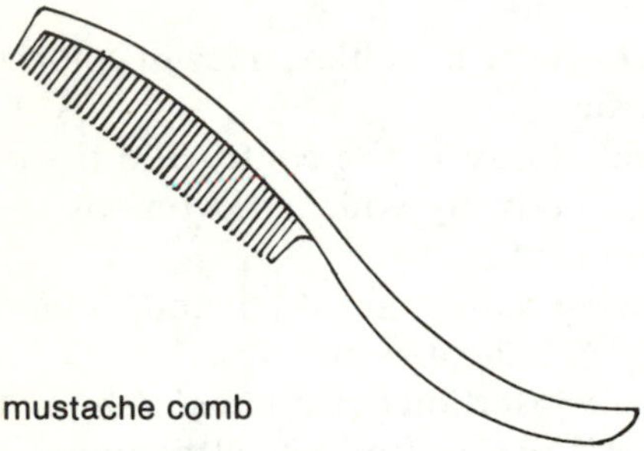

mustache comb

mustache styles (mŭs′tăsh stīlz): various designs of mustaches, some combined with beard and sideburn styles; usually styled to enhance the client's facial features or to conceal an undesired facial feature.

mutation (mū-tā′shûn): to change, as in quality, form or nature.

mutton chop (mŭt′'n chŏp): a beard style with side whiskers, narrow at the temples and widening at the lower cheeks.

myalgia (mī-ăl′jă): pain in the muscles.

myasthenia (mī-ăs-thēn′ē-ă): muscular weakness.

mycetoma (mī-sĕ-tō′mă): a chronic fungus infection usually of the feet.

mycosis (mī-kō′sĭs): any disease or infection caused by fungus.

myodystrophy (mī-ô-dĭs′trŭ-fē): degeneration of muscles.

myoedema (mī-ō-ĕ-dē′mă): edema of a muscle.

myology (mī-ŏl′ă-jē): the science of the nature, functions, structure and diseases of muscles.

myomalacia (mī-ō-mă-lā′shē-ă): degeneration with softening of muscle tissue.

myoneural (mī-ō-nū′râl): relating to nerve endings in muscle tissue.

myopalmus (mī-ō-păl′mûs): twitching and quivering of muscles.

myopathic (mī-ō-păth′ĭk): pertaining to disease of the muscles.

myoplasty (mī′ō-plăs-tē): plastic surgery on a muscle or group of muscles.

myositis (mī-ō-sī′tĭs): inflammation of muscle tissue.

myotasis (mī-ŏt′ă-sĭs): stretching and extending of a muscle.

myotrophy (mī-ŏt′ră-fē): nutrition of the muscles.

myrrh (mŭr): an aromatic gum resin from the myrrh shrub; used in perfumery, in some medicinal preparations, and in skin tonics.

M-N

N

naevus; nevus (nē′vŭs); pl., **naevi, nevi** (-vī): a birthmark; a congenital skin blemish.

nail (nāl): unguis; the horny protective plate located at the end of the finger or toe.

nail bed (nāl bĕd): that portion of the skin on which the body of the nail rests.

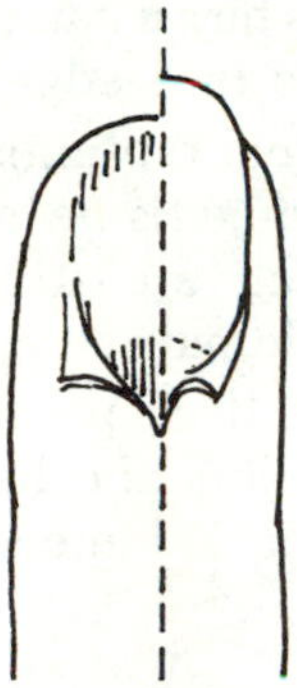

nail bed

nail biting (nāl bī′tĭng): the habit of biting off the tips of the nails to the nail bed; see onychophagia.

nail bleach (nāl blēch): a product used in manicuring to remove stains and to whiten the nails.

nail body (nāl bŏd′ē): the horny nail blade resting upon the nail bed.

nail brush (nāl brŭsh): a small brush used to clean under and around the nails.

nail buffer (nāl bŭf′ẽr): an instrument made of leather or chamois; used with a polishing powder to polish the nails to a high luster.

nail cap (nāl kăp): an artificial nail attached to the natural nail to make the nail stronger and more attractive.

nail emery (nāl ĕm′rē): a small flat stick coated with finely ground emery; used as a manicuring instrument; emery board.

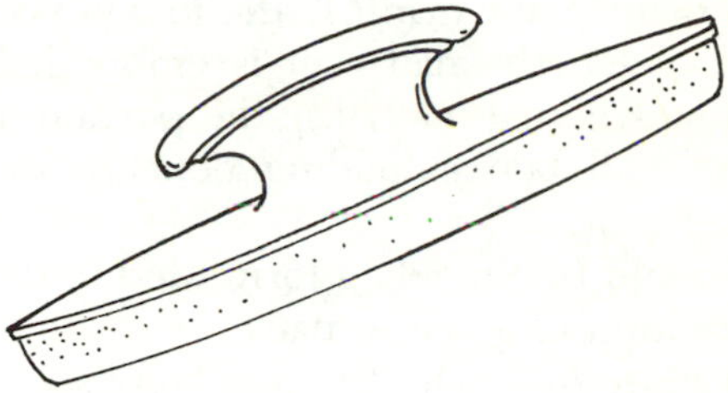

nail buffer

nail enamel (nāl ē-năm′ăl): a fingernail polish in liquid form, applied to protect and beautify the nails.

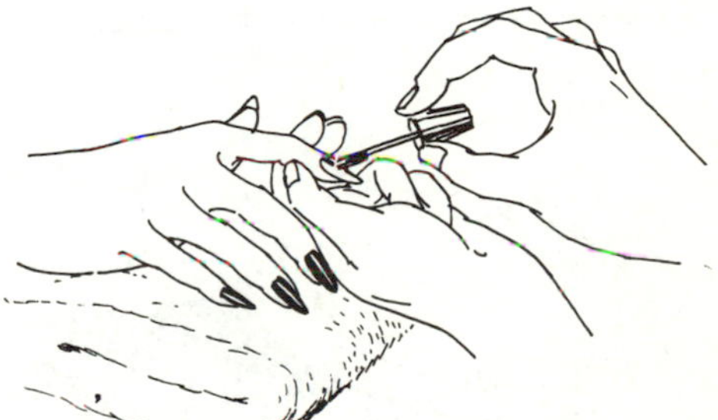

nail enamel

nail extender (nāl ĕk-stĕn′dẽr): a product applied to the natural nail over a fingernail form; when the mixture hardens, it is shaped to resemble a longer natural nail.

nail file (nāl fīl): a metal instrument with a specially prepared surface used to file and shape the nails.

nail fold (nāl fōld): nail wall.

M-N

nail grooves (nāl gro͞ovz): the slits or furrows on the sides of the nails upon which the nail moves as it grows.

nail lacquer (nāl lăk′ẽr): a thick liquid which forms a glossy film on the nail.

nail mantle (nāl mănt′'l): the fold of skin in which the nail root is embedded.

nail matrix (nāl mā′trĭks): the portion of the nail bed extending beneath the nail root.

nail mold (nāl mōld): a form used in the creation of artificial nails.

nail plate (nāl plāt): the nail body.

nail polish remover (nāl pŏl′ĭsh rē-mo͞ov′ẽr): a solution used to remove polish from the nails.

nail repair (nāl rē′pâr): the use of a special tape and cement to mend a broken nail.

nail root (nāl ro͞ot): the part of the nail located at its base; embedded underneath the skin.

nail shaper (nāl shāp′ẽr): a disk made of emery; used to shape the nails.

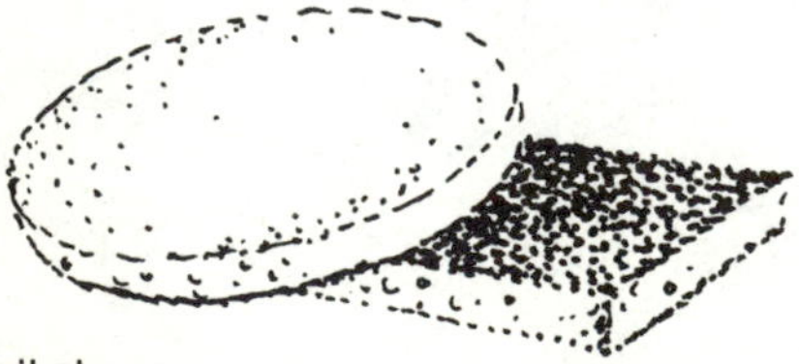

nail shaper

nail skin (nāl skĭn): cuticle.

nail tips (nāl tĭps): preformed artificial nails which are applied to the tips of the natural fingernails.

nail transplant (nāl trăns′plănt): the repairing of a broken nail by cementing the broken part to the natural fingernail.

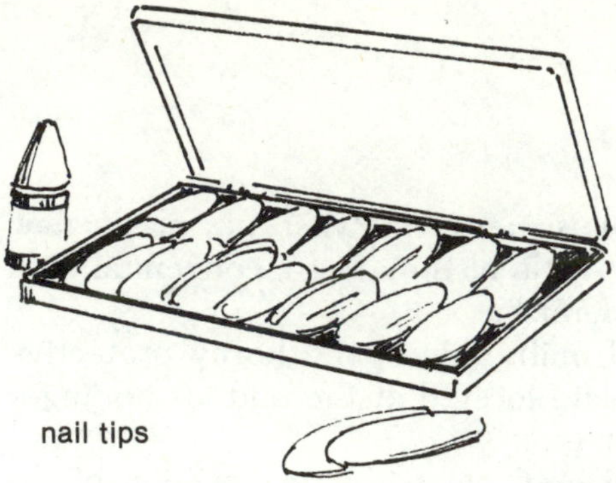

nail tips

nail wall (nāl wôl): cuticle covering the lateral and proximal edge of the nail.

nail white (nāl whīt): a nail cosmetic used to whiten the free edge of the nails.

nail wrapping (nāl răp′ĭng): a corrective treatment using tissue and sealer to form a protective coating for a damaged or fragile nail.

nape (nāp): the back part of the neck.

nape line (nāp līn): the hairline at the nape of the neck; nape section.

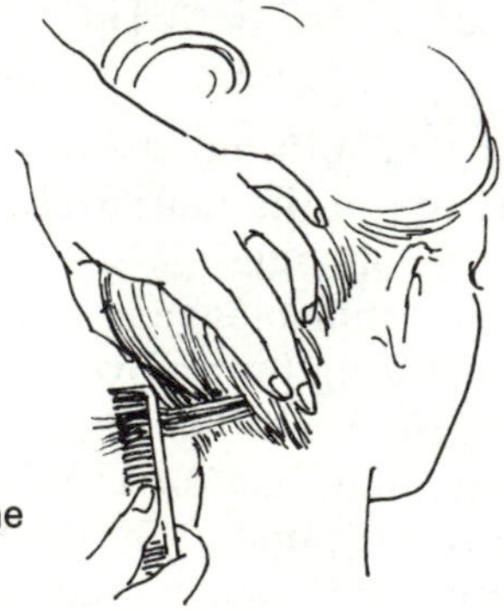

nape line

naris (nā′rĭs); pl., **nares** (-rēz): a nostril.

nasal (nā′zâl): pertaining to the nose.

nasal bones (nā′zâl bōnz): bones that form the bridge of the nose.

nasalis (nā-zā′lĭs): a muscle of the nose.

nasal nerve (nā′zâl nûrv): nerve which receives stimuli for the skin on the sides of the nose.

nasitis (nā-sī′tĭs): rhinitis; inflammation of nasal mucous membrane of the nose.

nasus (nā′sûs); pl., **nasi** (-sī): the nose.

natural bristle brush (năt′û-râl brĭst′'l brŭsh): a brush with bristles made from the hairs of an animal, not from synthetic hair.

natural distribution (năt′û-râl dĭs′tră-byōō′shûn): the direction hair assumes as it grows out from the scalp.

natural growth pattern (năt′û-râl grōth păt′ẽrn): the direction in which hair grows naturally, usually in a large circle from the crown.

natural neckline (năt′û-râl něk′līn): haircutting technique that allows the hair to follow its natural growth tendency rather than forcing a pattern into the hair.

navicular (nă-vĭk′û-lär): boat-shaped; a bone of the wrist.

neck (něk): the part of the body which connects the trunk and head.

neck duster (něk dŭs′tẽr): a brush used to remove hair from the neck after a haircut; in some states this procedure is prohibited as it is considered unsanitary.

neckline (něk-līn): in haircutting, the line where the hair growth of the head ends and the neck begins; hairline.

neck strips (něk strĭps): soft, flexible strips of paper placed around the client's neck to keep the shampoo cape from touching the skin while a service is being given.

negative pole (něg′ă-tĭv pōl): the pole from which negative galvanic current flows.

negative skin test (něg′ă-tĭv skĭn těst): having no reaction to a skin test for allergy, indicating the safety of performing the service.

negative terminal (něg′ă-tĭv tûr′mĭ-nâl): the end of the conducting circuit of the electric current manifesting alkaline reaction; the zinc plate in a battery.

nerve (nûrv): a whitish cord, made up of bundles of nerve fibers, through which impulses are transmitted.

nerve cell (nûrv sěl): a neuron; the fundamental cellular unit of the nervous system.

nerve center (nûrv sěn′tẽr): an aggregation of neurons with a specific function for a part of the body; command center.

nerve fiber (nûrv fī′bẽr): thread-like processes (axons and dendrites) arising from a neuron which make up a nerve.

nerve impulse (nûrv ĭm′pŭls): an electrical wave transmitted along a nerve that has been stimulated.

nervous cutaneous (nûr′vûs kû-tā′nē-ûs): a cutaneous nerve; any nerve supplying an area of the skin.

nervous system (nûr′vûs sĭs′têm): the body system composed of the brain, spinal cord, nerves, ganglia and other parts of the receptor.

net (nět): a fabric of thread or cord woven in an open pattern or meshwork; a fabric of this type used to cover the hair and hold the set in place while drying.

net foundation (nět faůn-dā′shûn): a mesh or other open weave material used for a foundation of a hairpiece.

nettle (nět′'l): an herb (genus urtica) used for its astringent qualities.

neuralgia (nû-râl′jē-ă): acute pain along the course of a nerve.

neurasthenia (nûr-ăs-thē′nē-ă): a condition of weakness and depression due to exhaustion which affects the nervous system.

neuritis (nû-rī′tĭs): inflammation of a nerve.

neurology (nû-rŏl′ă-jē): the science of the structure, function and pathology of the nervous system.

neuromuscular junction (nû-rô-mŭs′kû-lăr jŭnk′shûn): the point where the motor neuron and muscle join.

neuron (nû′rŏn): the basic unit of the nervous system, consisting of a nucleus, its processes, and extensions; a nerve cell.

neutral (nū′trâl): exhibiting no positive properties; indifferent; in chemistry, neither acid nor alkaline.

neutral blond (nū′trâl blŏnd): a beige-blond that is neither gold nor ash.

neutralization (nū-tră-lĭ-zā′shûn): that process that counterbalances or cancels another action; in chemistry, reaction forming a substance which is neither alkaline nor acid; a chemical reaction between an acid and a base; rehardening the hair in cold waving or in chemical hair relaxing.

neutralize (nū′tră-līz′): to render ineffective; to effect neutralization; counterbalance of an action or influence.

neutralizer (nū′trăl-īz′ẽr): an agent capable of neutralizing another substance.

neutralizing (nū′tră-līz-ĭng): the process of stopping the action of a permanent wave solution and hardening the hair in its new form by the application of a chemical solution.

neutralizing headband (nū′tră-līz-ĭng hĕd′bănd): an absorbent band placed around the client's hairline during a permanent to prevent dripping on the client's face during the neutralizing process.

nevus (nē′vûs): a birthmark.

nevus pilosus (nē′vûs pī-lō′sûs): hairy nevus; a birthmark characterized by hair growing from the dark area.

new growth (nū grōth): the part of the hair shaft between the scalp and the hair which had previously received treatment.

ninth cranial nerve (nīnth krā′nē-âl nûrv): the glossopharyngeal nerve.

nipper (nĭp′ẽr): a tool used in pedicuring and manicuring to trim the cuticle around fingernails or toenails.

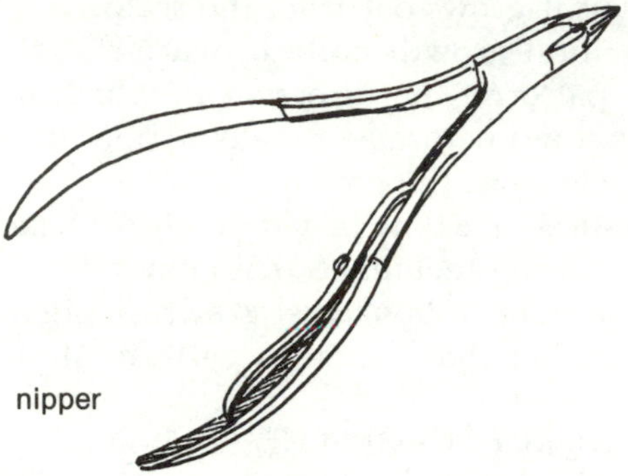

nipper

nit (nĭt): the egg of a louse, usually attached to a hair.

nitrazine (nī′tră-zēn pā′pẽr): a form of paper used to test the acidity or alkalinity of products.

nitrocellulose (nī′trô-sĕl′û-lōs): pyroxylin; gun cotton; a granular, yellowish mass formed in the chemical reaction between cellulose and nitric acid; used in nail polishes.

nitrogen (nī′tră-jĕn): a colorless gaseous element; tasteless and odorless; found in air and living tissue.

nitrous (nī′trûs): designating a compound of nitrogen.

no-base relaxer (nō-bās rē-lăks′ẽr): a preparation used to straighten the hair which does not require application of a protective base.

node (nōd): a knot or knob; a circumscribed swelling; a knuckle or finger joint.

nodose (nō′dôs): having nodes or knot-like swellings.

M-N

nodule (nŏd′ûl): a small node.
noma (nō′mă): a sore or ulcer, usually of the mouth.
non (nŏn): a prefix denoting not.
nonallergenic cosmetic (nŏn-ă-lẽr-jĕn′ĭk kŏz-mĕt′ĭk): a preparation formulated without certain ingredients that have been found to cause reaction in hypersensitive people.
nonconductor (nŏn-kôn-dŭk′tôr): any substance that does not easily transmit electricity light, heat or sound.
noninfectious (nŏn-ĭn-fĕk′shûs): not spread by contact; unable to spread disease.
nonpathogenic (nŏn-păth-ō-jĕn′ĭk): not harmful; not disease producing.
nonresistant (nŏn-rē-zĭs′tênt): porous hair; the condition of the hair which absorbs moisture readily.
nonstriated (nŏn-strī′āt-ĕd): without striations, as smooth muscle which acts involuntarily without the action of the will.
nonstripping shampoo (nŏn-strĭp′ĭng shăm-pōō′): a shampoo that cleanses the hair without removing tint.
normal (nôr′mâl): regular; natural; conforming to some ideal norm or standard.
normal hair condition (nôr′mâl hâr kôn-dĭ′shûn): an average condition in which hair is neither porous nor resistant, neither dry nor oily.
normal hair shampoo (nôr′mâl hâr shăm-pōō′): a shampoo formulated for hair that is neither too dry nor too oily.
normalize (nôr′mâl-īz): to make something conform to a norm or standard; to return the pH of the skin or hair to normal.
normalizer (nôr′mâl′īz-ẽr): a solution used to return the hair to its normal pH (4.5 to 5.5), or the skin to about 4.5 to 6.0.
normal skin (nôr′mâl skĭn): skin that is neither too dry nor too oily and is free of conditions such as blackheads, whiteheads, acne or disease.
nose (nōz): the organ of smell.
no stem (nō stĕm): a type of curl or roller that is placed directly on its base for maximum volume and minimum mobility.

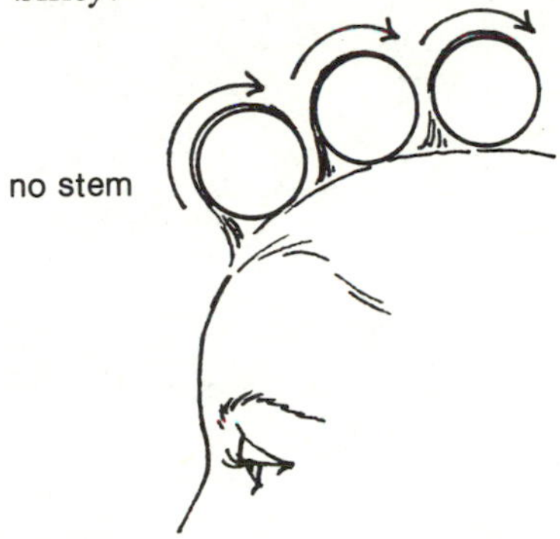

nostril (nŏs′trĭl): one of the two external openings of the nose.
nourish (nŭr′ĭsh): to feed; to furnish with whatever promotes growth.
nourishing cream (nŭr′ĭsh-ĭng krēm): a cream formulated to nourish the skin; used in massage and facial treatments.
nourishment (nŭr′ĭsh-mênt): anything which nourishes; nutriment; food.
novice (nŏv′ĭs): a beginner in any occupation; one who is learning a skill, trade or craft.
noxious (nŏk′shûs): harmful; poisonous.
nucha (nū′kă): the nape or back of the neck.
nucleic acid (nû-klē′ĭk ă′sĭd): one of a group of compounds found in cell nuclei and cytoplasm involved in building the proteins necessary to the formation of living matter.
nucleus (nū′klē-ûs); pl., **nuclei** (-ī): the active center of cells.
nutmeg (nŭt′mĕg′): the hard, aromatic

seed of the East Indian tree; used as a spice and to flavor mouthwashes and dentifrices.

nut oil (nŭt oyl): an oil from the kernals of walnuts often used in skin preparations.

nutrient (nū′trē-ênt): a nourishing substance; nutritious.

nutriment (nū′trĭ-mênt): that which nourishes; food.

nutrition (nû-trĭsh′ûn): the processes involved in taking in nutriments and assimilating and utilizing them.

nylon (nī′län): a synthetic thermoplastic polyamide from which fibers and bristles are made.

O

o: chemical symbol for oxygen.

oatmeal (ōt′mēl): a cereal made from oats that is sometimes mixed with other ingredients and used as a facial cleanser or mask.

obese (ô-bēs′): extremely overweight; stout; corpulent; fat.

obesity (ô-bē′sĭ-tē): the condition of having excessive body weight over what is considered to be normal for one's height and bone structure.

objective (ŏb-jĕk′tĭv): aim or goal; something observable or verifiable by scientific methods.

oblique (ŏb-lēk): slanting or inclined.

oblong (ŏb′lông): longer than broad; rectangle whose horizontal sides are longer than its vertical sides.

oblong face shape (ŏb′lông fās shāp): a face characterized by a long, thin structure.

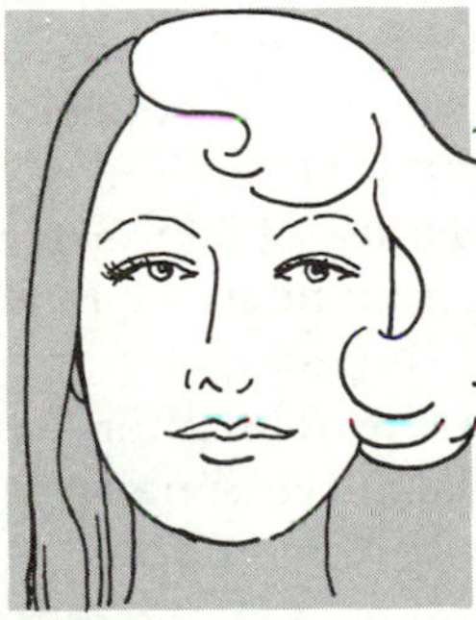

oblong face shape

obsolete (ŏb-sô-lēt′): out of date; no longer in use; not current.

occipita (ŏk-sĭp′ĭ-tă): the back of the head or skull.

occipital (ŏk-sĭp′ĭ-tâl): pertaining to the back part of the head; the bone which forms the back and lower part of the cranium.

occipital artery (ŏk-sĭp′ĭ-tâl är′tĭr-ē): the artery that supplies blood to the skin and muscles of the scalp, back of the head and the neck.

occipital bone (ŏk-sĭp′ĭ-tâl bōn): the hindmost bone of the skull below the parietal bones.

occipital frontalis (ŏk-sĭp′ĭ-tâl frŏn-tā′lĭs): epicranius; the scalp muscle.

occipitalis (ŏk-sĭp′ĭ-tā′lĭs): a muscle that draws the scalp backward.

occipital lobe (ŏk-sĭp′ĭ-tâl lōb): one of the lobes of the cerebrum.

occipital nerve (ŏk-sĭp′ĭ-tâl nûrv): major occipital nerve; nerve that receives stimuli for the skin of the posterior portion of the scalp.

occupational disease (ŏk-û-pā′shûn-âl dĭ-zīz′): illness resulting from conditions associated with an occupation such as coming in contact with certain chemicals, dyes, etc.

ocher (ō′kẽr): a hydrated iron oxide mixture; a dark yellow color derived from or resembling ocher; yellow ocher.

ocular (ŏk′û-lûr): pertaining to the eye; the eyepiece of a microscope; the lens at the upper end of the microscope.

oculist (ŏk′û-lĭst): a specialist in diseases of the eye.

oculofacial (ŏk′û-lō-fā′shâl): pertaining to the eyes and face.

oculomotor (ŏk′û-lō-mō′tẽr): pertaining to movement of the eyeball.

oculomotor nerve (ŏk′û-lō-mō′tẽr nûrv): third cranial nerve which controls the motion of the eye.

oculus (ŏk′û-lûs); pl., **oculi** (-lī): the eye.

odontic (ō-dŏn′tĭk): pertaining to the teeth.

odor (ō′dẽr): scent; the property of a substance that causes it to be perceptible to the sense of smell.

odorless (ō′dẽr-lês): having no odor.

off base (ŏf bās): in hairstyling, the position of a curl or a roller completely off its base for maximum mobility and minimum volume.

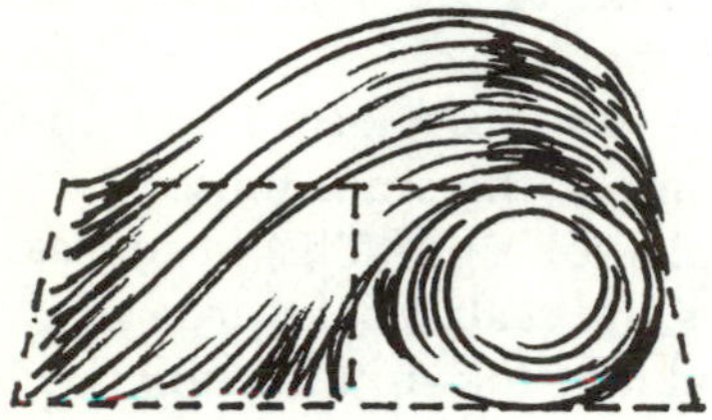

off base curl

O-P

off-color (ŏf-kŭl′ẽr): lacking the correct or acceptable standard of color.

off-white (ŏf-whīt): not pure white; white that has an undertone of gray or yellow.

ohm's law (ōmz lô): the simple statement that the strength of a current in an electric circuit is equal to the electromotive force divided by the resistance.

oil (oyl): a greasy liquid of vegetable, animal or mineral origin, soluble in alcohol and ether, but not in water; used in foods, cosmetics and many other products.

oil bleach (oyl blēch): a combination of sulphonated oil, ammonia water and hydrogen peroxide.

oiled silk (oyld sĭlk): silk material treated with oil; used to protect those parts of a man's hairpiece where adhesive is placed.

oil gland (oyl glănd): an oil-secreting gland; the sebaceous gland.

oily hair (oyl′ē hâr): hair that has an excessive amount of oil due to overactivity of the sebaceous glands.

oily hair shampoo (oyl′ē hâr shăm′po͞o): a preparation formulated for cleansing excessive oil from the hair and scalp.

oily skin (oyl′ē skĭn): skin that is excessively oily due to the overactivity of the sebaceous glands.

ointment (oynt′mênt): a medicated mixture applied externally; a preparation for the skin or scalp.

ol (ôl): a word termination denoting that the name of the substance to which the termination is added belongs to the series of alcohols or hydroxyl derivatives, such as glycerol.

oleaginous (ō-lē-ăj′ĭ-nûs): oily; greasy.

oleic acid (ō-lē′ĭk ăs′ĭd): an oily acid used in soaps, shampoos and some ointments.

oleum (ō′lē-ŭm); pl., **olea** (-ă): oil.

olfaction (ŏl-făk′shûn): the sense of smell; the act or process of smelling.

olfactory (ŏl-făk′tẽr-ē): relating to the sense of smell; first cranial nerve; the special nerve of smell.

olfactory glands (ŏl-fak′tẽr-ē glănz): serous glands found in the mucous membranes of the nose.

olfactory nerve (ŏl-făk′tẽr-ē nûrv): the first cranial nerve; sensory nerve fibers of the mucous membrane of the nose.

olfactory organ (ŏl-făk′tẽr-ē ôr′găn): the sense organ located in the nasal cavity responsible for the ability to detect pleasant or unpleasant odors.

oligocythemia (ŏl-ĭ-gō-sī-thēm′ē-ă): a deficiency of red corpuscles.

oligotrichia (ŏl′ĭ-gō-trĭk′ē-ă): scantiness or thinness of hair.

olive (ŏl′ĭv): a small oily fruit from which a rich oil is obtained.

olive green (ŏl′ĭv grēn): a yellow-green color resembling that of the green olive.

olive oil (ŏl′ĭv oyl): a light-yellow oil pressed from olives; used in some foods and in some cosmetic preparations.

oma (ō′mă): a word termination properly added to words derived from Greek roots, denoting a tumor, such as cystoma.

on base curl (ŏn bās kûrl): a curl placed directly on its base.

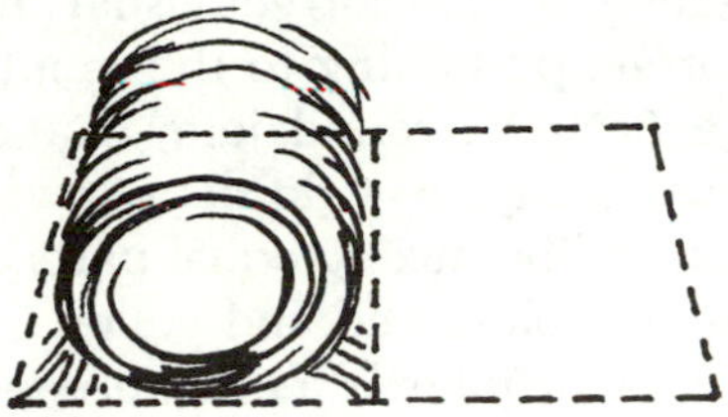

on base curl

oncogenic (ŏn-kō-jĕn′ĭk): tending to cause tumors; relating to tumor formation.

one application process (wŭn ăp-lĭ-kā′-shûn prŏ′sĕs): a hair coloring process which decolorizes and colors in a single application.

onych (ŏn′ĭck): prefix from the Greek word onyx meaning nail; the first syllable of many names for diseases and conditions affecting the nails.

onychatrophia (ŏn-ĭ-kă-trō′fē-ă): atrophy of the nails.

onychauxis (ŏn-ĭ-kôk′sĭs): enlargement of the nails.

onychia (ô-nĭk′ē-ă): inflammation of the matrix of the nail with formation of pus and shedding of the nail.

onychitis (ô-nĭ-kī′tĭs): inflammation of the area around the nails.

onycho (ŏn′ĭ-kô): a prefix meaning relating to the nails.

onychoclasis (ôn′ĭ-kŏk′lă-sĭs): breaking of a nail.

onychocryptosis (ŏn′ĭ-kō-krĭp-tō′sĭs): ingrowing nail.

onychogryposis (ŏn′ĭ-kō-grī-pō′sĭs): thickening and curvature of the nail.

onychohelcosis (ŏn′ĭ-kō-hĕl-kō′sĭs): ulceration of a nail.

onycholysis (ŏn′ĭ-kŏl′ĭ-sĭs): loosening of the nail without shedding.

onychomadesis (ŏn′ĭ-kō-mă-dē′sĭs): separation and falling off of a nail from the nailbed.

onychomycosis (ŏn′ĭ-kō-mī-kō′sĭs): disease of the nails due to fungi.

onychopathy (ŏn-ĭ-kŏp′ă-thē): any disease of the nails.

onychophagia (ŏn′ĭ-kō-fā′jē-ă): the habit of biting the fingernails.

onychophosis (ŏn-ĭ-kŏf-ō′sĭs): growth of horny epithelium in the nailbed.

onychophyna (ŏn-ĭ-kō-fī′mă): enlarged or thickened nails.

onychorrhexis (ŏn-ĭ-kō-rĕk′sis): abnormal brittleness with striation of the nail plate; fissures may or may not be present.

onychorrhiza (ŏn-ĭ-kō-rī′ză): the root of the nail.

onychosis, onychonosus (ŏn-ĭ-kō′sĭs, ŏn-ĭ-kō-nō′sûs): any deformity or disease of the nails.

onychostroma (ŏn-ĭ-kō-strō′mă): the matrix of the nail.

onychotrophy (ŏn-ĭ-kŏt′ră-fē): nourishment of the nails.

onyx (ŏn′ĭks): a nail of the fingers or toes.

onyxis (ôn′ĭk-sĭs): ingrowing toenail.

onyxitis (ŏn-ĭk-sī′tĭs): inflammation of the nail matrix.

ooze (o͞oz): to flow or leak out slowly; to gradually seep or trickle moisture.

opaque (ō-pāk′): impervious to light rays; neither transparent nor translucent.

open end (ō′pĕn-ĕnd): the concave, indented end of a wave or shaping.

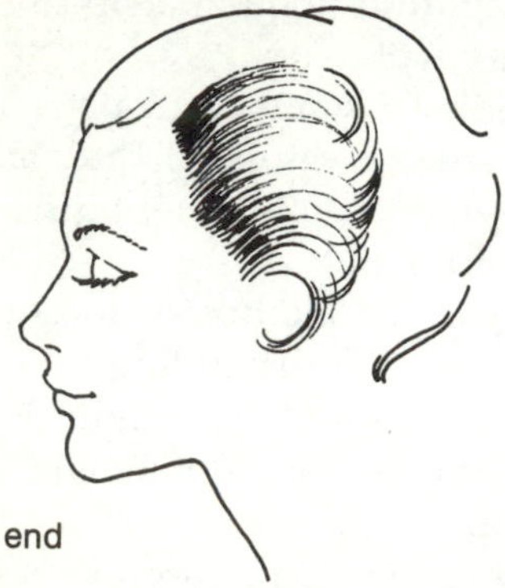

open end

open mesh net (ō′pĕn mĕsh nĕt): a wig net with large openings between the threads.

O-P

operator (ŏp′ĕr-ā-tĕr): one who is able to perform correctly any service rendered professionally in the care of the face, hair, etc.; term sometimes used to describe a cosmetologist.

ophthalmic (ŏf-thăl′mĭk): pertaining to the eye.

ophthalmic artery (ŏf-thăl′mĭk är′tĭr-ē): the main branch of the carotid artery supplying the eye and nearby structures.

ophthalmic nerve (ŏf-thăl′mĭk nûrv): a sensory nerve which innervates the skin of the forehead, the upper eyelids and interior portion of the scalp, orbit, eyeball and nasal passage.

ophthalmitis (ŏf-thăl-mī′tĭs): inflammation of the eye.

ophthalmology (ŏf-thăl-mŏl′ō-jē): the science dealing with the structure, functions and diseases of the eye.

ophthalmoplasty (ŏf-thăl′mō-plăs′tē): plastic surgery of the eye or its parts.

optic (ŏp′tĭk): pertaining to the eye or to vision.

optical illusion (ŏp′tĭ-kôl ĭ-lo͞o′zhûn): an image that appears different from what actually exists.

optician (ŏp-tĭsh′ûn): one who makes eyeglasses.

optic nerve (ŏp′tĭk nûrv): the second cranial nerve; the nerve of sight which conducts impulses from the retina of the eye to the brain.

optional (ŏp′shûn-âl): left to one's discretion or choice; not compulsory.

optometrist (ŏp-tŏm′ĕ-trĭst): a person who examines eyes and fits or prescribes glasses to correct visual defects.

oral (ôr′âl): pertaining to the mouth.

orange (ôr′ĕnj): a round, juicy fruit of the citrus family; a reddish-yellow color produced by mixing equal parts of the primary colors, red and yellow.

orange oil (ôr′ĭnj oyl): a deep orange colored liquid from the fresh peel of a ripe orange; used in soaps and perfumery.

orangewood stick (ôr′ĕnj wo͝od stĭk): a stick made from the wood of the orange tree; used in manicuring procedures.

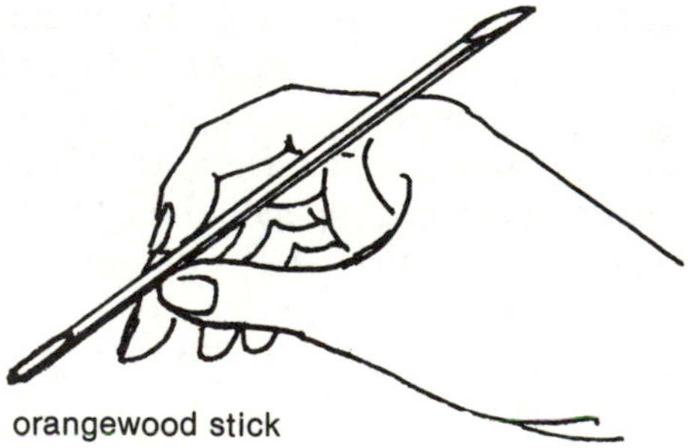

orangewood stick

orbicular (ôr-bĭk′û-lĕr): circular; a term applied to a muscle whose fibers are circularly arranged.

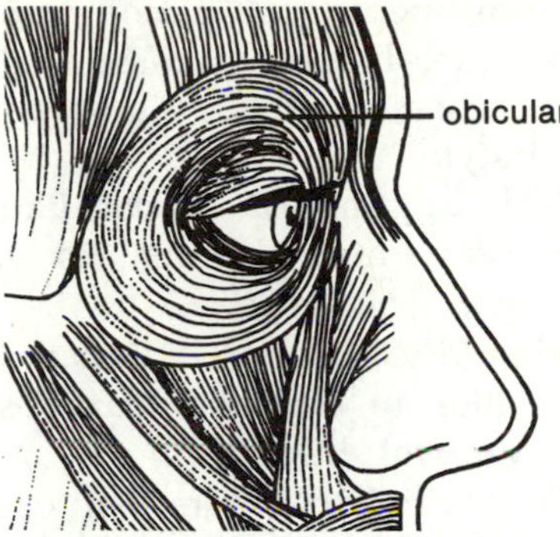

orbicularis oculi (ôr-bĭk-û-lăr′ĭs ŏk′û-lī): orbicularis palpebrarum; the ring muscle of the eye.

orbicularis oris (ôr-bĭk-û-lăr′ĭs ō′rĭs): orbicular muscle; muscle of the mouth.

orbicularis palpebrarum (ôr-bĭk-û-lăr′ĭs păl-pĕ-brâr′ŭm): a muscle of the face that closes the eyes.

orbit (ôr′bĭt): the bony cavity of the eyeball; the eye-socket.

orbital (ôr′bĭ-tâl): pertaining to the orbits.

orchid (ôr′kĭd): a distinctive flower of temperate regions from which essences for perfumes are derived; orchid color, a delicate light rosy purple.

organ (ôr′gan): in plants and animals, a structure composed of specialized tissues and performing specific functions.

organic (ôr-găn′ĭk): relating to an organ; pertaining to substances having carbon-to-carbon bonds.

organic chemistry (ôr-găn′ĭk kĕm′ĭs-trē): chemistry of carbon-based compounds.

organic compound (ôr-găn′ĭk kŏm′-poŭnd): a compound containing carbon exclusive of salts of carbonic acid.

organic cosmetics (ôr-găn′ĭk kŏz-mĕt′ĭks): cosmetics made from animal or vegetable products.

organism (ôr′gă-nĭz′m): any animal or plant with organs that function to maintain life.

oriental blends (ôr′ē-ĕn′t′l blĕnd): a basic perfume type usually including amber, musk, civet oils and special spices.

Oriental hair (ôr′ē-ĕn′tâl hâr): hair from Asian countries; used in the manufacture of wigs and hairpieces.

orifice (ŏr′ĭ-fĭs): an opening; a mouth.

origin (ŏr′ĭ-jĭn): the beginning; the starting point of a nerve; the place of attachment of a muscle to a bone.

original (ŏ-rĭj′ĭ-nâl): something that is new, different and creative.

originate (ŏ-rĭj′ĭ-nāt): to produce as new; to create.

ornament (ôrn-ă′mênt): in hairdressing, a ribbon, comb, pin or other accessory added to the finished hairstyle.

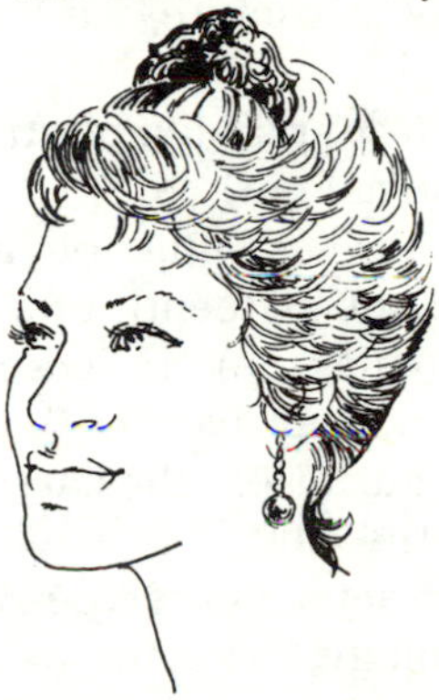
ornament

orris root (ôr′ĭs rōōt): a special powder used to give a dry shampoo.

orthopedics (ôrth-ă-pē′dĭks): the branch of surgery which deals with prevention and correction of problems of the skeletal system.

os (ŏs): a bone.

oscillate (ŏs′ĭl-lāt): to swing back and forth like a pendulum; to vibrate.

oscillation (ŏs-ĭ-lā′shûn): movement like a pendulum; a swinging or vibration.

oscillator (ŏs′sĭ-lā-tĕr): an apparatus that

O-P

produces vibrating movements used in massage.

osis (ō′sĭs): a word termination denoting an abnormal or a diseased condition.

os magnum (ŏs măg′nûm): bone in the lower row of the carpus.

osmidrosis (ŏz-mĭ-drō′sĭs): bromidrosis; foul smelling perspiration.

osmosis (ŏz-mō′sĭs): the diffusion of a fluid or solution through a semipermeable membrane; especially the passage of a solvent through a membrane from a dilute solution into a more concentrated one.

osseous; osseus (ŏs′ê-ûs): bony.

osteodermia (ŏs′tē-ō-dûr′mē-ă): a condition characterized by bony formations in the skin.

osteology (ŏs-tē-ŏl′ă-jē): science of the anatomy, structure, and function of bones.

O-P

otoplasty (ŏ′tō-plăs-tē): plastic surgery of the external ear.

ounce (oùns): a unit of measure of weight; one sixteenth of a pound.

outcrop (aùt′krŏp): in cosmetology, a new growth of hair.

outer ear (aùt′ĕr-ēr): the flared outer portion of the ear.

outer perimeter (aùt′ĕr pĕ-rĭm′ĭ-tĕr): in cosmetology, the outer area of the hair length.

outline (aùt′līn): the line that defines a shape; the boundary of a figure or a body; the defining of the eyes or lips by use of a cosmetic pencil.

outmoded (aùt-mō′dĭd): outdated; no longer in fashion.

outside curve (aùt′sīd kûrv): the convex, curving outward curve in which hair may be cut.

outside design line (aùt′sīd dĕ-zīn′ līn): the nape and face framing design of a hairstyle.

outside movement (aùt′sīd mo͞ov′mênt): the volume, height or mass of hair which creates the outer silhouette of the hairstyle.

oval (ō′vâl): egg-shaped; shaped like an elipse; something having an oval shape; oval facial type.

oval design (ō′vâl dê-zīn′): a hair design shaped like an elipse; a hair design having an oval shape.

overdirected (ō′vĕr-dĭ-rĕk′tĕd): in excess of the normal amount of direction.

overgrowth (ō′vĕr-grōth): excessive or abnormal growth.

overhydration (ō′vĕr-hī-drā′shûn): the presence of excess fluids in the tissues of the body.

overlap (ō-vĕr-lăp′): to extend over and cover a part of something; when tint or lightener is allowed to run onto the previously tinted or lightened hair during application.

overlapping (ō′vĕr-lăp′ĭng): in cosmetology, applying a chemical solution, such as tint or lightener, beyond the limits of the new growth of hair.

overlapping curl (ō′vĕr-lăp′ĭng kûrl): a pincurl which partially covers its adjacent curl.

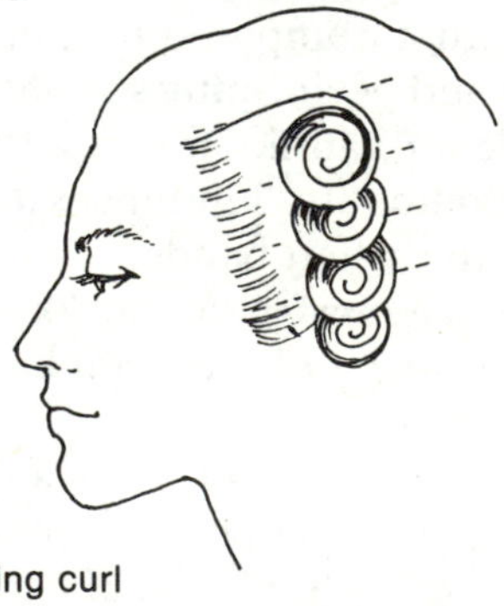

overlapping curl

overporosity (ō′vĕr-pô-rŏs′ĭ-tē): excessive ability of the hair to absorb moisture.

overprocessing (ō′vĕr-prŏs′ĕs-ĭng): overexposure of the hair to the chemical action of the wave solution, usually resulting in weakened or damaged hair.

ovular (ō'vû-lẽr): egg-like in shape; pertaining to the ovum, or egg.

o/w: abbreviation for oil in water.

o/w—oil in water

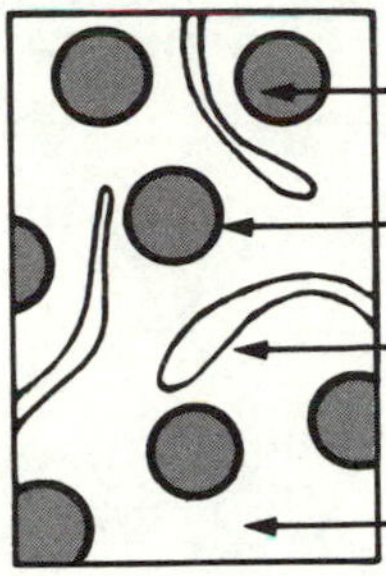

oxidation (ŏk-sĭ-dā'shûn): the act of combining or causing an element or compound to combine with oxygen; the loss of an electron in a chemical reaction.

oxidation dye (ŏk-sĭ-dā'shûn dī): aniline derivative dye; hair tint.

oxide (ŏk'sīd): a compound of oxygen with another element or radical.

oxidize (ŏk'sĭ-dīz): to combine or to cause an element or radical to combine with oxygen.

oxidizing agent (ŏk'sĭ-dīz'ĭng ā'jênt): a substance that releases oxygen, causing a chemical reaction; an example is hydrogen peroxide.

oxygen (ŏk'sĭ-jĭn): a gaseous element, essential to animal and plant life.

oxygenation (ŏk'sĭ-jĕ-nā'shûn): saturation with oxygen; to combine a substance with oxygen; the aeration of the blood with oxygen.

oxyhemoglobin (ŏk'sĭ-hē'mă-glō'bĭn): the combination of hemoglobin with oxygen.

oxymelanin (ŏk'sĭ-mĕl'ă-nĭn): a compound formed by a combination of an oxidizing agent with the dark melanin (color) pigments in the hair; generally found in the red to yellow shades.

oz: symbol for ounce.

ozone (ō'zōn): a pale blue gas which is another form of oxygen; used as a deodorizing and bleaching agent; a form of oxygen used as a disinfectant.

ozone spray (ō'zōn sprā): a fine mist produced by the combination of ozone and water.

P

pack (păk): a special cosmetic formula used to benefit the skin; see mask.

packet (păk′ĕt): a small package used for samples of skin and hair care products.

packing (păk′ĭng): heavy back combing, matted at the scalp and extended along the hair strand, giving the strand of hair almost a rigid quality.

pad (păd): a small, soft cushion-like item, usually of cotton or sponge; used to apply makeup, to remove nail polish, etc.

pageboy style (pāg′boy stīl): a hairstyle in which the ends of the hair are turned under.

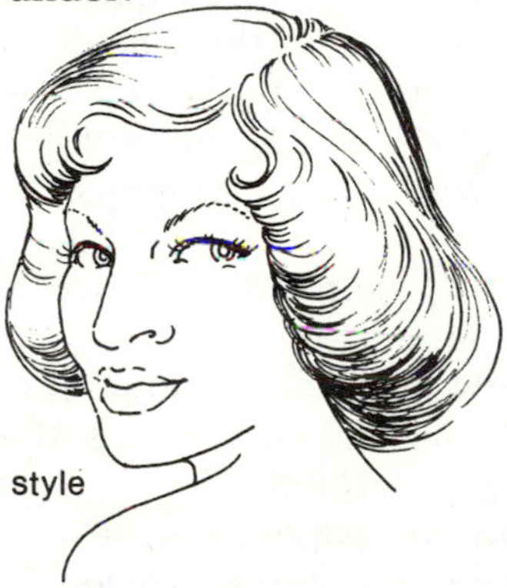

pageboy style

pain receptors (pān rē-sēp′tôrz): sensory nerve fibers that respond to pain-causing stimuli.

painting (pānt′ĭng): a technique in hair coloring in which the hair is darkened or lightened in thin strands with a brush.

palate (păl′ĕt): the roof of the mouth and the floor of the nose.

palatine (păl′ă-tĭn): referring to the roof of the mouth or palate.

palatine bones (păl′ă-tĭn bōnz): bones situated at the back part of the nasal fossae.

pale (pāl): deficient in color; light shade of any color; lacking brightness.

palette (păl′ĕt): a thin board with a hole for the thumb upon which the artist places an assortment of paint colors; the selection of colors for an individual.

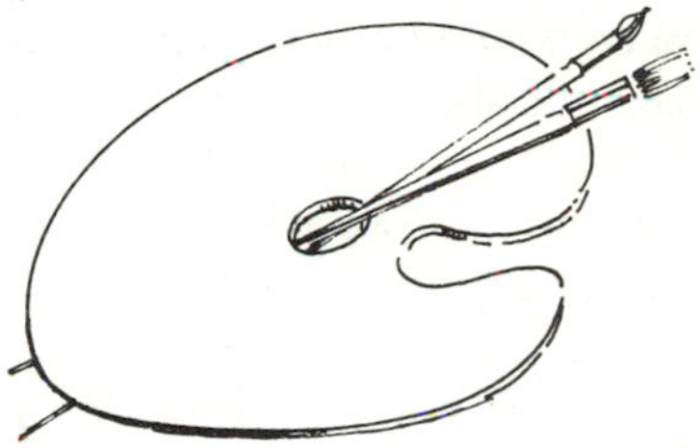

palette

palid (păl′ĭd): weak and lacking color.

pallor (păl′ĕr): paleness; deficiency of color, especially of the face.

palm (päm): the inner surface of the hand between the wrist and base of the fingers.

palmar (päl′mĕr): of or pertaining to the palm or hollow of the hand.

palmar arch (päl′mĕr ärch): the branches of arteries in the palm which supply blood to the bones, joints, muscles and skin of the palm of the hand and fingers.

palmar friction (päl′mĕr frĭk′shûn): a massage movement using the palm of the hand to apply pressure and a rubbing movement over underlying structures.

O-P

palmar kneading (päl′mẽr nēd′ĭng): a massage movement in which the flesh is grasped with palms and fingers, squeezed and released.

palmar manus (päl′mẽr măn′ûs): the palm of the hand.

palmar rotation (päl′mẽr rō-tā′shûn): a massage movement in which the palms are moved in a circle over underlying tissues.

palmar stroking (päl′mẽr strōk′ing): a massage movement in which the palms are used to stroke large areas of the skin; also called effleurage.

palm oil (päm oyl): palm butter; oil obtained from the fruit and seeds of the palm tree; used in soaps and lubricants.

palpebra (păl-pē′bră); pl., **palpebrae** (brē): the eyelid or eyelids.

palpebral artery (păl′pĕ-brâl är′tĭr-ē): the lateral artery that supplies blood to the upper and lower eyelids.

O-P

palpebral nerve, inferior (păl′pĕ-brâl nûrv): nerve that receives stimuli from the lower eyelid.

palpebral nerve, superior (păl′pĕ brâl nûrv): nerve that receives stimuli from the upper eyelid.

palpebrarum (păl-pĕ-brā′rŭm): of or pertaining to the eyelids.

panacea (păn-ă-sē′ă): a remedy that is claimed to be curative for all diseases; a universal remedy; a cure-all.

pancreas (păn′krē-ûs): a gland located in the abdomen that secretes an enzyme that digests proteins, fats, carbohydrates, and the hormone insulin.

panel (păn′′l): in hairdressing, the area between two parallel partings.

panhidrosis (păn′hĭ-drō′sis): generalized perspiration.

papain (pă-pā′ĭn): enzyme from the juice of papaya; used as a digestant and in some facial preparations.

papaya (pă-păy′ŭh): a fruit from the carico papaya tree from which papain is extracted; used in skin care preparations.

paper curl (pā′pẽr kûrl): a curl rolled up on a stick, encased in a triangle of special paper and pressed with a warm iron.

paper curling (pā′pẽr kûrl′ĭng): producing curls by dividing hair into strands which are formed into flat circle curls, covered with folded paper and heated by a pressing iron.

papilla (pă-pĭl′ă); pl., **papillae** (-ē): a small cone-shaped projecting body part.

papilla, hair (pă-pĭl′ă, hâr): a small, cone-shaped elevation at the bottom of the hair follicle in the dermis.

papillary (păp′ĭ-lẽr-ē): relating to, resembling, or provided with papillae.

papillary layer (păp′ĭ-lẽr-ē lā′ẽr): the outer layer of the dermis.

papilloma (păp-ĭ-lō′mă); pl., **papillomata** (păp-ĭ-lō′mă-tă): an epithelial tumor formed by hypertrophy of the papillae of the skin.

papular (păp′û-lẽr): characterized by papules.

papule (păp′ûl): a pimple; a small circumscribed elevation on the skin containing no fluid.

papulosis (păp-û-lō′sĭs): a condition involving multiple papules.

papulous (păp′û-lûs): covered with papulae or pimples.

para (pă′ră): a prefix denoting alongside of; beyond; beside; against or near; see paraphenylenediamine.

parabens (păr′ă-bēns): parabens (methyl-, propyl-, and parahydroxybenzoate) are preservatives that are the most commonly used in cosmetics; they are safe to use, nonpoisonous, and nonirritating.

paradye (păr′ă-dī): an aniline derivative hair tint.

paraffin (păr′ă-fĭn): a white mineral wax consisting of hydrocarbons and extracted from petroleum; used in hair removal products and in some types of facial masks.

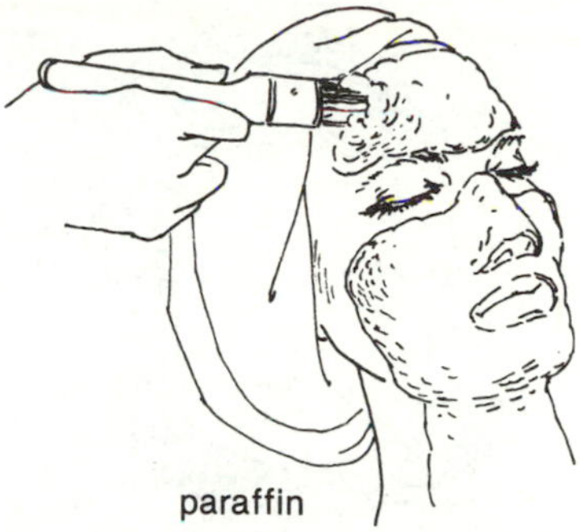
paraffin

paraffin wax mask (păr′ă-fĭn wăx măsk): a specially prepared facial mask containing paraffin and other beneficial ingredients.

parallel (păr′ă-lĕl): extending, as two lines, in the same direction and maintaining a constant distance apart.

paralysis (pă-răl′ĭ-sĭs): loss of muscle function or of sensation through injury to or disease of the nerves or neurons.

para-phenylene-diamine (păr′ă-fēn-′ĭ-lēn-dī-ăm′ĭn): an aniline derivative used in hair tinting.

parasite (păra′ă-sīt): a vegetable or animal organism which lives in or on another organism and draws its nourishment from that organism.

parasitic (păr-ă-sĭt′ĭk): pertaining to parasites.

parasitical (păr-ă-sĭt′ĭ-kôl): pertaining to living organisms which live upon or within some other living being.

parathyroid (păr-ă-thī′royd): an endocrine gland located near the thyroid.

para tint (păr′a tĭnt): a tint made from an aniline derivative.

para-toluene-diamine (păr′ă-tŏl′ū-ĕn-dī-ăm′ĭn): a variety of aniline derivative dyes commonly used in preparations compounded to provide red and blond tones.

parietal (pă-rī′ĕ-tâl): pertaining to the wall of a cavity; a bone at the side of the head.

parietal artery (pă-rī′ĕ-tâl är′tĭr-ē): the artery that supplies blood to the side and crown of the head.

paronychia (păr-ô-nĭk′ē-ă): felon; an inflammation of the tissues surrounding the nail.

parotid (pă-rŏt′ĭd): near the ear; a gland near the ear.

parsley oil (pärs′lē oyl): oil obtained from the ripe seeds of the herb of the parsley family; used as a fragrance and a preservative.

part (pärt): a line dividing the hair to the scalp.

part base (pärt bās): the part or line in the hair toward which the hair is rolled or curled.

parting silk (pär′tĭng sĭlk): strong, fine (white or flesh-colored) silk; used in wiggery for making drawn-through partings.

passive (păs′ĭv): inactive; inert; acted upon by causes from without.

passive massage (păs′ĭv mă-săzh′): a massage movement in which the part (hand, foot, finger, toe) is bent up, down or forward to flex the joints.

pastel (păs-tĕl′): a soft, delicate color or tint.

paste on (pāst ŏn): any item such as a jewel, flower, artificial lash or nail that can be glued or pasted on the skin, hair or nails as a decoration.

pat (păt): to tap lightly; to apply makeup by pressing lightly to the skin.

patch (păch): a blotch; an irregular spot or area.

patch test (păch tĕst): test for determining allergy to a specific substance;

O-P

made by applying a small amount of the substance to the skin and observing the reaction.

pate (pāt): top of the head.

patella (pă-tĕl′ă): the kneecap.

pathogenesis (păth-ô-jĕn′ĕ-sĭs): the origin of and course of development of a disease.

pathogenic (păth-ô-jĕn′ĭk): causing disease; disease-producing.

pathological (păth′ă-lŏj′ĭ-kâl): relating to pathology; morbid; diseased; due to disease.

pathology (pă-thŏl′ă-jē): the science which treats of modifications of the functions and changes in structure caused by disease.

pattern (păt′ẽrn): in hairstyling, a diagram showing where and in which direction hair rollers or pincurls are placed in order to achieve the finished style; a head shape or design from which a hairpiece is constructed.

O-P

peak (pēk): a point formed by the hair growth at the center of the forehead; also called a widow's peak, named after a bonnet styled with a center point at the forehead; worn by widows in the 19th century.

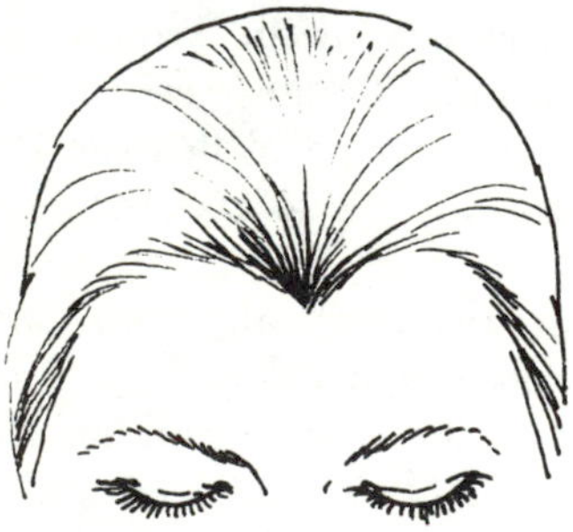

peak

peanut oil (pē′nŭt oyl): arachis oil; oil obtained from the seeds of the peanut; used in many cosmetics such as hair preparations, face creams, shampoos, and emollients.

pear-shaped face (pâr-shāpt fās): a facial structure characterized by a wide jaw and a narrow forehead.

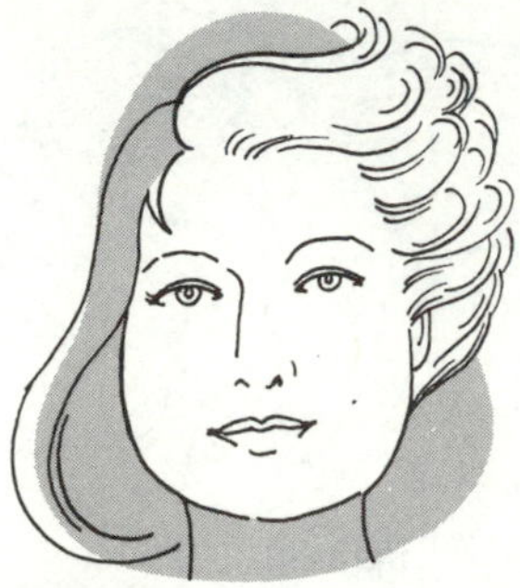

pear-shaped face

pectin (pĕk′tĭn): a carbohydrate contained in the cell walls of some fruits and vegetables, such as lemons, apples, and carrots, and used as the basis of gels; a substance used in facial masks.

pectoralis (pĕk-tô-rā′lĭs): a muscle of the chest.

pectoralis major (pĕk-tô-rā′lĭs mā′jôr): the muscle that flexes and rotates the arm forward and inward.

pectoralis minor (pĕk-tô-rā′lĭs mī′nôr): the muscle that draws the shoulder forward and rotates the scapula (shoulder blade) downward.

pectoral nerve (pĕk′tă-rûl nûrv): lateral pectoral nerve; the nerve that stimulates the pectoralis major and minor.

pedi (pĕd′ē): pertaining to the feet.

pedicare (pĕd-ĭ-kâr): care of the feet.

pediculosis (pĕ-dĭk-û-lō′sĭs): a skin disease caused by infestation of lice.

pediculosis capitis (pĕ-dĭk-û-lō′sĭs kăp′ĭ-tĭs): infestation of the hair of the head with lice.

pediculous (pĕ-dĭk′û-lûs): infested by pediculi; lousy.

pedicure (pĕd′ĭ-kûr): the care of the feet and toenails.

peel (pēl): a technique in facial treatments in which a product is applied to the face to remove dead cells from the surface of the skin.

peeling treatment (pēl′ĭng trēt′mênt): a facial treatment using a chemical agent to remove the surface layer of skin, the epidermis, to eliminate lines and acne scars.

pelada (pĕ-lă′dă): a disease of the hair causing circumscribed patches of baldness; alopecia areata.

pelage (pĕl′ĭdj): the hair covering of the body of humans and animals.

pellagra (pĕ-lăg′ră): a syndrome due to niacin deficiency; characterized by dermititis, and in later stages, by nervous and mental disorders.

pencil sharpener (pĕn′sĭl shärp′ĕn-ẽr): a tool designed to sharpen writing pencils or makeup pencils.

pencils, makeup (pĕn′sĭls, māk′ŭp): pencils manufactured with a wide assortment of colored leads; used for making up the eyes, lips and for facial contouring.

penetrate (pĕn′ĕ-trāt): to pass into or through; to enter by overcoming resistance.

penetrating tint (pĕn′ĕ-trāt-ĭng tĭnt): a tint which penetrates into the cortex and deposits color permanently.

penetration (pĕn-ĕ-trā′shûn): act or power of penetrating.

pep bag (pĕp băg): a trade term which designates a product which speeds up the action of a lightener and hydrogen peroxide.

peppermint oil (pĕp′ẽr-mĭnt′ oyl): an aromatic plant of the mint family whose leaves produce an oil used in flavorings, toothpaste, mouthwashes and various lotions.

pepsin (pĕp′sĭn): an enzyme which digests protein.

peptide (pĕp′tīd): a compound of two or more amino acids containing one or more peptide groups; continuous filaments in the case of fiber protein or keratin.

peptide bond (pĕp′tīd bŏnd): the joining together of amino acids.

peptones (pĕp′tōnz): any of various water-soluble products of partial hydrolysis of proteins.

per (pẽr): a prefix denoting through; throughout; by; for.

percussion (pẽr-kûsh′ûn): a form of massage consisting of repeated light blows or taps of varying force.

perforate (pẽr′fă-rāt): to pierce with holes.

perfume (pẽr′fūm): a fragrant substance, usually a volatile liquid, which emits a pleasant odor or scent.

peri (pĕr′ĭ-): a prefix denoting about; near; around.

pericardium (pĕr-ĭ-kär′dē-ûm): the membranous sac around the heart.

perimeter (pĕ-rĭm′ĭ-tẽr): the outer line of a hairstyle; the silhouette line.

perimysium (pĕr-ĭ-mĭs′ē-ûm): the sheath that encases bundles of muscle fibers.

perionychium (pĕr′ē-ô-nĭk′-ē-ûm): the epidermis surrounding a nail.

periosteum (pĕr-ē-ŏs′tē-ûm): the fibrous membrane covering the surface of the bones.

peripheral nervous system (pĕ-rĭf′ē-râl nûr′vûs sĭs′tĕm): system of nerves and ganglia that connect the peripheral parts of the body to the central nervous system; it has both sensory nerves and motor nerves.

periphery (pĕ-rĭf′ẽr-ē): the part of the

body away from the center; the outer part or surface.

peristalsis (pĕr-ĭ-stăl′sĭs): muscular movements of the digestive tract.

periwig (pĕr′ĭ-wĭg): an old fashioned name for a wig.

perm (pûrm): a permanent wave or a straightening treatment.

permalite (pûr′mă-līt): a light for drying the permanent wave after the wave has been set.

permanent (pûr′mă-nĕnt): lasting; enduring; not changing; see permanent wave.

permanent, cold wave (pûr′mă-nĕnt, kōld wāv): a system of permanent waving employing chemicals rather than heat.

permanent color (pûr′mă-nĕnt kŭl′ĕr): permanent tint; a hair color which is enduring and remains in the hair until the new growth of hair.

O-P

perm cap (pûrm kăp): a plastic head covering used during the processing time of a permanent wave to help speed up the action of the product being used.

permeable (pûr′mē-ă-b'l): permitting the passage of liquids.

perm rod (pûrm rŏd): a cylindrical or concave rod used for winding the hair for permanent waves.

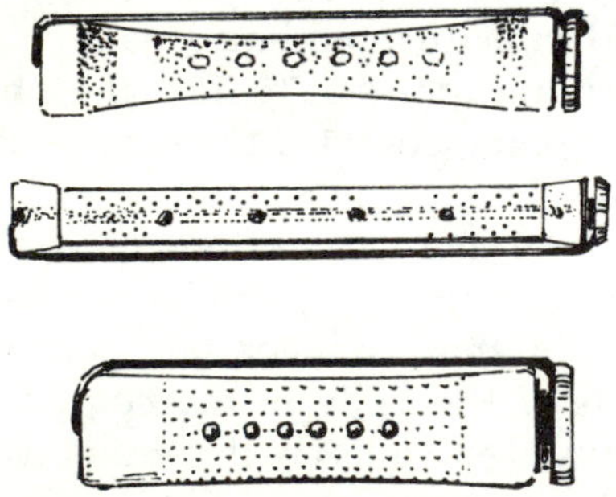

perm rods

peroneal brevis (pĕr-ô-nē′âl brĕ′vĭs): muscle that allows the foot to be flexed downward and outward.

peroneal longus (pĕr-ô-nē′âl lŏng′ûs): muscle that flexes the foot and supports the arches.

peroneal muscle (pĕr-ô-nē′âl mŭs′'l): muscle located on the outer portion of the lower leg which assists in turning the foot downward and outward.

peroneal nerve (pĕr-ô-nē′âl nûrv): nerve that receives stimuli from the skin of the lateral aspect of the leg.

peroxide (pẽr-ŏk′sīd): common term for hydrogen peroxide; see hydrogen peroxide.

peroxometer (pẽr-ŏks-ŏm′ē-tẽr): a device which measures the strength of hydrogen peroxide.

perpendicular (pẽr-pĕn-dĭk′û-lăr): being perfectly upright; being at right angles to a given line on a plane.

personality (pẽr-sûn-âl′ĭ-tē): the distinctive characteristics or qualities of a person.

perspiration (pẽr-spĭ-rā′shûn): sweat; the fluid excreted from the sudoriferous glands of the skin.

perspire (pẽr-spīr′): to emit perspiration from the pores of the skin; to sweat.

peruke (pĕ-rōōk′): a wig popular from the 17th-19th century.

peruke

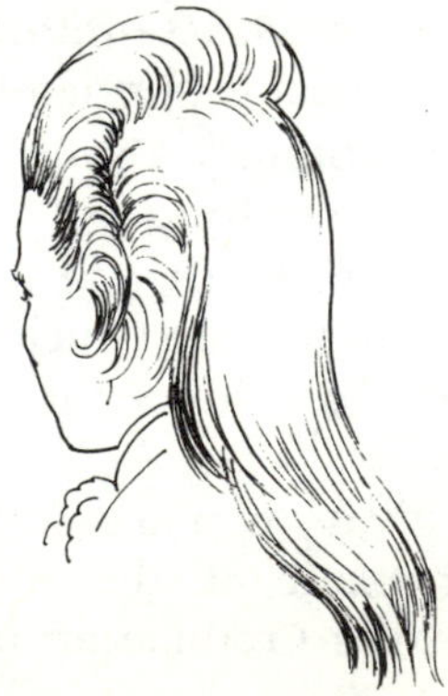

peruquer; perukier (pĕr-o͞ok′ĕr): a wig maker.

petrissage (pā-trĭ-säzh′): the kneading movement in massage.

petrolatum (pĕt-rô-lā′tûm): petroleum jelly; vaseline; a purified, yellow mixture of semisolid hydrocarbons obtained from petroleum.

petroleum (pĕ-trô′lē-ûm): an oily liquid coming from the earth and consisting of a mixture of hydrocarbons.

pH: symbol for hydronium-ion concentration in water; the relative degree of acidity or alkalinity; pH values are arranged on a scale from 1 to 14; above 7, represents alkalinity, below 7, represents acidity.

phalanx (fā′lănks); pl., **phalanges** (fă-lăn′-jēz): one of the bones of the fingers or toes.

pharmacologist (fär-mă-kŏl′ă-jĭst): one versed in the science of the nature and properties of drugs.

pharynx (făr′ĭnks): the upper portion of the digestive tube, behind the nose and mouth.

phenol (fē′nōl): carbolic acid; caustic poison; in dilute solution is used as an antiseptic and disinfectant.

pH number (pē-āch nŭm′bĕr): also pH factor a measure of the degree of acidity or alkalinity of a solution.

phoresis (fôr-ĕ′sĭs): a combining form meaning transmission; the process of introducing solutions into tissues through the skin by use of galvanic current.

phosphoric (fŏs-fôr′ĭk): pertaining to or derived from phosphorus.

phosphorous (fŏs′fôr-ûs): an element found in the bones, muscles and nerves; a mineral element required in the diet of humans.

photodermatitis (fō′tō-dĕr mă-tī′tĭs): a skin condition caused by exposure to light, cosmetics, drugs or irritants.

pH paper (pH pā′pĕr): a special type of paper used to test the pH factor in a product; the paper changes color according to the degree of acidity or alkalinity, thus indicating its pH factor.

pH pencil (pH pĕn′sĭl): a pencil used to indicate the degree of acidity or alkalinity of a solution or product.

pH scale (pH skāl): scale numbered from 0 to 14; used to indicate the degree of acidity or alkalinity of a solution; 7.0 indicates neutral, below 7 indicates acid and above 7 indicates alkaline.

phyma (fī′mă); pl., **phymata** (fī′mă-tă): a circumscribed swelling on the skin, larger than a tubercle.

physi; physio (fĭz′ē; fĭz′ē-ō): combining form indicating relationship to nature.

physical (fĭz′ĭ-kâl): relating to the body, as distinguished from the mind.

physical change (fĭz′ĭ-kâl chānj): altering or changing the form or appearance of a substance without changing its chemical composition.

physics (fĭz′ĭks): the branch of science that deals with matter, energy, motion, light, heat, electricity, sound, mechanics and their interactions.

physiognomical haircutting (fĭz-ē-ŏg-nŏ′mĭ-kâl hâr′kŭt-ĭng): cutting and styling hair in accordance with the facial features of the client.

physiognomy (fĭz′ē-ŏg′nă-mē): the physical appearance of a person; especially his or her facial features thought to reveal certain traits or characteristics.

physiological (fĭz-ē-ă-lŏj′ĭ-kâl): of or relating to the functions of an organism and its parts during life.

physiology (fĭz-ē-ŏl′ă-jē): the science of

the function of living things and their parts.

physiotherapy (fĭz′ē-ō-thĕr′ă-pē): the use of physical means, such as light, heat, air, water and exercise, in the treatment of diseases and injuries.

phytotherapy (fī′tō-thĕr-ă-pē): treatment by use of plants; herbal therapy.

picealis (pĭs-ê-ă′lĭs): a type of acne caused by an allergy to tar products.

picric acid (pĭk′rĭk ăs′ĭd): an organic acid used as an antiseptic.

pie shape (pī shāp): the triangular shape of the subsections used when setting hair with conoid rollers, and for curls when it is necessary to avoid splits in the finished style.

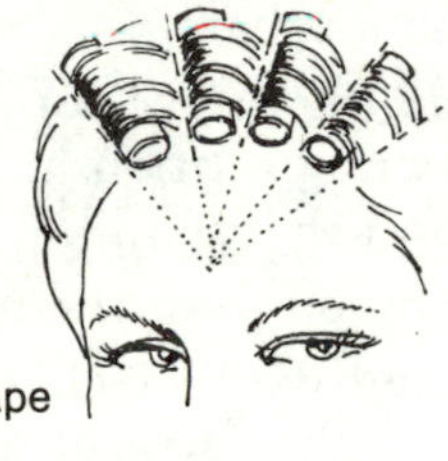

pie shape

piggyback (pĭg′ê-băk′): the double rod method used in perming long hair; two rods are used for a strand of hair.

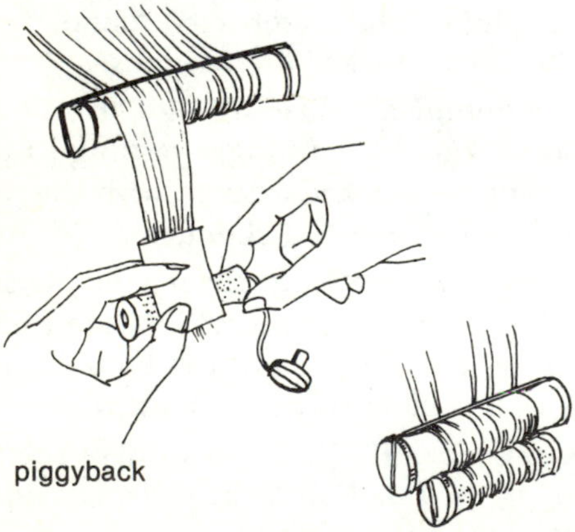

piggyback

O-P

pigment (pĭg′mênt): any organic coloring matter; as that of the red blood cells, of the hair, skin, iris, etc.

pigmentary (pĭg′mĕn-tĕr-ē): pertaining to producing or containing pigment.

pigmentation (pĭg′mĕn-tā′shûn): the deposition of pigment in the skin or tissues.

pileous (pī′lē-ûs, pĭl′ē-ûs): pertaining to hair; hairy.

pili; pilar (pī-lĕ; pī′lẽr): hair; related to hair.

piliation (pĭ-lē-ā′shûn): the formation and production of hair.

pili incarnati (pī′lĕ ĭn-kär-nā′tī): ingrown hairs.

pili multigemini (pī′lĕ mŭl′tĭ-jĭm′ĭ-nī): several hairs growing from a single follicle opening.

pili tactiles (pī′lĕ tăk′tĭ-lēz): tactile hairs; associated with the sense of touch.

pili torti (pī′lĕ tôr′tī): a congenital deformity of the hair, characterized by short, broken hairs that resemble stubble.

pilocarpine (pī-lô-kär′pĭn; -pēn): an alkaloid obtained from the leaves of pilocarpus; a syrupy liquid; stimulates the tissues and increases secretion of the glands.

piloerection (pī′lô-ĭ-rĕk′shûn): the condition known as gooseflesh, characterized by erection of hair and a bump around the follicle.

pilomotor (pī-lô-mō′tẽr): causing movement of the hair; as the pilomotor muscles.

pilomotor muscle (pī-lô-mō′tẽr mŭs′′l): the arrector pili muscle.

pilomotor nerve (pi′lo-mō′ter nûrv): a nerve causing contraction of one of the arrectores pilorum muscles.

pilomotor reflex (pī-lô-mō′tẽr rē′flĕks): erection of hairs of the skin (gooseflesh) as a response to cold or emotional stimuli.

pilonidal (pī′lō-nī′dāl): pertaining to hair growing within a cyst.

pilose (pī′lōs): covered with hair; hairy.

pilosebaceous (pī′lō-sĕ-bā′shûs): pertaining to the hair follicles and the sebaceous glands.

pilosis (pī-lō′sĭs): abnormal or excessive development of hair.

pilosity (pī-lŏs′ĭ-tē): the state of being pilose or hairy.

pilous gland (pī′lûs glănd): the sebaceous gland of a hair follicle.

pilus (pī′lûs); pl., **pili** (-lī): a hair.

pilus cuniculatus (pī′lûs kû-nĭk-û-lā′tûs): a burrowing hair.

pilus incarnatus (pī′lûs ĭn-kär-nā′tûs): an ingrown hair.

pilus incarnatus recurvus (pī′lûs ĭn-kär-nā′tûs rĕ-kûr′vûs): caused by a curved hair re-entering the skin; ingrown hair.

pimple (pĭm′p'l): any small pointed elevation of the skin; a papule or small pustule.

pin (pĭn): a small curved device designed to hold the hair in place; bobpins; hairpins.

pincurl (pĭn′kûrl): a strand of hair combed smooth and wound into a circle with the ends on the inside of the curl; a flat curl.

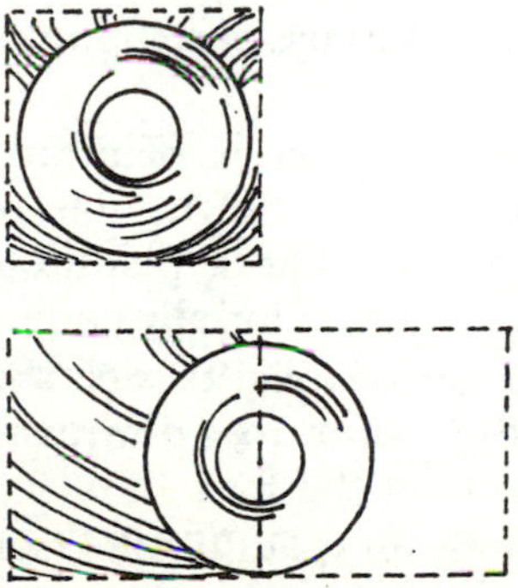

pincurl

pincurl base (pĭn′kûrl bās): the area of the scalp where a pincurl is secured; the base may be sectioned into a square, a slanted oblong, or an arc or C-shaped base.

pincurl direction (pĭn′kûrl dī-rĕk′shûn): the line in which a pincurl is moved or designed to move.

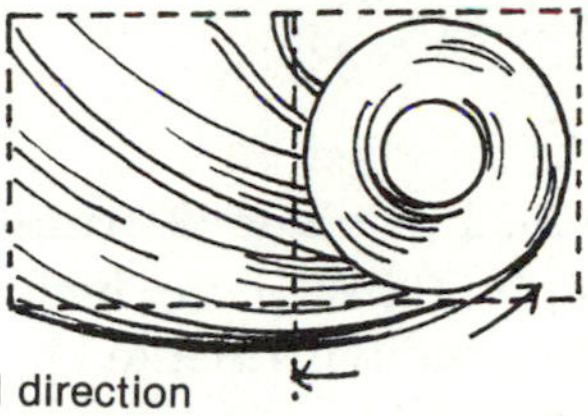

pincurl direction

pincurl foundation (pĭn′kûrl faùn-dā′shûn): the area at the scalp where the pincurl is secured; pincurl base.

pincurling (pĭn′kûrl-ĭng): the forming of circles or ringlets by winding the hair and fastening the circles in place with clips.

pincurl permanent wave (pĭn′kûrl pĕr′-mă-nênt wāv): a cold wave achieved by setting the hair in pincurls instead of rollers.

pincurl stem (pĭn′kûrl stĕm): the part of the pincurl between the base and the first arc of the circle of hair.

pincurl wave (pĭn′kûrl wāv): the technique of alternating the direction of the rows of pincurls to form a wave when the hair is combed.

pineal body (pĭn′ē-âl bŏd′ē): a ductless gland attached to the brain.

pine tar (pīn tär): tar obtained from the wood of the palm tree; used in soaps, shampoos and medications for skin ailments.

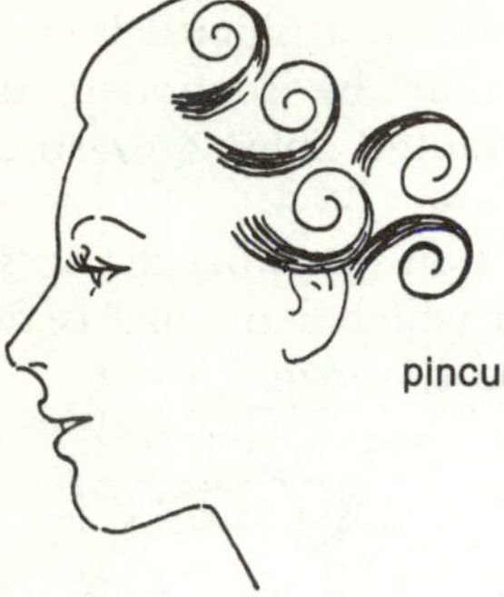

pink (pĭnk): a pale hue of crimson.

pinkeye (pĭnk′ī): an acute, highly contagious conjunctivitis marked by redness of the eyeball.

pinna (pĭn′ă): the external ear, exclusive of meatus.

pint (pīnt): a liquid or dry measure, equal to half a quart.

pipette (pī-pĕt′): a slender tube used for measuring liquids.

O-P

pisiform (pī′sĭ-fôrm): pea-shaped; a bone of the wrist.

pit (pĭt): a surface depression or hollow.

pith (pĭth): center; the marrow of the bones; the center of the hair.

pit scar (pĭt skär): a scar that heals with a hollow pit; usually caused by acne.

pituitary (pĭ-tū′ĭ-tĕr-ē): a ductless gland located at the base of the brain.

pityriasis (pĭt′ĭ-rī′ă-sĭs): dandruff; an inflammation of the skin characterized by the formation and flaking of fine, thin scales.

pityriasis capitis simplex (pĭt′ĭ-rī′ă-sĭs kăp′ĭ-tĭs sĭm′pleks′): a scalp inflammation marked by dry dandruff or thin scales.

pityriasis pilaris (pĭt′ĭ-rī′ă-sĭs pī-lâr′ĭs): a skin disorder characterized by an eruption of papules surrounding the hair follicles: each papule pierced by a hair and tipped with a horny plug or scale.

pityriasis steatoides (pĭt′ĭ-rī′ă-sĭs stē-ă-toy′dēz): a scalp inflammation marked by fatty type of dandruff; characterized by yellowish to brownish waxy scales or crusts on the scalp.

pityroid (pĭt′ĭ-royd): pertaining to a condition of the skin or scalp characterized by thin scales.

pityrosporum ovalli (pĭt′ĭ-rō-spō′rŭm ō-vā′lē): a species of fungus found on the skin or hair follicle and associated with infectious seborrheic dermatitis.

pivot point (pĭv′ŏt poynt): pivot hair shaping; the exact point from which the hair is directed in forming a curvature or shaping.

placental extract (plă-sĕn′tâl ĭk-străkt′): the nourishing substance surrounding an embryo or fetus; after birth; used in some facial preparations.

plait (plāt): to interweave strands of hair into an intricate pattern; to braid.

plankton extract (plānk′tŏn ĭk′străkt′): the microscopic animal and plant life found in the oceans and in fresh water; algae or seaweed; used in certain cosmetic preparations, usually in facial and body treatment preparations.

planta pedis (plăn′tă pēd′ĭs): the undersurface or sole of the foot.

plantar (plăn′tär): pertaining to the sole of the foot.

plantar arterial arch (plăn′tär är-tĭr′ē-âl ärch): the arch in the sole of the foot made by the lateral plantar artery and branch of the dorsalis pedis artery.

plantar flexion (plăn′tär flĕk′shûn): bending the foot or toes downward toward the sole of the foot.

plantar flexor (plăn′tär flĕk′sẽr): muscle that bends the foot downward.

plantar reflex (plăn′tär rē′flĕks): flexing of the toes in response to stroking massage movements on the outer sides of the soles.

plant extracts (plănt ĕk′străkts): organic substances extracted from leaves, roots and flowers of various plants for use in such products as perfumes and grooming aids.

plasma (plăz′mă): the fluid part of the blood and lymph.

plastic applicator (plăs′tĭk ăp′lĭ-kā-tēr): a squeeze bottle used for applying tints and lighteners.

plastic cap (plăs′tĭk kăp): a cap made of plastic employed as a head covering to help retain body heat during a number of cosmetology techniques, such as permanent waving and coloring.

plasticizer (plăs′tĭ-sī-zēr): a compound which keeps a substance soft and thick, as in nail polishes.

plastic surgeon (plăs′tĭk sûr′jûn): a surgeon who builds up or molds tissue and bones to repair physical defects.

plastic surgery (plăs′tĭk sûr′jēr-ē): surgical repair of defects or deformities.

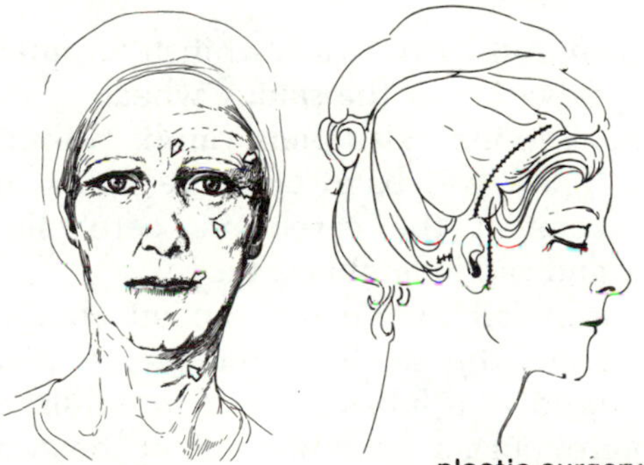

plastic surgery

platelets (plāt′lĕts): blood cells which aid in the forming of clots.

platinum (plăt′ĭ-nûm): a heavy steel-gray metal; the color resembling platinum; a silver-gray.

platinum blond (plăt′ĭ-nûm blŏnd): very light, almost white blond hair.

platysma (plă-tĭz′mă): a broad thin muscle of the neck.

pledget (plĕdj′ĕt): a compress or small, flat mass of absorbent cotton.

plexus (plĕk′sûs): a network of nerves or veins.

pliability (plī-ă-bĭl′ĭ-tē): flexibility.

pluck (plŭk): to pull with sudden force.

plume (plūm): a cluster of feathers or hair generally seen in showy headdresses.

plump (plŭmp): full, rounded; as a plump, full face or figure.

podiatrist (pō-dī′ă-trĭst): one who treats diseases of the feet.

point (poynt): a sharp end or apex; an abcess, the wall of which becomes thin and is about to break.

point knotting (poynt nŏt′ĭng): a method of attaching hair, in the formation of a hairpiece, which assures that only the points of the hair remain as part of the finished work.

point of distribution (poynt of dĭs-trĭ-bû′shûn): radial motion; the central point from which hair is distributed in a preplanned manner.

point of origin (poynt of ôr-ĭ′jĕn): in hairdressing, place where a motion starts or the beginning of a design.

points (poynts): wigpoints; headless nails used for attaching the wig foundation to the wooden block in order to assure a custom fit.

poison (poy′z'n): a substance which when taken internally is injurious to health or dangerous to life.

poisoning, blood (poy′z'n-ĭng, blŭd): septicemia; the invasion of pathogenic bacteria into the blood, causing infection.

poison ivy (poy′z'n ī′vē): a climbing plant

O-P

which produces an irritating oil that may cause an intensely itching skin rash.

poisonous (poy′z'n-ûs): having the quality or effects of poison.

polarity (pō-lăr′ĭ-tē): the property of having two opposite poles, as that possessed by a magnet or galvanic current.

pole (pōl): an electrical terminal.

poliosis (pō-lē-ō′sĭs): a condition characterized by absence of pigment in the hair.

polish (pŏl′ĭsh): nail enamel formulated to strengthen, protect and beautify the nails; clear or colored lacquer.

polish dryer (pŏl′ĭsh drī′ĕr): a chemical preparation which speeds the drying process of freshly applied nail polish.

polish remover (pŏl′ĭsh rē-mōōv′ĕr): a product which is used to dissolve and remove nail polish.

O-P

polish thinner (pŏl′ĭsh thĭn′ĕr): a chemical preparation formulated to thin nail polish that has become too thick.

pollex (pŏl′ĕks): the thumb.

polychromatic (pŏl′ē-krō-măt′ĭk): having many colors.

polyglycerol (pŏl′ē-glĭs′ĕr-ōl′): a substance prepared from fats, oils and esters; derived from vegetables such as corn soy beans and from peanuts, palm, sesame, tallow and pure lard.

polymer (pŏl′ē-mĕr): substance formed by combining many small molecules (monomers) usually in a long chain-like structure; examples are hair, plastic, rubber, and human tissue.

polyp (pŏl′ĭp): a smooth growth extending from the surface of the skin; polyps may also grow within the body.

polypeptide bonds (pŏl′ē-pĕp′tīd bŏnz): bonds that link peptide chains together to form protein.

polypeptide chain (pŏl′ē-pĕp′tīd chān): amino acid chains joined together by peptide bonds; the prefix "poly" meaning many.

polyunsaturated (pŏl-ē-ŭn-săch′ă-rā-tĭd): pertaining to any of a class of fats having more than two double bonds in its molecule, or to fats used in diets to reduce blood cholesterol.

pomade (pō-măd′; -mäd′): a perfumed ointment for the hair or scalp.

pompadour (pŏm′pă-dôr): a hairstyle that is combed up from the forehead; a style using a pad or roller to create a puffed arrangement of the hair above the forehead.

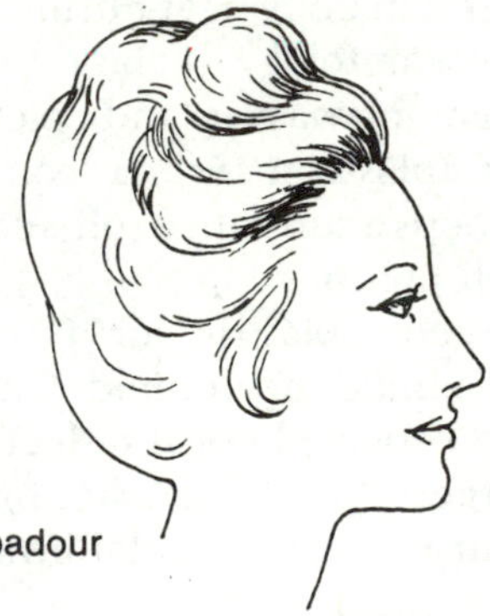

pompadour

pomphus (pŏm′fûs): a whitish or pinkish elevation of the skin; a wheal.

pons (pŏnz): also **pons varolii** (vă-rō′lē-ī): a broad band of nerve fibers that connect the cerebrum, cerebellum, and medulla oblongata.

poppy oil (pop′ē oyl): an oil obtained from the seeds of the poppy plant; used as a lubricant and in emulsions.

pore (pôr): a small opening of the sweat glands of the skin.

porosity (pô-rŏs′ĭ-tē): ability of the hair to absorb moisture.

porous (pô′rûs): full of pores.

porous hair (pô′rûs hâr): hair which is characterized by lifted cuticle scales which allow faster absorption of moisture or chemicals into the hair.

portable (pôr′tă-b'l): easily carried or moved from one place to another.

portable hair dryer (pôr′tă-b'l hâr drī′ẽr): a compact hair dryer in a case that can be carried from place to place.

positive (pōz′ĭ-tĭv): affirmative; not negative; the presence of abnormal conditions; having a relative high potential in electricity.

positive pole, P or + (pŏz′ĭ-tĭv pōl): the pole from which positive electricity flows.

positive skin test (pŏz′ĭ-tĭv skĭn tĕst): direct proof that the substance involved in a test is hostile to the body; having a reaction to a skin test for allergy; showing signs of redness, swelling, irritation.

positive terminal (pŏz′ĭ-tĭv tẽr′mĭ-nâl): the end of a conducting circuit manifesting acid reaction; the carbon plate in a battery.

post (pōst): a prefix denoting back; after.

posterior (pŏs-tēr′ē-ẽr): situated behind; coming after or behind.

posterior auricular artery (pŏs-tēr′ē-ẽr ô-rĭk′û-lẽr är′tĭr-ē): the artery that supplies blood to the scalp.

posterior auricularis (pŏs-tēr′ē-ẽr ô-rĭk-û-lăr′ĭs): muscle that draws the ear backward.

posterior auricular nerve (pŏs-tēr′ē-ẽr ô-rĭk′û-lẽr nûrv): nerve that supplies stimuli to muscles in the posterior surface of the ear.

posterior cerebral artery (pŏs-tēr′ē-ẽr sĕ-rē′brâl är′tẽr-ē): artery that supplies blood to the cortex and the temporal and occipital bones.

posterior cutaneous nerve (pŏs-tēr′ē-ẽr kû-tā′nē-ûs nûrv): nerve that stimulates the skin of the posterior aspect of the forearm.

posterior interosseous artery (pŏs-tēr′ē-ẽr ĭn-tẽr-ŏs′ē-ûs är′tĭr-ē): artery that supplies blood to the muscles and skin of the forearm.

posterior tibial artery (pŏs-tēr′ē-ẽr tĭb′ē-âl är′tĭr-ē): artery that supplies blood to ankles and dorsum of the foot.

postiche (pôs-tēsh′): artificial hairpiece; curls, braids, or other extra hairpiece used in creating coiffures.

posticheur (pô-stēsh-ūr′): one who designs and dresses hairpieces.

postnasal (pōst-nā′zâl): situated behind the nose.

posture (pŏs′tūr): the position or carriage of the body when standing, sitting, walking or posing.

potassium (pô-tăs′ē-ûm): an element, the salts of which are used in medicine; an essential mineral found in vegetables and fruits and necessary to the health of the skin; potassium and sodium regulate the water balance within the body.

potassium bromate (pô-tăs′ē-ûm brō′-māt): a metallic element of the alkali group; used in medicines as a sedative.

potassium carbonate (pô-tăs′ē-ûm kär′-bă-nāt): a white salt which forms a highly alkaline solution; used to make soap and other cleansing products.

potassium chloride (pô-tăs′ē-ûm klôr′īd): a colorless, crystalline salt; used as a buffer in solid perfumes and in some eye washes.

potassium hydroxide (pô-tăs′ē-ûm hī-drŏk′sīd): a powerful alkali, used in the manufacture of soft soaps.

potassium permanganate (pô-tăs′ē-ûm pẽr-măn′gă-nāt): a salt of permanganate acid, used as an antiseptic and deodorant.

potential (pō-tĕn′shâl): indicating possibility of power; tension in an electrical source enabling it to do work under suitable conditions.

poultice (pōl′tĭs): a soft mass of some substance mixed with water, sometimes medicated; applied to the skin to supply heat and moisture.

powder (paů′dẽr): a finely ground substance forming a mass of loose particles; used as a cosmetic and in some medicines.

powder base (paů′dẽr bās): term sometimes used to describe a foundation cream or lotion that is applied to the face before powder.

powder bleach (paů′dẽr blēch): a strong fast-acting bleach in powdered form; used for off-the-head lightening.

powder dry shampoo (paů′dẽr drī shăm-pōō′): a substance composed of a mixture of orris root, borax, etc., which is employed to clean hair without using soap or water.

O-P

powder puff (paů′dẽr pŭf): a small fluffy circle or square of cotton, sponge or silk used to apply powder.

prebleaching (prē-blēch′ing): see prelightening.

precaution (prē-kô′shûn): a written or verbal warning whose purpose is to prevent harm and to assure safety.

precipitate (prê-sĭp′ĭ-tāt): in chemistry, to cause a substance in a solution to settle in solid particles; to separate from solution or suspension by chemical or physical change.

precipitation (prê-sĭp-ĭ-tā′shûn): in chemistry, the process of separating the constituents of a solution by reagents or by mechanical means; the process of precipitating.

precision (prē-sĭzh′ûn): the state or quality of being accurate and precise; exactness.

predispose (prē-dĭs-pōz): to make susceptible; to render vulnerable to a disorder or disease.

predisposition (prē-dĭs-pă-zĭsh′ûn): a condition of special susceptibility to disease; allergy.

predisposition test (prē-dĭs-pă-zĭsh′ûn tĕst): see patch test.

prelightening (prē-lit′ĕn-ĭng): a decoloring process, preliminary to the application of toner.

preliminary (prê-lĭm′ĭ-nẽr-ē): introductory; preparatory.

premature (prē′mă-tūr′): happening, arriving, existing, or performed before the usual time.

premature canities (prē′mă-tūr′ kă-nĭsh′ē-ēz): premature graying of the hair.

prescribe (prê-scrīb′): to set or lay down, authoritatively, a course or a rule to be followed.

presenile (prē-sĕn′īl): prematurely old.

presoftener (prē-sŏf′′nẽr): a chemical solution applied to the hair in order to make easier the penetration of additional chemicals to the hair.

pressing (prĕs′ĭng): a temporary method of straightening overcurly hair with a heated comb or iron.

pressing irons (prĕs′ĭng ī′ûrns): an implement resembling a curling iron; used to straighten hair.

pressure receptors (prĕsh′ẽr rē-sĕp′tôrz): nerves supplying the skin that register pressure or touch; nerve fibers that respond to pressure.

prickle cell layer (prĭk′′l sĕl lā′ẽr): the layer of cells between the granular cell layer and the basal cell layer of the epidermis.

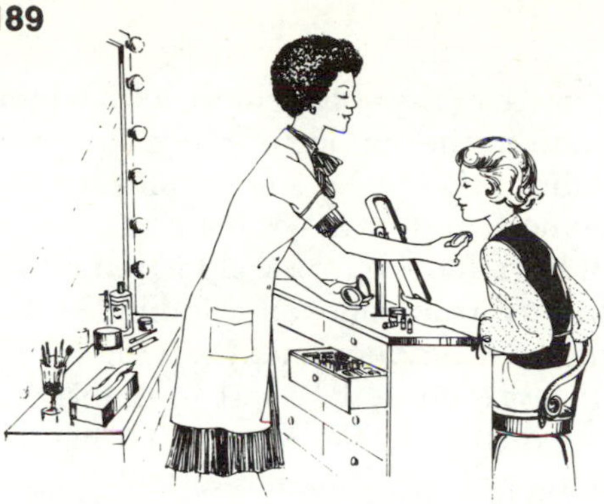

professional

prickly heat (prĭk′lē hēt): also called miliaria rubra; a cutaneous eruption of red vesicles accompanied by burning and itching; usually caused by overexposure to heat.

primary (prī′mă-rē): first; basic; fundamental; principal.

primary colors (prī′mă-rē kŭl′ẽrz): not obtained from a mixture; primary colors are red, yellow and blue.

primary hair (prī′mă-rē hâr): the baby-fine hair that is present over almost the entire smooth skin of the body.

primer (prĭ′mẽr): see: filler.

prism (prĭz′'m): a transparent solid with triangular ends and two converging sides; it breaks up white light into its component colors.

procedure (prō-sē′jẽr): a series of definite steps to follow in a certain order to achieve desired results.

procerus (prō-sē′rûs): pyramidalis nasi muscle.

process (prŏ′sĕs): a course of development; a series of actions to bring about a particular result or condition.

processed hair (prŏs′ĕst hâr): hair that has been lightened, stripped, tinted, permanently waved or chemically relaxed.

processing (prŏs′ĕs-ĭng): the action of a chemical solution in cold waving, hair straightening, or hair coloring.

processing time (prŏs′ĕs-ĭng tīm): the time or period required for the chemical solution to act upon the hair.

profession (prô-fĕsh′ûn): an occupation that requires a liberal, scientific or artistic education, or related equivalent.

professional (prô-fĕsh′ûn-âl): one who pursues as a business or livlihood, a particular occupation or vocation.

profile (prō′fīl): the outline of a face, head, figure or an object seen in a side view.

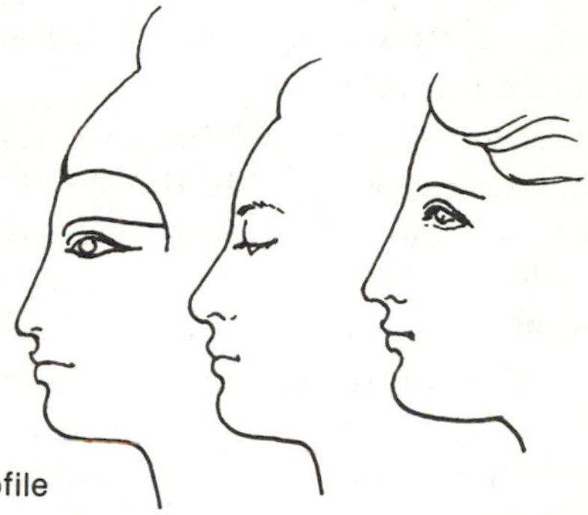

profile

profile base (prō′fīl bās): a profile section of a hairform used in practical exercises.

progressive dye (prŏ-grĕs′ĭv dī): hair restorer; color that develops gradually; metallic dye.

projection angle (prä-jĕk′shûn an′g'l): the angle at which the hair is held while cutting.

proliferate (prô-lĭf′ẽr-āt): to grow by reproduction of new parts, cells or offspring.

prominence (prŏm′ĭ-nĕnts): a projection.

prominent (prŏm′ĭ-nênt): especially noticeable or conspicuous.

prong (prŏng): the round rod of the marcel iron; a slender pointed or projecting part of an implement.

O-P

pronounced (prô-naŭnst): strongly marked or clearly indicated.

properties (prŏp′ẽr-tēz): the identifying characteristics of a substance which are observable; a peculiar quality of anything such as color, taste, smell, etc.

prophase (prō′fāz): the first stage in mitosis.

proportion (prô-pôr′shûn): a harmonious relationship between parts or things; balance or symmetry; comparative relation of one thing to another.

propylparaben (prō′pĭl-pâr-ă′bēn): esters of p-hydroxybenzoate are widely used in cosmetics as a preservative and to destroy bacteria and fungus.

protective cream (prō-tĕk′tĭv crēm): a base cream applied to the skin to protect it against chemicals used during a perm, color or straightening treatment.

O-P

protein (prō′tēn): a complex organic substance present in all living tissues, such as skin, hair and nails; necessary to sustain life; also used in some skin and hair conditioners.

proteinaceous (prô-tē-nā′shûs): pertaining to or resembling protein.

protein filler (prō′tēn fĭl′ẽr): a conditioning filler.

protinator (prō′tĭn-ā-tẽr): an agent which accelerates the release of oxygen in hair lightening.

protoplasm (prō′tô-plăz′m): the material basis of life; a substance found in all living cells.

proximal (prŏk′sĭ-mâl): nearest; located near the center of the body.

pruritus (prōō-rī′tûs): itching.

psoriasis (sô-rī′ă-sĭs): a skin disease characterized by red patches; covered with adherent white-silver scales.

pterygium (tĕ-rĭd′ē-ûm): a forward growth of the eponychium with adherence to the surface of the nail.

ptyalin (tī′ă-lĭn): a starch-splitting enzyme found in the saliva.

pull burn (pōōl bûrn): scalp irritation resulting from uneven winding of the hair during permanent waving.

pull test (pōōl tĕst): a test to determine the degree of elasticity of the hair.

pulmonary (pōōl′mă-nẽr-ē): relating to the lungs.

pulmonary circulation (pul′mă-nẽr′ē sûr′kū-lā′shûn): blood circulation from heart to lungs and back to heart.

pumice (pŭm′ĭs): hardened volcanic substance, white or gray in color; also called pumice stone; used for smoothing and polishing.

punctata, acne (pŭnk-tā′tă, ăk′nē): a form of acne in which the lesions are pointed papules with a comedone in the center.

pungent (pŭn′jênt): acrid; of odors, sharp or irritating.

pupil (pyōō′p'l): the small opening in the iris of the eye through which light enters.

purple (pûr′p'l): any of a variety of colors combining equal or unequal portions of red and blue; a secondary color produced by combining equal parts of red and blue.

purpura (pûr′pū-ră): a disease characterized by the formation of purple patches on the skin and the mucous membranes.

pus (pŭs): a fluid product of inflammation, consisting of a liquid containing leucocytes and the debris of dead cells and tissue elements.

pusher (pōōsh′ẽr): a steel instrument used to loosen the cuticle from the nail.

push wave (pōōsh wāv): a wave which is pushed into place with the hands.

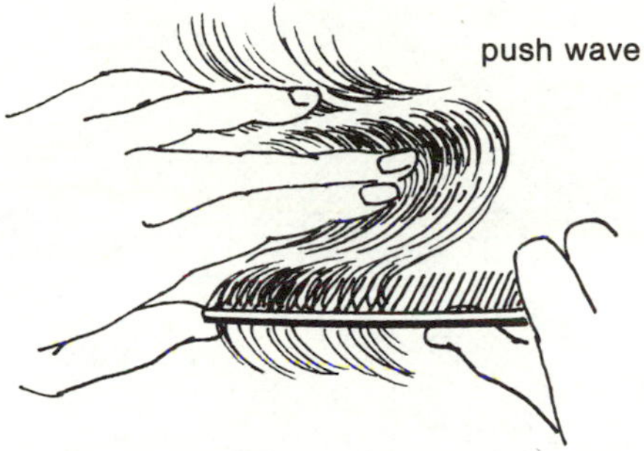

pustular (pŭs′tû-lẽr): pertaining to or characterized by pustules.

pustule (pŭs′tūl): an inflamed pimple containing pus.

pustulosa, acne (pŭs-tû-lō′să, ăk′nē): a form of acne characterized by pustules.

putrefaction (pû′trê-făk′shûn): decomposition; decay; the splitting up of the molecule of a protein into less complex substances by bacteria and fungi along with the formation of foul smelling products.

PVP abbreviation for polyvinyl pyrrolidone (pŏl-ē-vī′nĭ pĭr-rōl′ĭ-dŏn): a synthetic polymer incorporated in hair sprays and some conditioning products.

pyogenic (pī-ô-jĕn′ĭk): pus-forming.

pyosis (pī-ō′sĭs): the formation of pus.

pyramidal bone (pĭ-răm′ĭ-dâl bōn): the wedge-shaped bone of the carpus.

pyramidalis nasi (pĭ-răm-ĭ-dā′lĭs nā′sī): procerus; muscle of the nose.

pyrogallol (pī-rô-găl′ōl): pyrogallic acid; antiseptic hair dye for hair restorers; used medicinally in the treatment of psoriasis, ringworm and other skin infections.

Q

quadrant (kwŏd′rênt): a quarter of a circle, subtending an arc of 90°; anything resembling the quarter section of a circle.

quadratus (kwŏd-rā′tûs): a square-shaped muscle; a muscle of the lower jaw.

quadratus labii inferioris (kwŏd-rā′tûs lā′bē-ī ĭn-fĭr-ē-ŏr′ĭs): a muscle of the lower lip.

quadratus labii superioris (kwŏd-rā′tûs lā′bē-ī sū-pĭr-ē-ŏr′ĭs): a muscle of the upper lip.

quadriceps femoris (kwŏ′drĭ-sĕps fĕm′ŏ-rĭs): the large extensor muscle of the thigh.

quality of hair (kwŏl′ĭ-tē of hâr): the form, length, elasticity, size and texture of the hair.

quantitative analysis (kwŏn′tĭ-tā-tĭv ă-năl′ĭ-sĭs): the process of finding the amount or percentage of an element or ingredient present in a material or compound.

quart (kwôrt): a measure of capacity; the fourth part of a gallon, or two pints; the dry quart is equal to 1.10 liters and a liquid quart is equal to 0.946 liter.

quarter (kwôr′tẽr): one of four equal parts.

quartz lamp (kwôrtz lămp): a glass bulb lamp used for cosmetic purposes; the cold quartz lamp produces mostly short ultraviolet rays, and the hot quartz lamp is an all-purpose lamp used for tanning and for germicidal purposes.

quaternary ammonium compounds (quats) (kwă-tẽr′nă-rē ă-mō′nē-ûm kŏm′paŭndz): a group of compounds of organic salts of ammonia employed very effectively as disinfectants, conditioners and other surface-active agents.

quaternium (kwă-tẽr′nē-ûm): pertaining to a quaternary ammonium compound; used as an ingredient in hair conditioners.

quince seeds (kwĭnts sēdz): the dried seeds of Pyrus Cydonia which yield a mucilage used in the making of hand lotions.

quinine (kwī′nīn): an alkaloid from cinchona bark that enters into the composition of some hair lotions and medicines.

quininoderma (kwin-ĭ-nō-dûr′mă): a form of dermatitis caused by the ingestion of quinine.

R

radial artery (rā′dē-âl är′tĭr-ē): artery that supplies blood to the muscles of the skin, of the hands and fingers, and to the wrist, elbow and forearm.

radial motion (rā′dê-âl mō′shûn): see: point of distribution.

radial nerve (rā′dê-âl nûrv): a nerve which affects the arm and hand.

radial pulse (rā′dē-âl pŭls): the pulse in the radial artery as felt at the wrist near the base of the thumb.

radiation (rā-dê-ā′shûn): the process of giving off light or heat rays; energy radiated in the form of waves or particles.

radiation burn (rā-dē-ā′shûn bûrn): a burn resulting from overexposure to radiant energy, such as X rays, radium or strong sunlight.

radiation therapy (rā-dē-ā′shûn thĕ′ră-pē): the treatment of disease and skin conditions by any type of radiation, most commonly with ionizing radiation such as beta and gamma rays and by X rays.

radical (răd′ĭ-kâl): extreme; in chemistry, a group of atoms passing as such from one compound to another, acting thus like a single atom.

radium (rā′dē-ûm): a radioactive metallic element; the rays from this metal are used in the treatment of some skin diseases.

radius (rā′dē-ûs): a line extending or radiating from a center point to the circumference or outer limit of a circle; the outer and smaller bone of the forearm.

ragged (răg′ĭd): having an irregular edge or outline; uneven.

raise (rāz): to make higher; to elevate or lift.

raised scar (rāzd skär): scar tissue that has healed and formed above the level of the surrounding skin.

rake (rāk): a high frequency electrode used in scalp treatments.

rake comb (rāk kōm): a large toothed comb designed to remove tangles.

rash (răsh): a skin eruption having little or no elevation; a superficial, often localized condition of the skin.

rat (răt): a cushion or small pad over which the hair is combed to create body and volume.

ratio (rā′shē-ō): a proportion; the relationship between two items with respect to quantity, size or amount.

rat-tail comb (răt′tāl kōm): a comb designed with teeth on one end and a long, slender tail at the other; used to section and subsection the hair; also called "fantail" comb.

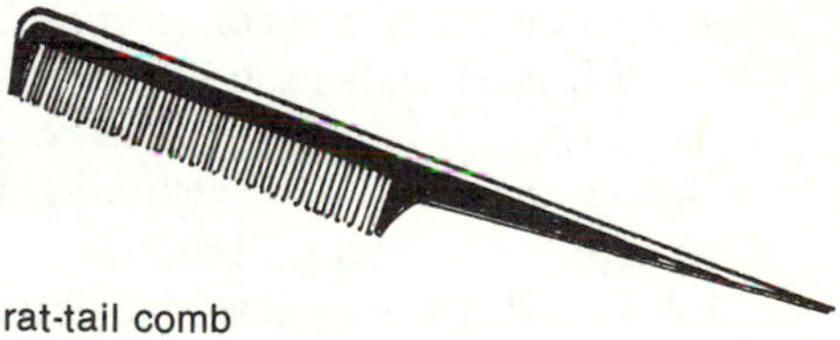

rat-tail comb

ratting (răt′ĭng): the technique of back combing sections of hair from ends to-

Q-R

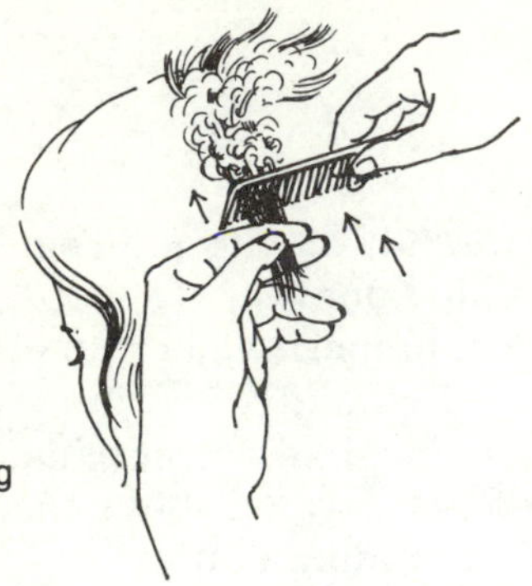

ratting

ward the scalp forming a cushion or base over which longer hair is combed.

raw (rô): irritated; chafed; abraded.

ray (rā): a beam of light or heat.

razor (rā′zẽr): an instrument with a keen cutting edge used for shaving and haircutting; hair shaper.

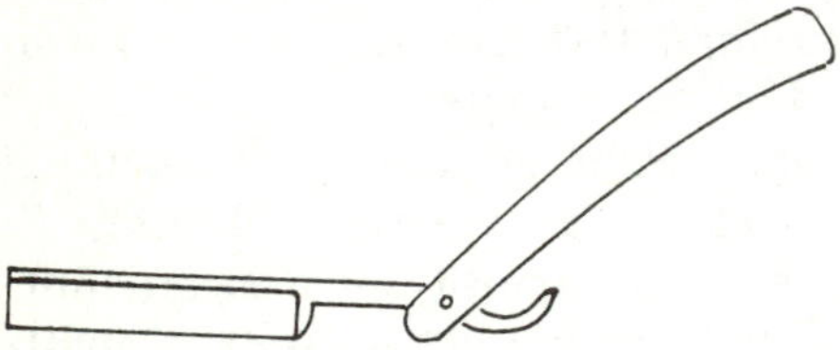

razor

razor blade (rā′zẽr blād): the cutting edge or part of the razor; disposable blade for insertion into the back of the razor.

razor hone (rā′zẽr hōn): a rectangular block of abrasive material such as a fine grained hard stone used to sharpen razor blades.

razor strop (rā′zẽr strŏp): a strap-like device made of leather and/or canvas; used to bring the razor blade to a smooth, whetted edge.

re (rē): a prefix denoting again; back to the original or former state or position.

reactant (rē-ăk′tênt): a substance that is affected or altered during the course of a chemical reaction.

reaction (rê-ăk′shûn): a response.

reagent (rê-ā′jênt): a substance used in detecting, examining or measuring other substances because of its chemical or biological activity.

real (rēl): genuine; not artificial; as real hair.

rebuild (rē-bĭld′): in treating hair, to replace damaged protein structure by conditioners.

recede (rē-sēd′): to move back; to slope backward as a receding hairline.

receptacle (rē-sĕp′tă-k'l): a container used for storage; a basin.

receptive (rē-sĕp′tĭv): able or inclined to receive; open and responsive to ideas or suggestions.

receptor (rē-sĕp′tôr): a cell or group of cells that receive stimuli, as a pain or sensation receptor of the skin.

recess (rē′sĕs): a hollow, depression or indentation.

recline (rê-klīn′): to lie down or back; to cause to assume a recumbent position.

recognize (rĕk′ŏg-nīz): to avow knowledge of; identify.

recondition (rē-kôn-dĭ′shûn): in cosmetology, to restore the hair to its natural healthy state by conditioning.

reconditioner (rē-kôn-dĭ′shûn-ẽr): a product formulated to improve the condition of hair by replacing lost protein, moisture, oil, etc.

reconditioning (rē-kôn-dĭ′shûn-ĭng): the application of a special product to the hair in order to improve its condition.

reconstructing (rē-kôn-strŭkt′ĭng): in cosmetology, replacing internal and external protein structure in the hair.

reconstruction perm (rē-kôn-strŭk′shûn

pûrm): permanent wave procedure that first removes excessive curl and then reconstructs desired curl pattern.

reconstructive surgery (rē-kôn-strŭk′tĭv sûr′jẽr-ē): plastic surgery and cosmetic surgical procedures to build and repair facial and body structures damaged by accidents and disease; surgery to correct and beautify.

record card (rĕk′ôrd kärd): card designed with a special form to keep a record of the services rendered, formulas, supplies used, and any condition pertaining to the client.

recover (rē-kŭv′ẽr): to bring back; to be restored to normal condition.

rectangle (rĕk′tăn′g'l): a four sided figure with two sets of parallel sides.

rectangular (rĕk-tăng′ū-lăr): having edges or surfaces that meet at right angles.

rectifier (rĕk′tĭ-fī-ẽr): an apparatus to change an alternating current of electricity into a direct current.

rectum (rĕk′tûm): the terminal portion of the digestive tube.

rectus (rĕk′tûs): straight; any of several straight muscles.

rectus capitis anterior (rĕk′tûs kăp′ĭ-tĭs ăn-tĭr′ē-ẽr): the muscle that flexes the head.

rectus capitis lateralis (rĕk′tûs kăp′ĭ-tĭs lăt-ĕ-rā′lĭs): muscle that assists in lateral movements of the head.

rectus capitus posterior (rĕk′tûs kăp′ĭ-tûs pŏs-tēr-′ē-ẽr): muscle that functions to extend the head.

red (rĕd): the color of the spectrum farthest from violet; one of the primary colors; a warm hue.

red corpuscle (rĕd kôr′pŭs'l): the blood cell whose function is to carry oxygen to the cells; called erythrocyte.

redhead (rĕd′hĕd): a person having red hair.

red-on-red (rĕd-ŏn-rĕd): the technique of prelightening strands of red hair to orange, then toning to produce a lighter, medium or deeper red color.

reduce (rĭ-dūs′): to diminish in amount, extent or number.

reducing agent (rĭ-dūs′ĭng ā′jênt): a substance that is capable of adding hydrogen to a chemical compound or subtracts oxygen as a cold wave solution.

reduction (rĭ-dŭk′shûn): the subtraction of oxygen from or the addition of hydrogen to a substance; to make smaller; to lessen.

refined hair (rē-fīnd′ hâr): hair that has been chemically treated to make it more pliable.

reflect (rē-flĕkt′): to project back a light or image.

reflex (rē′flĕks): an involuntary nerve reaction; an automatic response to a stimulus that does not involve the conscious mind.

reflexology (rē-flĕks-ŏl′ă-jē): the study of body reflexes; the study of the various areas of the feet as they affect and are affected by other parts of the body.

refresh (rē-frĕsh′): to restore to normal or previous vitality.

regimen (rĕj′ĕ-măn): a systematic course of action or a plan to improve health or a particular condition.

rehydration (rē-hī-drā′shûn): the restoration of water to the skin or other parts of the body when it has become dehydrated.

rejuvenate (rê-jo͞o′vă-nāt): to make young or vigorous again.

relapse (rē′lăps): the return of symptoms and signs of a disease or condition after apparent recovery has taken place.

relax (rê-lăks′): to loosen or slacken; to make less tense or rigid.
relaxation (rê-lăk-sā′shûn): the act of relaxing.
relaxer (rē-lăk′sēr): a chemical applied to the hair to remove the natural curl.
relaxer testing (rê-lăk′sēr tĕst′ĭng): checking the action of the relaxer in order to determine the speed at which the natural curl is being removed.
release (rē-lēs): to free; to let go; a form signed by the client before a service for insurance purposes.
remedy (rĕm′ĕ-dē): a medicine or treatment that relieves or cures a condition.
remover (rē-mo͞ov′ĕr): hair color remover; a chemical compound formulated to remove color from the hair; tint stain remover, a product to remove tint stains from the skin; nail polish remover, a product formulated to remove nail polish.
renal (rē′nâl): relating to a kidney.
reprocess (rê-prŏ′sĕs): to repeat a chemical service due to unsatisfactory results.

reproductive (rē-prô-dŭk′tĭv): pertaining to reproduction or the process by which plants and animals produce offspring.
research (rē-sûrch): a careful search for facts or principles.
residue (rĕz′ĭ-dū): that which remains after a part is taken; remainder.
resilience (rê-zĭl′yêns): property of the hair enabling it to retain curl formation and spring back into curled shape after being extended.
resin (rĕ′zĭn): mixture of organic compounds used in hair sprays and setting preparations, for their holding properties.
resistance (rē-zĭst′êns): an opposing or slowing force; the characteristics of the hair shaft that makes penetration by moisture or chemicals difficult.
resistive massage (rē-sĭs′tĭv mă-säzh′): a massage movement to develop strength in the joints of the client's hands and wrists.
resorcinal (rĕ-zôr′sĭn-ōl): a chemical obtained from various resins; chiefly used as an external antiseptic in psoriasis, eczema seborrhea and ringworm.
respiration (rĕs-pĭ-rā′shûn): the act of breathing; the process of inhaling air into the lungs and expelling it.
respiratory (rĕs′pĭr-ă-tō-rē): relating to respiration.
respiratory system (rĕs′pĭr-ă-tō-rē sĭs′-têm): the system of organs consisting of the nose, pharynx, larynx, trachea, bronchi and lungs, which assist in breathing.
restorative (rĭ-stôr′ă-tĭv): a food or medicine given to restore health and vigor.
restorative art (rĕ-stôr′ă-tĭv ärt): the craft of restoring the features of a deceased person through corrective and artistic techniques; see desairology.
restore (rê-stōr′): to bring back to former strength; repair; rebuild; to heal or cure.
restructuring (rê-strŭk′chēr-ĭng): rebuilding and bringing back into alignment the structural layers of the hair.
retard (rê-tärd′): to hinder or delay.
retention (rē-tĕn′shûn): keeping; maintaining.
retention papers (rē-tĕn′shûn pā′pērz): special papers used to control the ends of the hair in wrapping, e.g., in winding hair on rods or rollers.
reticular (rē-tĭk′ū-lēr): sponge-like structure associated with the medulla of the hair and the lower layer of the dermis.
reticular layer (rĕ-tĭk′ū-lēr lā′ĕr): the

deeper layer of the derma, made up of collagenous and elastic fibers.

retina (rĕt′ĭ-nă): the sensitive membrane of the eye which receives the image formed by the lens.

retouch (rē′tŭch): application of hair color, lightener or chemical hair relaxer to new growth of hair.

retral (rē′trâl): posterior; situated toward the back.

retro (rĕt′rō): a prefix denoting backward or located behind.

reverse (rē-vûrs′): to go in the opposite direction.

reverse back hand (rē-vûrs′ băk hănd): a hand position with the palm up using a downward stroke when shaving the face.

reverse curl (rē-vûrs′ kûrl): a curl formed for a style to move away from the face.

reverse elevation (rē-vûrs′ ĕl-ĕ-vā′shûn): a haircut in which hair is shortest at the top of the head and longest at the lower hairline.

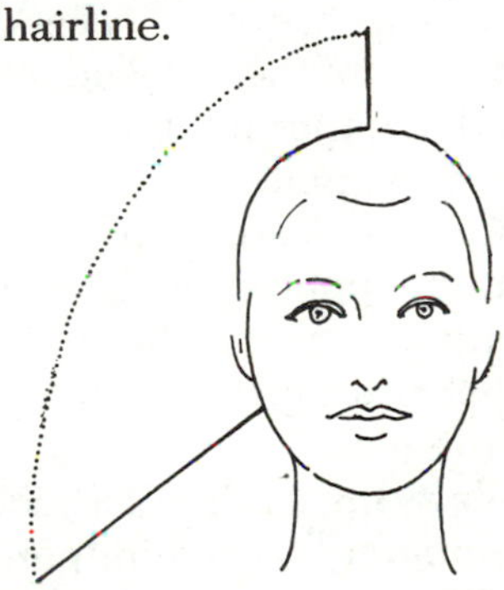

reverse elevation

reverse free hand (rē-vûrs′ frē hănd): a hand position with upward palm and upward stroke, used when shaving the face.

reverse graduation (rē-vûrs′ grăj-ōō-ā′shûn): down angle cutting of the hair.

reverse stack wave (rē-vûrs′ stăk wāv): permanent wave wrap pattern with rods at top of each section wrapped to the scalp, and subsequent rods wrapped further from the scalp.

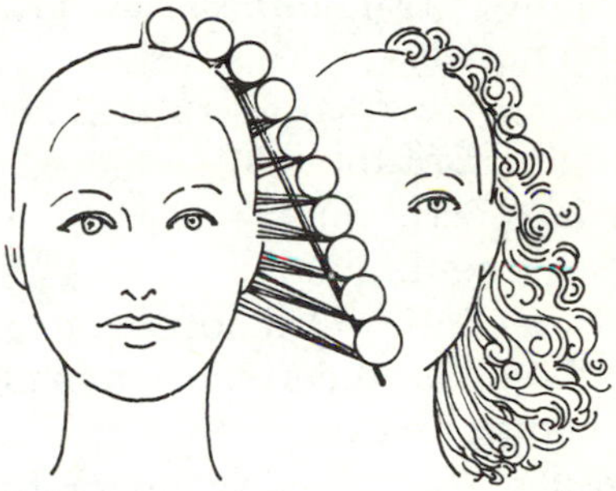

reverse stack wave

reversible (rê-vērs′ĭ-b'l): capable of going through a series of changes in either direction, forward or backward, as a reversible chemical reaction.

revert (rē′vûrt): to return to a previous condition.

rewave (rē-wāv): in permanent waving, giving a permanent wave to a head of hair which still retains some of the former permanent.

rheostat (rē′ô-stăt): a resistance coil; an instrument used to regulate the strength of an electric current or intensity of light.

rheumatism (rōō′mă tĭz'm): a painful disease of the muscles and joints, accompanied by swelling and stiffness.

rhinitis (rī-nī′tĭs): inflammation of the nasal mucous membrane.

rhinocheiloplasty (rī-nō-kī′lō-plăs-tē): plastic surgery of the nose and upper lip.

rhinokyphosis (rī-nō-kī-fō′sĭs): the condition of having an abnormal hump or bump in the bridge of the nose; a prominent bridge.

rhinophyma (rī-nō-fī′mă): a form of acne rosacea characterized by redness and swelling of the skin of the nose, sometimes accompanied by nodules.

rhinoplasty (rī′nō-plăs-tē): plastic surgery on the nose.

rhinothrix (rī′nō-thrĭks): hair growth in the nostrils.

rhysema (rī-sē′mă): a wrinkle line or corrugation of the skin.

rhythm (rĭth′'m): regularly recurring movement.

rhythmic (rĭth′mĭk): movements marked by regular recurrence; moving in a definite rhythm.

rhytidectomy (rĭt-ĭ-dĕk′tō-mē): the excision of skin to eliminate wrinkles; facelift.

ribboning (rĭb′ôn-ĭng): hair setting technique in which hair is forced between thumb and back of comb to create tension.

ribcage (rĭb′kāj): the skeletal framework of the chest made up of the sternum, the ribs and the thoracic vertebrae.

riboflavin (rī′bō-flā-vĭn): the heat stable factor of the vitamin B complex; a water soluble vitamin and essential nutrient; used in emollients and conditioning agents.

ribonucleic acid (RNA) (rī′bō-nū-klē′ĭk ă′sĭd): a nucleic acid of high molecular weight found in the cytoplasm and nuclei of cells; aids synthesis of cell proteins.

ribs (rĭbz): the twelve pairs of bones forming the wall of the thorax.

ridge (rĭdj): crest of a wave.

ridge curl (rĭdj kûrl): a pin curl placed immediately behind or below a ridge to form a wave.

right angle (rīt ăng′'l): a 90° (degree) angle; an angle formed by intersection of two perpendicular lines.

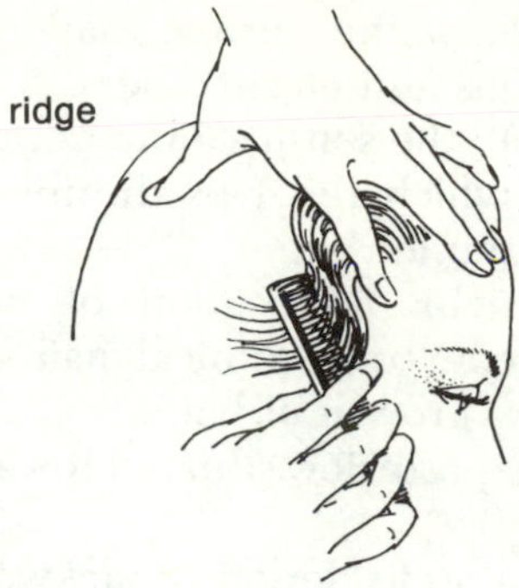

rigid (rĭj′ĭd): inflexible; fixed; not moving; resisting change of form.

rim (rĭm): the border or edge.

ringed hair (rĭng'd hâr): a variety of canities in which the hair appears white or colored in the rings.

ring finger (rĭng fĭn′gĕr): the third finger, next to the little finger of the left hand, on which a wedding ring is customarily worn.

ringlet (rĭng′lĕt): a small curl.

ringworm (rĭng′wûrm): a vegetable parasitic disease of the skin and its appendages which appears in circular lesions and is contagious.

rinse (rĭns): to cleanse with a second or repeated application of water after washing; a prepared rinse water; a solution that temporarily tints or conditions the hair.

rinse, color (rĭns, kŭl′ĕr): see: color rinse.

rinse, temporary (rĭns, tĕm′pôr-âr-ē): an artificial coloring for the hair which coats the shaft and is removed with a single shampoo.

risorius (rĭ-zôr′ē-ûs): muscle at the side of the mouth.

RNA : abbreviation for ribonucleic acid.

rod (rŏd): the round, solid prong of a waving iron; curler used for permanent waving.

Q-R

rod selector chart (rŏd sē-lĕk′tôr chärt): a chart designed for the selection of the proper size and circumference of permanent wave rods.

rolfing (rŏlf′ĭng): a method of massage using heavy pressure from the knuckles and elbows on areas of the body.

roll (rōl): to move forward or on a surface by turning over and over; to form by turning over.

rolled cotton (rōld kŏt′'n): cotton of the absorbent type packaged in rolls for use in cosmetology service procedures.

roller (rōl′ĕr): a cylindrical object varying in diameter and length, around which hair may be wound.

roller clip (rōl′ĕr klĭp): a metal pin, about three inches in length, used to secure a hair roller.

roller control (rōl′ĕr kŏn′trōl): the size of the base, in relation to the diameter of roller to be used, and the position of the roller to the base.

roller curl (rōl′ĕr kûrl): a means of setting hair by winding a damp strand around a cylindrical object in croquignole fashion and securing it in that position until the hair is dry.

roller direction (rōl′ĕr dī-rĕk′shûn): the direction or line in which a roller is moved.

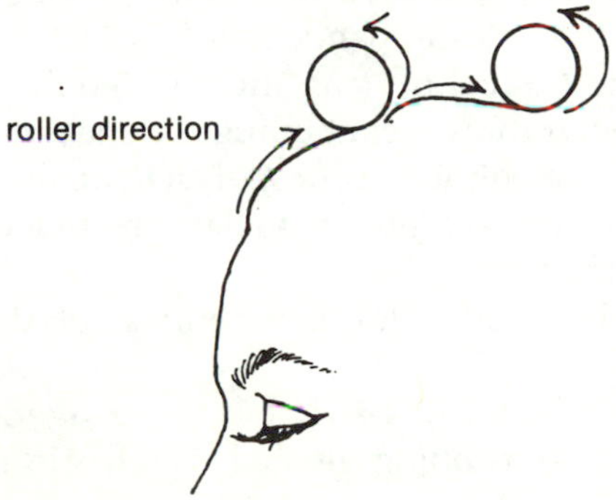

roller pick (rōl′ĕr pĭk): also called a roller pin; a plastic pin about three inches in length, used to secure a hair roller to the scalp.

roller placement (rōl′ĕr plās′mênt): the positioning of a roller in relation to its base; ½ off or on base.

roller set (rōl′ĕr sĕt): setting the hair entirely with rollers.

roller tray (rōl′ĕr trā): an open plastic receptacle with bins or trays on different levels, used to hold and store various sized hair rollers.

rolling (rōl′ĭng): a massage movement in which the tissues are pressed and twisted.

root (ro͞ot): the base; the foundation or beginning of any part.

root of hair (ro͞ot ŏf hâr): structure of the hair below the scalp.

root of the nail (ro͞ot ŏf thē nāl): base of the nail embedded underneath the skin.

root sheath (ro͞ot shēth): the tough membrane covering the root of a hair.

ropy (rō′pē): pertaining to hair that is stringy, sticky, and resembles a rope or cord.

rosacea, acne (rô-zā′shē-ă, ăk′nē): a chronic dermatitis appearing primarily on the cheeks, nose and forehead.

rose color (rōz kŭl′ĕr): a pinkish-red or purplish-red.

rosemary (rōz′mâr-ē): an essence made from an evergreen shrub of the mint family; used in conditioning rinses and tonics for the skin.

rose oil (rōz oyl): attar of roses; an essential oil distilled from fresh roses; used in perfumes and powders.

roseola (rō-zē-ō′-lă): pertaining to a rose-colored eruption such as rubella or German measles.

rose water (rōz wôt′ẽr): a fragrant preparation made from the oil distilled from rose petals and pure water.

rotary (rō′tă-rē): turning on an axis like a wheel; moving in a circular pattern; a movement used in massage.

rotate (rō′tāt): to turn; to revolve.

rotation (rō-tā′shûn): a massage movement for the joints using circular movements; used for fingers, hands, arms, toes and ankles.

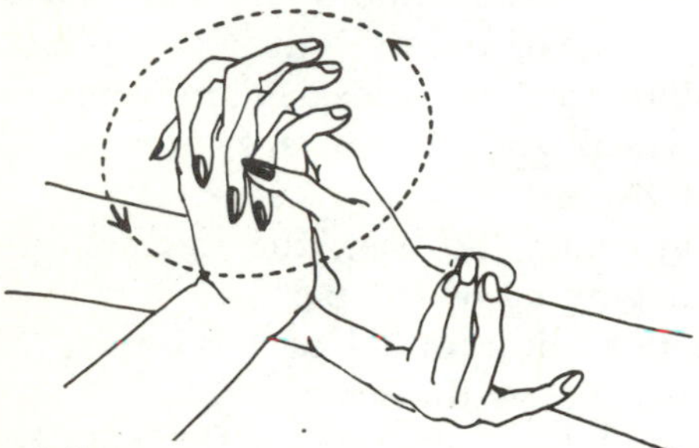

rotation

rouge (ro͞ozh): a pink to red cosmetic used to color the skin, especially the cheeks; cheek color.

rough (rŭf): not smooth or polished; having an uneven texture; coarse.

round (round): spherical; having a contour that is circular or nearly ring-shaped; not flat or angular.

round brush (raund brush): a hairbrush with a circular row of bristles on a round handle, designed for styling hair with a hand-held hair dryer; styling brush.

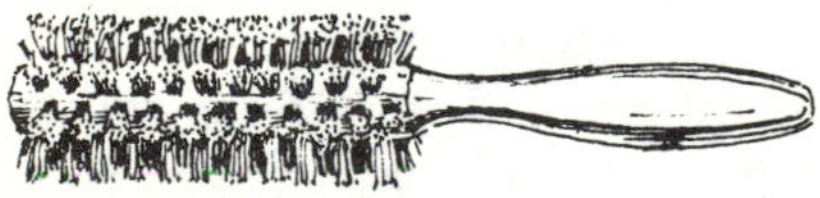

round brush

round-shaped face (raund-shāpt fās): a facial structure characterized by fullness at the cheekbones and jawline but shorter than an oval.

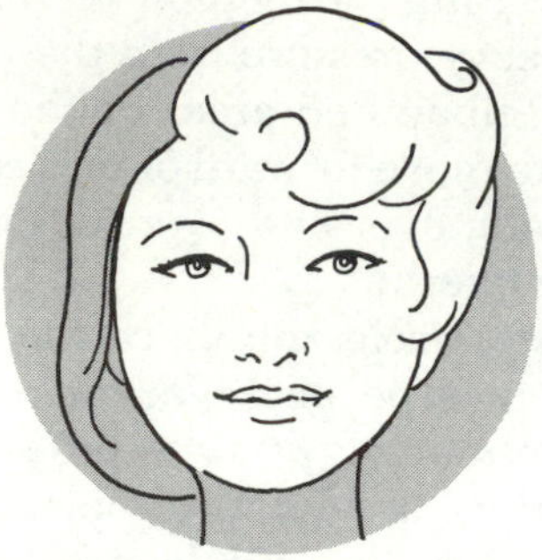

round-shaped face

row (rō): an arrangement or series of items or people in a continuous line; a series of pin curls or rollers placed one after the other in a line.

royal jelly (roy′ăl jĕl′ē): a white, concentrated food produced in the stomachs of worker honeybees, and used as an ingredient in some cosmetic preparations.

rub (rŭb): to move or pass over a surface with pressure and friction.

rubber (rŭb′ẽr): a resinous, elastic material obtained from the latex of the rubber tree and used in various products such as elastic bands and fabrics.

rubbing alcohol (rŭb′ĭng ăl′kô-hôl): a preparation containing denatured ethyl alcohol or isopropyl alcohol; used as a rubefacient to stimulate the tissues of the skin.

rubedo (ro͞o-bē′dō): any redness of the skin.

rubefacient (ro͞o-bă-fā′shênt): an agent, such as rubbing alcohol which stimulates blood to the surface of the skin, causing a reddish color.

ruffing (rŭf′ĭng): back combing; teasing of the hair.

ruffle (rŭf′'l): to comb back the shortest hairs.

rupia (rōō′pē-ă): thick, dark, raised crusts on the skin.

russet (rŭs′ĭt): a reddish or yellowish brown color.

S

sable (sā′b'l): the hair from the sable (marten); animal used for fine quality makeup brushes; the color sable brown, a dark brown-black.

Sabouraud, Rousseau (să′bo͞o-rō, ro͞o-sō′): a discoverer of a 24-hour skin test used in hair coloring to determine whether a client can tolerate an aniline derivative hair tint.

sacral (sā′krăl): pertaining to or located near the sacrum; the five fused vertebrae in humans.

sacular (săk′û-lẽr): shaped like a sac, such as oil glands.

safety razor (sāf′tē rā′zẽr): a straight razor or shaper with a removable guard for the cutting edge of the blade.

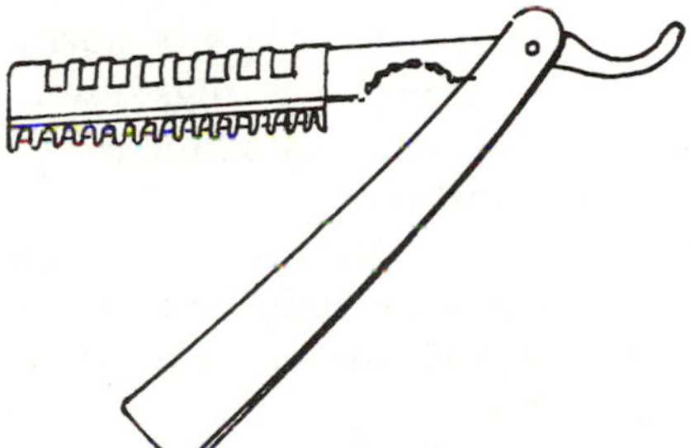

safety razor

safflower (săf′laủ-ẽr): a thistlelike herb from which oil is expressed for use in creams and lotions to soften the skin.

saffron (săf′răn): an old world plant of the iris family; the dried, aromatic stigmas are used as coloring matter in cosmetics; also used as a food flavoring; saffron yellow, an orange-yellow color.

safrole (săf′rōl): a substance found in the oil of sassafras; used in medicinal and fragrant preparations.

sage oil (sāj oyl): an oil obtained from a plant of the mint family, reputed to have healing powers; used in skin freshening lotions and in some types of hair rinses.

salad oil (săl′ăd oyl): any edible vegetable oil such as olive oil and corn oil; used in many cosmetic preparations including: cleansers, creams, hair dressings, shampoos and setting lotions.

salicylic acid (săl-ĭ-sĭl′ĭk ăs′ĭd): white crystalline acid used as an antiseptic, and its salts in some medicinal preparations.

saline (sā′lēn): salty; containing salt.

saliva (să-lī′vă): the secretion of the salivary glands; spittle.

salivary gland (săl′ĭ-vĕ-rē glănd): a gland in the mouth that secretes saliva.

sallow (săl′ō): a yellowish hue or complexion.

salmon (săm′ĭn): a reddish or pinkish orange color named after the color of the flesh of a fresh salmon; salmon pink.

salon (să-lŏn′): an establishment or shop devoted to a specific service or purpose, as a beauty salon.

salt (sôlt): the union of a base with an acid; sodium chloride.

salve (säv): a thick ointment that heals and soothes the skin.

sample (săm′p'l): a portion, piece or part to use in testing or as an example of the whole.

sandalwood oil (săn′d'l wo͝od oyl): oil expressed from the wood of a type of evergreen tree; used in perfumes.

sandpaper (sănd′pā-pĕr): paper coated with fine sand; used for smoothing and polishing; used to make emery boards for manicuring.

sanitary (săn′ĭ-tĕ-rē): pertaining to cleanliness in relation to health, or to the absence of any agent that may be injurious to health.

sanitation (săn-ĭ-tā′shûn): the maintenance of sanitary conditions to promote hygiene and the prevention of disease.

sanitize (săn′ĭ-tīz): to make sanitary.

sanitizer (săn′ĭ-tīz-ĕr): a chemical agent or product used to sanitize implements; a tall glass or plastic jar filled with a sanitizing agent in which implements are kept in a sanitary condition.

saphena (să-fē′nă): either of two large superficial veins of the leg.

saponification (să-pŏn′ĭ-fĭ-kā′shûn): act, process or result of converting into soap.

saponify (să-pŏn′ĭ-fī): to make into soap.

saponin (săp′ô-nĭn): any of a group of glucosides, found in soapwort or soapbark, which form a soapy foam when dissolved in water; used as detergents and in shampoos.

saprophyte (săp′rô-fīt): a microorganism which grows normally on dead matter, as distinguished from a parasite.

sarcoid (sär′koyd): resembling flesh.

sarcothlasis (sär-kō-thlā′sĭs): a bruise or hematoma.

sarcous (sär′kûs): pertaining to flesh or muscle.

saturate (săch′ă-rāt): to cause to become soaked or completely penetrated; to absorb all that is possible to hold.

saturated solution (săch′ă rāt-ĭd sō-lū′shûn): a solution that contains the maximum amount of substance able to be dissolved.

S-bonds: see sulfur bonds.

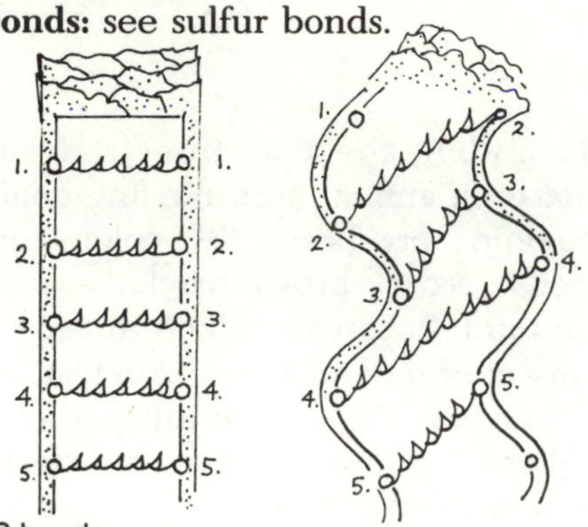

S-bonds

scab (skăb): a crust of hardened blood, serum and dead cells formed over the surface of a wound.

scabies (skā′bēz): a skin disease caused by an animal parasite, attended with intense itching.

scald (skôld): to burn with hot liquid or steam.

scale (skāl): any thin plate of horny epidermis; regular markings used as a standard in measuring and weighing; see: imbrications.

scaling (skāl′ĭng): the sectioning and subsectioning of the hair to obtain the desired proportions; loss of dead epidermal cells.

scalp (skălp): the skin covering the cranium.

scalp antiseptic (skălp ăn-tĭ-sĕp′tĭk): a liquid used to relieve itching scalp and arrest the growth of microorganisms.

scalp conditioner (skălp kôn-dĭsh′ă-nĕr): a product used to improve the health of the scalp.

scalp electrode (skălp ê-lĕk′trōd): a rake-shaped electrode used in some scalp massage procedures.

scalpette (skăl-pĕt-ā′): a hairpiece designed to cover an irregularly shaped

S-T

bald area on the front and/or the crown of the head.

scalpial (skăl′pē-âl): the technical term for general all-around treatment of the scalp.

scalp lotion (skălp lō′shûn): a liquid solution used to treat a dry scalp and/or dandruff.

scalp massage (skălp mă-säzh′): circular movements of the fingertips on the scalp to stimulate blood to the surface.

scalp movement (skălp mo͞ov′mênt): a procedure that moves the scalp gently as part of a treatment.

scalp steamer (skălp stēm′ĕr): an apparatus used to steam the scalp.

scalp treatment (skălp trēt′mênt): a procedure to improve the health of the scalp.

scaly (skāl′ē): covered with or having scales.

scaphoid bone (skăf′oyd bōn): the boat-shaped bone of the tarsus and the carpus.

scapula (skăp′û-lă): one of a pair of shoulder blades; a large flat triangular bone of the shoulder.

scar (skär): a mark remaining after a wound has healed.

scarfskin (scärf′skĭn): the epidermis or cuticle.

scarlet (skär′lĕt): a brilliant red-orange color.

scarlet fever (skär′lĕt fē′vĕr): a contagious disease accompanied by fever and a red rash.

scent (sĕnt): a distinctive odor or fragrance given off by a substance.

schedule (skĕd′ûl): a timetable for a preplanned program.

sciatica (sī-ăt′ĭ-kă): a painful inflammation of the nerve running down the back of the leg, called the sciatic nerve.

science (sī′êns): a body of knowledge arranged and systemized; based on observation and experiment to determine the basic nature or principles of the subject studied.

scientific (sī-ên-tĭf′ĭk): pertaining to, or used in science.

scissors (sĭz′erz): a two bladed instrument used to cut and trim.

scleroderma (sklĕr-ō-dûr′mă): a disease of the skin characterized by hard, thick patches.

scleroid (sklĕr′oyd): hard or bony in texture.

sclerosis (sklĕr-ō′sĭs): pathological hardening of tissues, especially by outgrowth of fibrous tissues.

scoliosis (skō-lē-ō′sĭs): abnormal lateral curvature of the spine.

scratch (skrăch): a slight wound in the form of a tear on the surface of the skin.

scratch patch test (skrăch păch tĕst): a test that consists of application of the test patch to an abraded skin area rather than to normal skin.

scrub (skrŭb): to rub briskly.

scrupulous (skro͞o′pû-lûs): extremely exact; careful and painstaking.

sculpture curl (skŭlp′chĕr kûrl): a curl placed close to the head to appear as if it were carved; another term for pin curl.

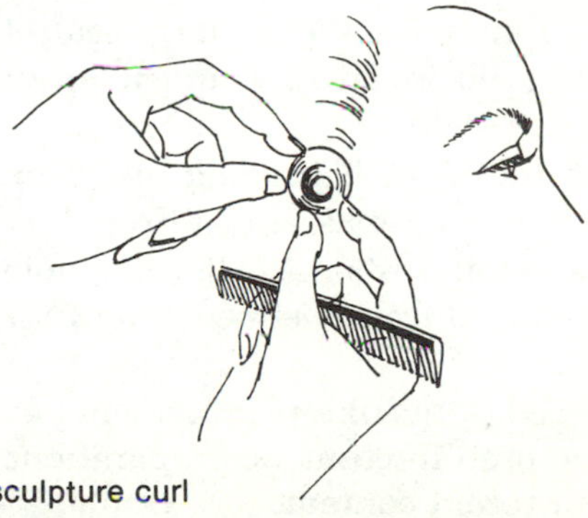

sculpture curl

sculptured nails (skŭlp′chẽrd nālz): artificial nails made by combining a liquid and powder mixture and painting it over a nail form attached to the natural nail; the new nail is then shaped to the desired length.

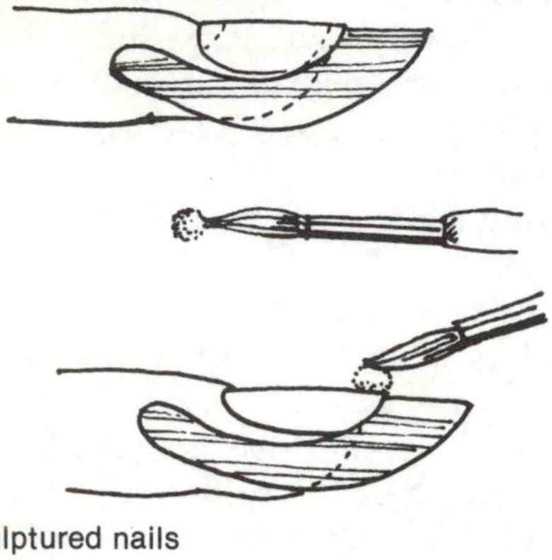

sculptured nails

sculpturing (skŭlp′chẽr-ĭng): the formation of a hair shape and silhouette by creating volume or volume and indentation.

scurf (skûrf): thin dry scales or scabs on the body, especially on the scalp; dandruff.

S-T

scurvy (skûr′vē): a nutritional disorder caused by deficiency of vitamin C (ascorbic acid); characterized by extreme weakness, spongy gums and bleeding under the skin.

scutellum (skū-tĕl′ŭm): a large scab often observed in favus; a fungal infection of the scalp.

seam (sēm): in hairstyling, an overlapping of two ends, as in a French twist.

seasame oil (sĕs′ă-mē oyl): the emollient produced from the seed of an East Indian herb.

seaweed (sē′wēd): a plant growing in the sea; used in cosmetic preparations for its protein content.

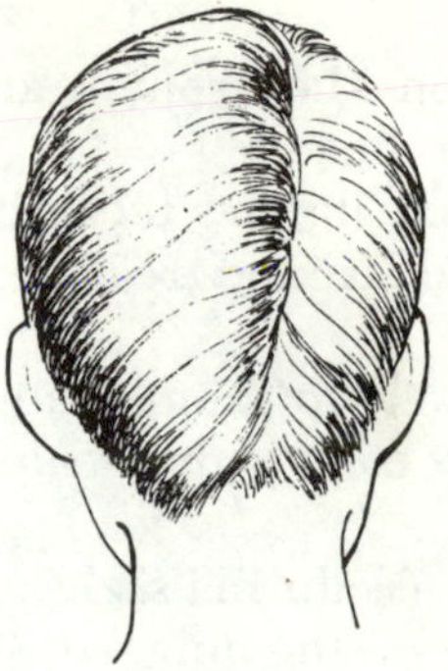

seam

sebaceous (sĭ-bā′shûs): pertaining to or having the nature of oil or fat.

sebaceous cyst (sĭ-bā′shûs sĭst): a distended oily or fatty follicle or sac.

sebaceous gland (sĕ-bā′shûs glăndz): oil glands of the skin; any glands in the corium of the skin that secrete sebum.

seborrhea (sĕb-ô-rē′ă): an abnormal increase of secretion from the sebaceous glands.

seborrhea capitis (sĕb-ô-rē′ă kăp′ĭ-tĭs): seborrhea of the scalp, commonly called dandruff; pityriasis.

seborrhea oleosa (sĕb-ô-rē′ă ō-lê-ō′să): excessive oiliness of the skin, especially of the forehead and nose.

seborrhea sicca (sĕb-ô-rē′ă sĭk′ă): an accumulation, on the scalp, of greasy scales or crusts, due to overaction of the sebaceous glands; dandruff or pityriasis.

seborrheic (sĕb-ô-rē′ĭk): seborrheal; pertaining to the overactivity of the sebaceous glands.

seborrheic, alopecia (sĕb-ô-rē′ĭk ăl-ô-pē′shē-ă): baldness caused by diseased sebaceous glands.

sebum (sē′bûm): the fatty or oily secretions of the sebaceous glands.

secondary (sĕk′ûn-dĕ-rē): second in rank, importance or value, or in the order of time or development.

secondary color (sĕk′ŭn-dĕ-rē kûl′ẽr): a

color obtained by mixing equal parts of two primary colors.

secondary hair (sĕk′ûn-dĕ-rē hâr): the stiff, short, coarse hair found on eyelashes, eyebrows and within the openings or passages of the nose and ears.

second degree burn (sĕk′ûnd dă-grē′ bûrn): a burn characterized by pain, blistering and destruction of the epidermis.

secrete (sê-krēt′): to separate from blood, form into new materials and emit as a secretion.

secretion (sê-krē′shûn): the process by which materials are separated from the blood, usually by glandular function, and formed into new substances used to carry out special functions.

secretory (sê-krē′tô-rē): relating to secretion or to the secretions.

section (sĕk′shûn): to divide the hair by parting into separate areas for control.

sedative (sĕd′ă-tĭv): tending to quiet or allay nervous excitement; any drug that produces a quieting effect on the central nervous system.

sedentary (sĕd′ĕn-tĕ-rē): settled; inactive.

seep (sēp): to ooze out slowly.

segment (sĕg′mênt): to separate into constituent parts; one of the constituent parts of something.

selector switch (sê-lĕk′tĕr swĭch): an apparatus used to select the kind of current desired for a treatment.

selenium (sĕ-lē′nē-ûm): in nutrition, an essential mineral found in cereals, vegetables and fish; preserves tissue elasticity and aids in promotion of body growth.

selenium sulphide (sĕ-lē′nē-ûm sŭl′fīd): a bright orange powder used in preparations for the treatment of seborrheic dermatitis and common dandruff.

SEM abbreviation for **scanning electron microscope** (skăn-ĭng ē-lĕk′trŏn mī′krô-skōp): an analytical instrument which bombards an object with electrons to produce an image; an instrument capable of magnification from 50 to 75,000 or more.

semilunar bone (sĕm-ē-lū′nĕr bōn): a crescent-shaped bone of the wrist.

semipermanent hair coloring (sĕ′mē-pûr′mă-nênt hâr kŭl′ĕr-ĭng): the process of hair coloring which is formulated to last through four to six shampoos.

semipermanent rinse (sĕ′mē-pûr′mă-nênt rĭns): a nonpermanent hair rinse that is removed after several shampoos.

semipermanent shampoo hair color (sĕ′mē pûr′mă-nênt shăm-pōō′ hâr kŭl′ĕr): a shampoo that imparts a semipermanent color that lasts several weeks.

semistand-up curl (sĕ′mē-stănd′ŭp kûrl): the placement of a curl on its base in such a manner as to allow it to partially stand away from the scalp; this produces a slightly directional volume in the combout; also known as a flare curl.

semitransformation (sĕ′mē-trăns-fôr-mā′shûn): a frontal hairpiece extending to just above or behind the ear.

senile (sē′nīl): relating to, or characteristic of old age or the infirmities of old age; exhibiting loss of mental faculties associated with old age.

senile canities (sē′nīl kă-nĭsh′ē-ēz): grayness of the hair in elderly people.

sensation (sĕn-sā′shûn): a feeling or impression arising as the result of the stimulation of an afferent nerve.

sense (sĕns): the faculty of sensation by which an individual perceives impressions such as taste, touch, smell, sight and hearing.

sense organ (sĕns ôr′găn): a living structure that receives sense impressions, (the eye, ears, nose, skin, tongue and mouth).

sensitive (sĕn′sĭ-tĭv): easily affected by outside influences.

sensitive skin (sĕn′sĭ-tĭv skĭn): skin that is easily damaged or reactive to substances.

sensitivity (sĕn-sĭ-tĭv′ĭ-tē): the state of being easily affected by certain chemicals or external conditions.

sensory (sĕn′să-rē): relating to or pertaining to sensation.

sensory nerve (sĕn′să-rē nûrv): afferent nerve; a nerve carrying sensations.

sentient (sĕn′shĭ-ĕnt): sensitive; capable of sensation; feeling.

sepia (sē′pē-ă): a reddish-brown color.

sepsis (sĕp′sĭs): the presence of various pus-forming and other pathogenic organisms, or their toxins, in the blood or tissues; septicemia.

septal artery (sĕp′tâl är′tĭr-ē): the artery that supplies the nostrils.

septic (sĕp′tĭk): relating to or caused by sepsis.

septicemia (sĕp-tĭ-sē′mē-ă): the condition which exists when pathogenic bacteria enter the bloodstream and circulate throughout the body, causing a general infection.

septum (sĕp′tûm): a dividing wall; a partition, especially between bodily spaces or masses of soft tissue.

sequestering agent (sĭ-kwĕs′tĕr-ĭng ā′jênt): a preservative used to prevent changes in the chemical and physical composition of certain products.

serous (sē′rûs): relating to or containing serum.

serrated (sĕr-rāt′ĕd): having saw-like notches along the edge.

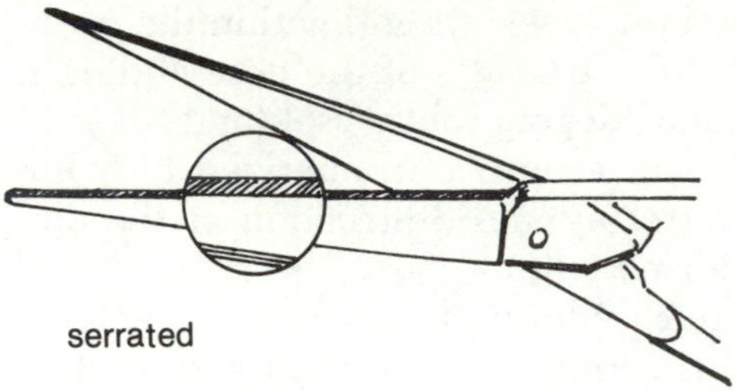

serrated

serratus anterior (sē-rā′tûs ăn-tĭr′ĭ ĕr): a muscle of the chest assisting in breathing and in raising the arm.

serum (sē′rûm): the clear portion of any bodily fluid; the fluid portion of the blood obtained after coagulation; an antitoxin as prepared for therapeutic use.

set (sĕt): to form and secure the hair into a pattern of curls or waves to meet the requirements of a specific hairstyle.

setting (sĕt′ĭng): an arrangement of the hair to meet the requirements of a specific hairstyle.

setting gel (sĕt′ĭng jĕl): a semi-solid holding agent used to set the hair.

shade (shād): the gradation in color value by adding black to a color; a color slightly different from the one under consideration.

shading (shā′dĭng): adding depth of color to strands of hair; in makeup, shadowing a feature to create the illusion of receding or becoming less prominent.

shadow (shă′dō): the low area of a circle in a hairstyle.

shadow wave (shă′dō wāv): a shaping which resembles the outline of a finger wave but does not have a definite ridge and formation.

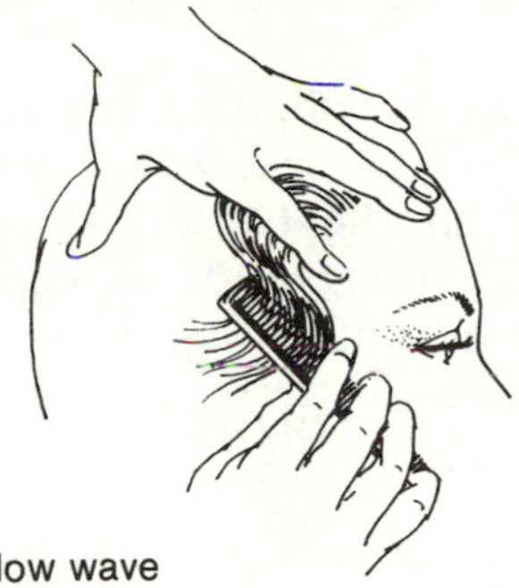
shadow wave

shaft (shăft): slender stem-like structure; the long slender part of the hair above the scalp.

shaking (shāk′ĭng): in massage a vibrating movement in which the hand is pressed on the body part and firmly moved from side to side.

shampoo (shăm-poo′): to subject the scalp and hair to washing and massaging with some cleansing agent such as soap or detergent; a product formulated for cleansing the hair and scalp.

shampoo bleach (shăm-pōō′blēch): a hair lightener containing peroxide and shampoo.

shampoo bowl (shăm-pōō′ bōl): a specially designed basin with a "U" shaped construction to allow the client to lie back in a comfortable position during the shampoo.

shampoo brush (shăm-pōō′ brŭsh): a firm-bristled brush used to section the hair and apply shampoo near the scalp.

shampoo cape (shăm-pōō′ kāp): a plastic or cloth cape used to protect the client's clothing during the shampoo procedure.

shampoo comb (shăm-pōō′ kōm): a large, wide-toothed comb used to comb shampoo or other products through the hair and to remove tangles; rake.

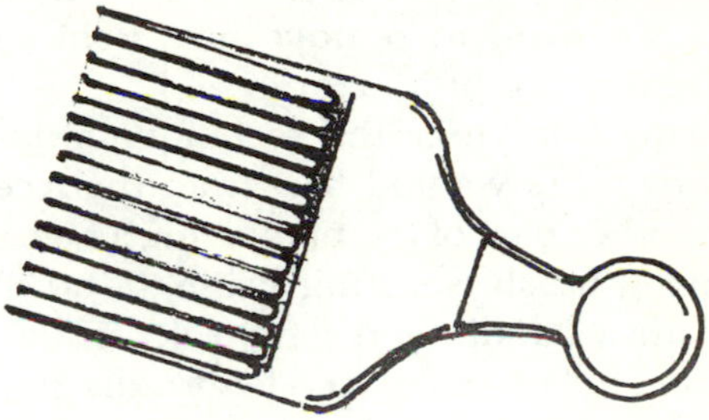
shampoo comb

shampooing (shăm-pōō′ĭng): the act of cleaning the hair and scalp.

shampoo station (shăm-pōō′ stā′shŭn): the area where shampoo chairs and equipment are located.

shampoo tint (shăm-pōō′ tĭnt): a shampoo product that cleans and adds color to the hair.

shape (shāp): the contour of an object; in hair sculpture, shape implies two dimensions.

shaper (shā′pẽr): a razor-like device used for shaping or cutting hair.

shaping (shāp′ĭng): the molding of a section of hair in a circular movement, in preparation for the formation of curls or a finger wave.

shaping, haircutting (shāp′ĭng, hâr′kŭt-ĭng): the process of shortening and thinning the hair to a particular style or to the contour of the head.

shaping, hairstyling (shāp′ĭng, hâr′stīl-ĭng): the formation of uniform arcs or curves in wet hair, thus providing a base for various patterns in hairstyling.

shaping, pivot (shāp′ĭng, pĭv′ŭt): see pivot, hair shaping.

shark-liver oil (shärk-lĭv′ẽr oyl): a brown fatty oil obtained from the livers of

S-T

sharks; a rich source of vitamin A; used in some types of creams and lotions.

shave (shāv): to cut hair or beard close to the skin; to remove hair from an area by use of a razor.

shaving (shā′vĭng): the technique of removing unwanted hair from the face or other part of the body using a razor.

shaving brush (shāv′ĭng brŭsh): a brush with a handle and long, soft bristles, used to lather the face before shaving.

shaving cream (shāv′ĭng krēm): an emollient cream used to soften the beard before shaving.

shaving soap (shāv′ĭng sōp): a soap formulated to soften the beard before shaving.

shears (shērz): an instrument which is used for cutting hair.

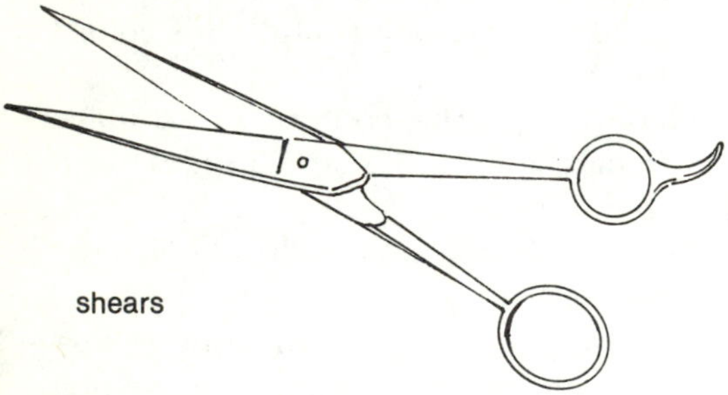

shears

sheath (shēth): a covering enclosing or surrounding some organ.

sheen (shēn): gloss; shininess.

shellac (shĕ-lăk′): a resinous substance dissolved in alcohol which was used in hair sprays.

shiatsu (shē-ă′tzōō): a Japanese therapeutic massage technique similar to acupuncture, except the thumbs and tips of the fingers are used on the special areas instead of needles.

shift (shĭft): to move the hair away from its natural fall position.

shin (shĭn): the frontal part of a leg below the knee; the shinbone.

shine (shīn): to reflect light; gloss or sheen.

shingle (shĭng′′l): a short haircut, particularly at the nape area, where the haircut starts at the hairline from zero length, becoming gradually longer toward the crown.

shingle

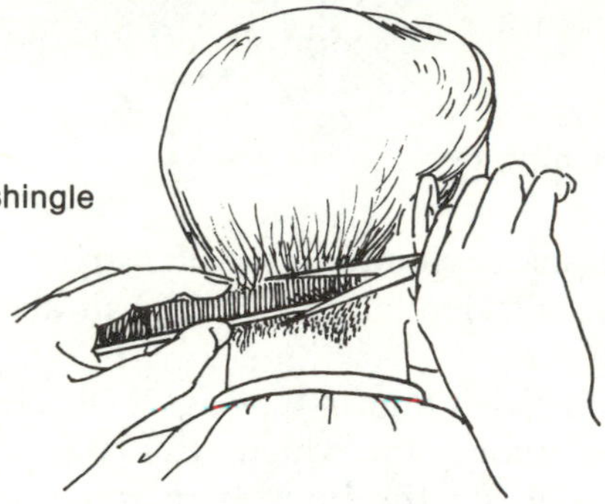

short (shôrt): low; brief; not long.

short circuit (shôrt sûr′kĭt): to shut or break off an electric current before it has completed its course.

shorten (shôrt′′n): to reduce in length or duration.

shortwave (shôrt′wāv′): a form of high-frequency current used in permanent hair removal.

shoulder (shōl′dẽr): the part of the body which connects the arms to the trunk.

shoulder length (shōl′dẽr lĕngth): the length of hair that reaches the top part of the shoulder.

shrink (shrĭnk): to contract into a smaller area.

shrivel (shrĭv′′l): to shrink into wrinkles, especially due to loss of moisture.

siccant; siccative (sĭ′kănt; sĭk′ŭ-tĭv): drying; tending to make dry.

side (sīd): the right or left half of a body or object.

S-T

sideburn (sīd′bûrn): continuation of the hairline in front of the ears.

side height (sīd hīt): that area of the hair from the end of the sideburns up to the point at which the vertical and horizontal bone structures meet.

side part (sīd pärt): a part in the hair that is on the side, not the center.

sienna (sē-ĕn′ă): an earth pigment containing iron and maganese oxides; it is yellowish-brown in the raw state and when burned turns a deep reddish brown; used as a coloring ingredient.

silhouette (sĭl-ōō-ĕt′): an outline or outer dimension.

silica (sĭl′ĭ-kă): dioxide of silicon.

silicon (sĭl′ĭ-kŏn): a very abundant nonmetallic element.

silicone (sĭl′ĭ kōn): a water resistant lubricant for the skin.

silicote (sĭl′ĭ kōt): a silicone oil used in some cosmetic products.

silk (sĭlk): a strong, glossy, natural fiber used in making better-quality wigs and hairpieces.

silk gauze (sĭlk gôz): a fine gauze silk material used in toupee work or for ventilated parts of hairpieces.

silking (sĭlk′ĭng): hair pressing.

silver hair (sĭl′vĕr hâr): hair that has grayed to resemble the metallic white of silver metal; silver gray hair.

silver nitrate (sĭl′vĕr nī′trāt): a white, crystalline salt; used as an antiseptic, germicide and astringent in cosmetics and as a coloring agent in hair dyes.

simplex (sĭm′plĕks): common; simple; single.

simplex, acne (sĭm′plĕks, ăk′nē): common pimple.

simulated (sĭm′ū-lāt′ĕd): fake; made to look genuine.

sinew (sĭn′ū): a fibrous cord; a tendon.

singe (sĭnj): in hairdressing; to burn the hair ends; to burn lightly on the surface.

singeing (sĭnj′ĭng): process of lightly burning hair ends with a lighted wax taper.

single application coloring (sĭng′′l ăp-plĭ-kā′shûn kŭl′ĕr-ĭng): a process that lightens and colors the hair in a single application.

single application tints (sĭng′′l ăp-lĭ-kā′-shûn tĭnts): products which lighten and add color to the hair in a single application; also called one process tints or one step tints.

single floral (sĭng′′l flôr′âl): a basic type of perfume containing the fragrance of one flower, such as rose, gardenia, violet or carnation.

single prong clip (sĭng′′l prŏng klĭp): a clip having only one prong, designed to hold small curls on thin hair.

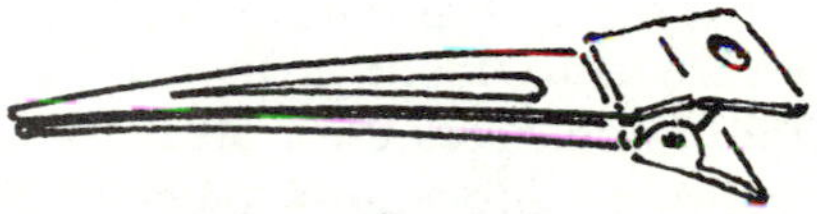

single prong clip

sinus (sī′nûs): a cavity or depression; a hollow in bone or other tissue.

sinusoid (sī′nûs-soid): resembling a sinus; a blood space in certain organs, as the liver, pancreas, etc.

sinusoidal current (sīn-ă-soid′âl kûr′ênt): an induced, interrupted current similar to faradic current.

sizing (sī′zĭng): the fitting of a wig to the client's head size.

S-T

skeletal muscles (skĕl′ĕ-tâl mŭs′'lz): muscles connected to the skeleton.
skeleton (skĕl′ĕ-tûn): the bony framework of the body; see chart.
skill (skĭl): the mastery of an art or technique; dexterity in doing learned physical tasks.
skin (skĭn): the external covering of the body.
skin abrasion peel (skĭn ă brā′zhûn pēl): a process that rubs or wears away the surface of the skin, usually done with pumice stone powder; must be done only by a qualified professional person.
skin analysis (skĭn ă-nâl′ĭ-sĭs): the examination and study of the skin to determine the appropriate treatment.
skin antiseptic (skĭn ăn-tĭ-sĕp′tĭk): a liquid product formulated to relieve excessive oiliness or irritations.
skin astringent (skĭn ă-strĭn′jênt): a liquid product formulated to contract organic tissue; used to help control excessive oiliness and to invigorate the skin.
skin bleach (skĭn blēch): a preparation formulated to lighten dark pigmentation spots on the skin.
skin care equipment (skĭn kâr ĭ-kwĭp′mênt): apparatus used during a facial treatment procedure (lamps, atomizer, receptacles, machines, etc.).
skin color (skĭn kŭl′ẽr): the color of skin as determined by the four types of pigment that determine skin color: melanin, hemoglobin (oxygenated and reduced) and carotenes.
skin freshener (skĭn frĕsh′ĕn-ẽr): a liquid product used to invigorate the skin following the use of cleansing cream or lotion; a mild astringent.
skin graft (skĭn grăft): skin taken from one part of the body to replace damaged skin on another part of the body; a service performed by a surgeon.
skin peel (skĭn pēl): mechanical skin peel; the use of rotating brushes to remove dead surface cells and debris from the skin.
skin peel (skĭn pēl): product peel; a procedure using a mild product to remove dead surface cells from the skin; also called epidermabrasion and not to be confused with dermabrasion.
skin peel product (skĭn pēl prŏ′dŭkt): a product such as vegetable enzymes in creams or lotions that give the face a mild surface peeling treatment.
skin pigmentation (skĭn pĭg-mĕn-tā′shûn): the deposition of pigment by the cells; color pigment.
skin scope (skĭn skōp): a magnifying glass-lamp combination used to analyze skin conditions; a magnifying lamp.
skin test (skĭn tĕst): a test to determine the existence or nonexistence of extreme sensitivity to certain things: foods, chemicals, etc., which do not adversely affect most individuals.
skin texture (skĭn tĕks′chẽr): the general feel and appearance of the skin, such as coarse, fine, smooth, rough, etc.
skin toner (skĭn tō′nẽr): a preparation that serves to freshen and tone the skin.
skin treatment (skĭn trēt′mênt): a procedure, such as a massage, to improve the health and appearance of the skin of the face and neck.
skip waving (skĭp wāv′ĭng): a setting method featuring a ridge following a shaping, against which is placed a series of overlapping pin curls, then repeating the shaping and curl placement.
skull (skŭl): the bony case or the framework of the head.
slack (slăk): loose; not tight.
slant (slănt): at an angle or incline; in

hairdressing, to make a hair parting on an angle.

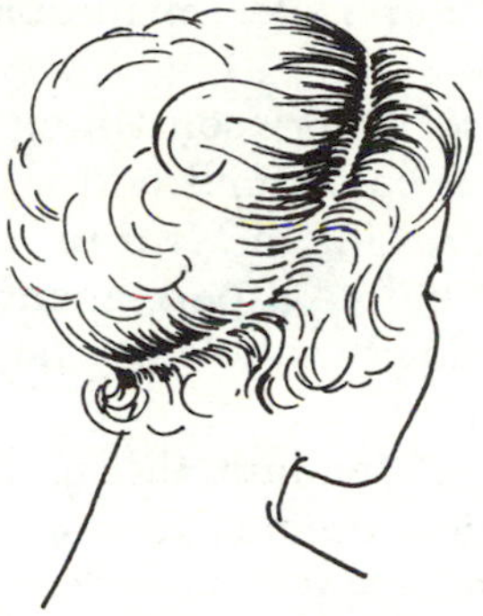

slant

slap (slăp): a movement in massage using the open hand, palm side down, to strike a part of the body abruptly.

sleek (slēk): smooth and glossy.

slicing (slīs′ĭng): carefully removing a section of hair from a shaping in preparation for making a pin curl (the remainder of the shaping is not disturbed).

slim (slĭm): small in thickness; slender, as a human figure, a hair or thread.

slip (slĭp): a smooth and slippery feeling imparted by talc to face powder.

slip on (slĭp′ŏn): a hollow rubber or plastic head with facial features and hair that can be slipped over a slip on mannequin head form; used to practice hairstyling techniques.

slippage (slĭp′ăj): the shifting and changing of position of sulfur bonds.

slithering (slĭth′ẽr-ĭng): tapering the hair to graduated lengths by sliding down the surface of hair with scissors.

slough (slŭf): to separate, as dead matter from living tissues; to discard.

smacking (smăk′ĭng): a massage movement in which the palm of the hand is used to slap the skin.

smaller occipital nerve (smôl′ẽr ŏk-sĭp′ĭ-tâl nûrv): sensory nerve affecting skin behind the ear.

small intestine (smôl ĭn-tĕs′tĭn): the part of the intestine lying between the stomach and the colon, consisting of the duodenum, jejunum and ileum.

smock (smŏk): a loose, lightweight garment worn to protect other clothing.

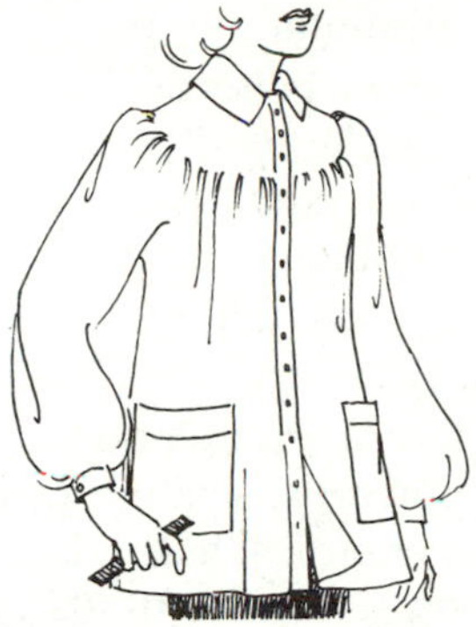

smock

smocking (smŏk′ĭng): in wig making, a length of weft sewn in triangles, diamonds or loops to create a flat, airy base.

smooth (smo͞oth): continuous and unroughened; lacking blemishes; being without hair; lacking irregularities.

smooth face (smo͞oth fās): a shaven face or face that is unblemished.

smooth muscle (smo͞oth mŭs′′l): muscle having nonstriated fibers.

smudge (smŭj): to spread or blur makeup or nail polish; to stain or smear.

snarls (snärlz): tangles, as of hair.

soak (sōk): to place in a liquid to saturate or soften.

soap (sōp): a compound of fatty acid, derived from fats and oils, chemically combined with an alkaline base; used as a cleaning agent.

soap cap (sōp kăp): a combination of prepared tint and shampoo which is applied to the hair like a regular shampoo; this is used to add some color and brightness to faded hair.

soapless shampoo (sōp′lĕs shăm-pōō′): a shampoo made with a synthetic detergent; it can be formulated at nearly any pH but is usually slightly acidic in reaction.

sodium (sō′dē-ûm): a metallic element of the alkali metal group.

sodium carbonate (sō′dê-ûm kär′bôn-ât): washing soda; used to prevent corrosion of metallic instruments when added to boiling water.

sodium chloride (sō′dê-ûm klôr′īd): table salt (NaCL).

sodium hydroxide (sō′dê-ûm hī-drŏk′-sīd): a powerful alkaline product used in some chemical hair relaxers; caustic soda; powerful alkali used in the manufacture of liquid soaps.

sodium lauryl sulfate (sō′dê-ûm lô′rêl sŭl′fāt): a metallic compound of the alkaline group, in white or light yellow crystals; used in detergents; a detergent, wetting agent, and emulsifier; used in shampoos for its degreasing qualities.

S-T

sodium nitrate (sō′dê-ûm nī′trāt): a clear, ordorless crystalline salt used to manufacture nitric acid; sodium nitrite; used as an oxidizing agent.

sodium perborate (sō′dê-ûm pē-bō′rāt): a compound formed by treating sodium peroxide with boric acid; on dissolving the substance in water, peroxide of hydrogen is generated; used as an antiseptic and bleaching agent.

sodium sulphite (sō′dê-ûm sŭl′fīt): a soft, white metallic salt of sulphurous acid; antiseptic, preservative and antioxidant used in hair color.

sodium thiosulphate (sō′dê-ûm thī-ô-sŭl′-fāt): a compound used in solutions for impetiginous conditions and parasitic alopecias of the beard.

soft (sôft): pliable; malleable; easily worked.

softener (sôf′ên-ẽr): something that softens, as a compound added to water; in hairdressing, a term for a product applied before a permanent wave or color to lower cuticle resistance; a presoftener.

softening (sŏf′ên-ĭng): the application of a chemical product to hair, making it more receptive to hair coloring or permanent waving.

soft press (sôft prĕs): pressing the hair to remove 50 to 60 percent of the curl.

soft soap (sôft sōp): fluid or semifluid soap.

soft water (sôft wô′tẽr): water which readily lathers with soap; water which is free from calcium or magnesium compounds.

sole (sōl): the bottom surface of the foot.

solid (sŏl′ĭd): any substance which does not flow; form of matter with definite shape, volume, and weight.

solid form (säl′ĭd fôrm): in hairdressing, an unbroken surface; unactivated texture.

solid peroxide (sŏl′ĭd pẽr-ŏk′sīd): sodium perborate and mild acid in tablet form which is dissolved in water before using.

solubility (sŏl-û-bĭl′ĭ-tē): the extent to which a substance (solute) dissolves in a liquid (solvent) to produce a homogeneous system (solution).

soluble (sŏl′û-b'l): capable of being dissolved.

solute (sŏl′ūt): the dissolved substance in a solution.

solution (sô-lū′shûn): a homogeneous mixture of solid, liquid or gaseous substances; the act or process by which a substance is homogeneously mixed with a liquid, gas or solid.

solvent (sŏl′vênt): a liquid which dissolves another substance without any change in chemical composition.

sorbic acid (sôr′bĭk ăs′ŭd): a white crystalline solid from the berries of the mountain ash; also produced synthetically; used in a wide variety of cosmetics as a binder, humectant and preservative.

soybean (soy′bēn): a leguminous herb which produces oil used in the manufacture of soaps, shampoos, and bath oils.

sparse (spärs): thinly diffused; not dense; consisting of a few or scattered elements; thin, irregular eyebrows; balding areas of the head.

spasm (spăz′′m): an involuntary muscular contraction.

spasmodic (spăz-mŏd′ĭk): pertaining to spasm; convulsive; intermittent.

spat (spăt): a slight blow or slap on the skin, used in some massage procedures.

spatula (spăt′û-lă): a flexible implement with a blunt blade, used for removing creams from their containers.

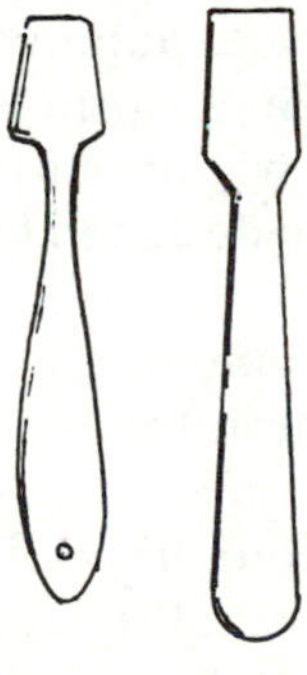

spatula

spearmint oil (spĭr′mĭnt′ oyl): a fragrant plant of the mint family; used as a flavoring agent, in perfumes and in toothpastes.

specialist (spĕsh′ă-lĭst): one who devotes himself or herself to some special branch of learning such as art, cosmetology or business.

spectrum (spĕk′trûm): an arrangement of colored bands produced by the passage of white light through a prism.

speed (spēd): a rate of motion: fast, medium, slow; fast speed: the closest rate of motion from its point of origin within its shape; medium speed: the rate of motion in the middle area of a shape, between fast and slow; slow speed: the furthest rate of motion from its point of origin within its shape.

sphenoid (sfē′noid): wedge-shaped; the wedge-shaped bone at the base of the skull.

sphere (sfĭr): a geometric figure generated by the revolution of a semicircle about its diameter.

spherical (sfĕr′ĭ-kâl): relating to or having the shape of a sphere.

spinal (spī′nâl): pertaining to the spine or vertebral column.

spinal accessory (spī′nâl ăk-sĕs′ô-rē): eleventh cranial nerve.

spinal column (spī′nâl kŏl′ûm): the backbone or vertebral column.

spinal cord (spī′nâl kôrd): the portion of the central nervous system contained within the spinal or vertebral canal.

spinal nerves (spī′nâl nûrvz): the nerves arising from the spinal cord.

spindle-shaped (spĭn′d′l-shāpt): shaped like a spindle; tapering toward each end.

spine (spīn): a sharp process of bone; the backbone.

spiral (spī′râl): coil; winding around a center, like a watch spring.

spiral curl (spī′râl kûrl): also called helical

wind; a method of curling hair by winding a strand around a rod; spiral winding.

spiral perm (spī′râl pûrm): a method in permanent waving in which hair is wound on perm rods from the scalp toward the ends.

spiral rod (spī′râl rŏd): a rod upon which the hair is wound in a spiral manner for a permanent wave.

spirillum (spī-rĭl′ûm); pl., **spirilla** (-ă): spiral bacterium.

spirit gum (spĭr′ĭt gŭm): gum used to attach false hair to skin or scalp.

splash neutralizer (splăsh nū′tră-lī-zẽr): a chemical agent capable of stopping the action of the cold waving solution and setting or hardening the hair in its new form.

split end (splĭt ĕnd): visible separation at end of the hair due to cuticle damage.

sponge (spŭnj): an elastic, porous substance that serves as an absorbent; the skeleton of an aquatic organism (phylum) cultivated for use as cosmetic and cleansing pads.

spongy hair (spŭn′jē hâr): hair that is overporous, due to overbleaching or abuse.

spool rod (spōōl rŏd): a straight cold wave rod.

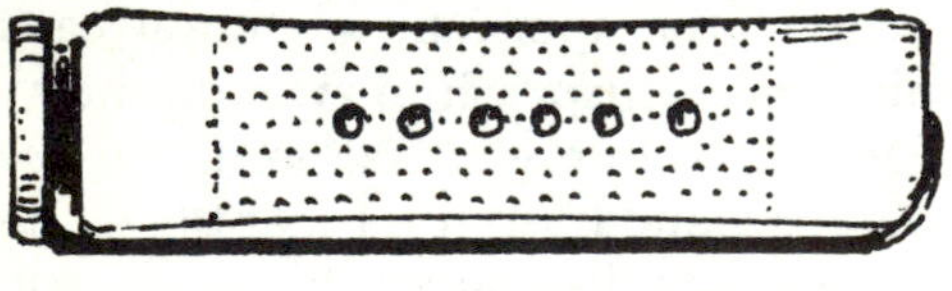

spool rod

spore (spôr): a tiny bacterial body having a protective wall to withstand unfavorable conditions.

spot bleaching (spŏt blēch′ĭng): applying bleach (lightener) to areas insufficiently lightened in order to produce even results.

spot tinting (spŏt tĭnt′ĭng): applying tint to areas insufficiently colored in order to achieve even results.

spray (sprā): to discharge liquid in the form of fine vapor.

spray gun (sprā-gŭn): an applicator used to spray a fine mist.

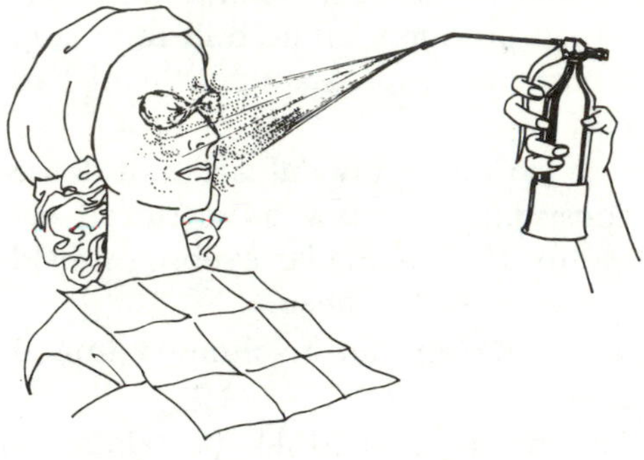

spray

spray machine (sprā mă-shēn′): a device employed to apply a very fine spray or mist of astringent to massage the nerve ends in the skin.

spring grip irons (sprĭng grĭp ī′ûrnz): thermal curling irons with a spring to enable it to close automatically.

springs; wig springs (sprĭngs): springs inserted into a wig or hairpiece foundation which are designed to hold it close to the head.

spur (spŭr): a pointed, horny outgrowth usually found on the feet.

squama (skwā′mă): an epidermic scale made up of thin, flat cells.

squamous (skwā′mûs): scaly; covered with scales; thin and flat like fish's scales.

square shaped face (skwâr shāpt fās): facial structure characterized by a wide forehead and jaw; usually shorter in length than an oval.

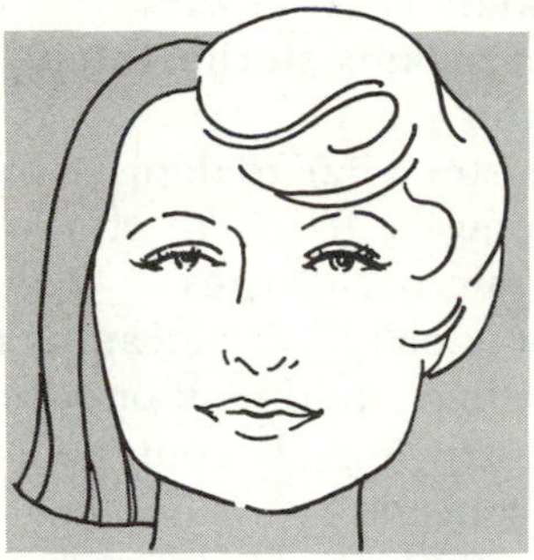

square-shaped face

stabilized (stā′-bĭ-līzd): made stable or firm, preventing changes.

stabilizer (stā′bĭ-lī-zẽr): a retarding agent or a substance that preserves a chemical equilibrium; see fixative.

stable (stā′b'l): in a balanced condition; not readily destroyed or decomposed; resisting molecular change.

stacking (stăk′ĭng): a haircutting technique using a slight gradation to achieve volume; an end permanent technique where one roller is stacked and extended above the other.

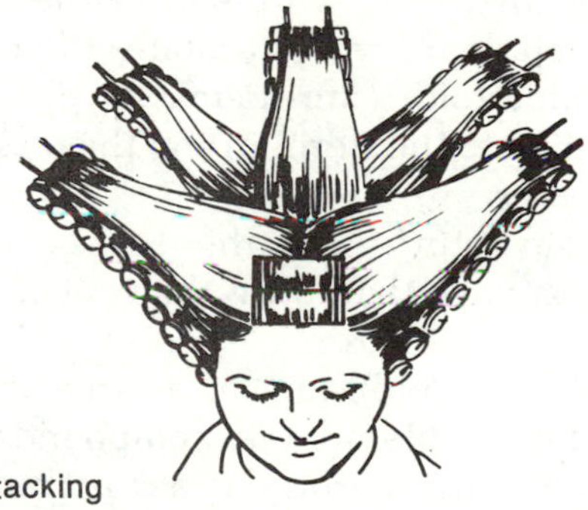

stacking

stack, permanent wave (stăk, pûr′mă-nênt wāv): a wrapping technique to curl ends of long hair; wrapping begins at the hairline and progresses to the crown with sticks used to maintain an even design.

stages (stā′jĕs): the term describing the seven colors the hair passes through during a lightening process.

stagger (stăg′ẽr): to arrange rollers on rods in a zigzag order.

stain (stān): an abnormal skin discoloration; hair color technique using a tint alone or mixed with conditioner rather than peroxide.

stand up curl (stănd ŭp kûrl): cascade curl; a strand of hair held directly up from the scalp and wound with a large center opening in croquignole fashion and fastened to the scalp in a standing position.

stand up curl

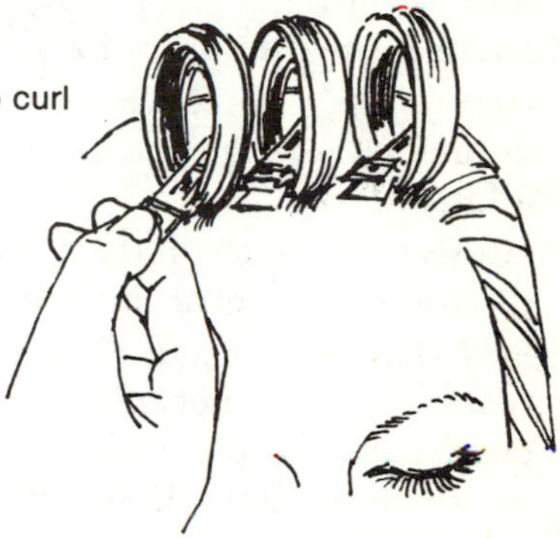

S-T

staphylococcus (stăf-ĭ-lô-kŏk′ûs); pl., **staphylococci** (-kŏk′sī): cocci which are grouped in clusters like a bunch of grapes; found in pustules and boils.

starch (stärch): a white, tasteless, odorless substance found in potatoes, corn, rice and similar vegetables; used in powders, dentifrices, hair colorings and many other cosmetic preparations.

starting knot (stärt′ĭng nŏt): the procedure in weaving and securing the first strand of hair.

static electricity (stăt′ĭk ê-lĕk-trĭs′ĭ-tē): a form of electricity generated by friction.

staying power (stā′ĭng paŭ′ẽr): the holding ability or power of a perm or set.

steam (stēm): water changed into vapor form when its temperature is raised to boiling.

steamer, facial (stēm′ẽr, fā′shâl): an apparatus, used in place of hot towels, for steaming the scalp or face.

steamer, scalp (stēm′ẽr, skălp): an apparatus, used in place of hot towels, for steaming the scalp.

stearate (stē′ă-rāt): a salt of stearic acid.

stearic acid (stê-ăr′ĭk ăs′ĭd): a white, fatty acid, occurring in solid animal fats and in some of the vegetable fats; used in powders, creams, lotions, and soap as a lubricant.

stearrhea (stē-ă-rē′ă): a form of seborrhea.

steatoma (stē-ă-tō′mă): a sebaceous cyst; a fatty tumor.

steatosis (stē-ă-tō′sĭs): fatty degeneration; disease of the sebaceous glands.

stem (stĕm): the strand of hair from the scalp up to but not including the first curvature of a pin curl.

stem direction (stĕm dĭ-rĕk′shûn): the direction in which the stem moves from the base to the first arc: up, down, forward, and back.

S-T

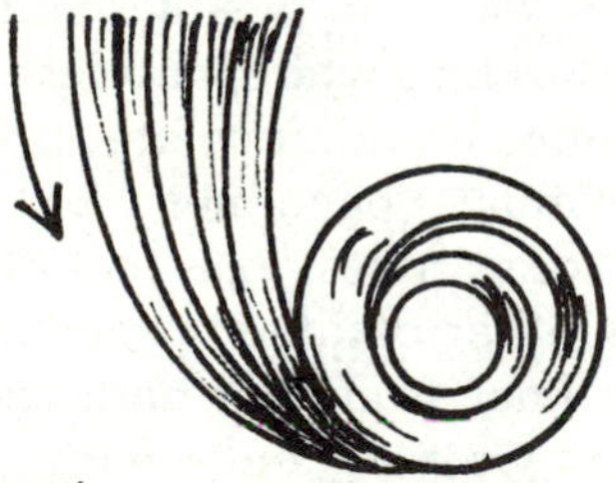

stem direction

steps (stĕps): irregular layers in a haircut.

sterile (stĕr′ĭl): barren; free from all living organisms.

sterilization (stĕr-ĭ-lĭ-zā′shûn): the process of making sterile; the destruction of germs.

sterilize (stĕr′ĭ-līz): to deprive of production power; to make sterile or free from microorganisms.

sterilizer (stĕr′ĭ-lī-zẽr): an apparatus used to sterilize equipment or other objects by destroying all contaminating microorganisms.

sterilizer cabinet, dry (stĕr′ĭ-lī-zẽr kăb′ĭ-nĕt, drī): a closed receptacle containing chemical vapors to keep sterilized objects ready for use.

sterilizer, wet (stĕr′ĭ-lī-zẽr, wĕt): a receptacle containing a disinfectant for the purpose of sterilizing implements.

sterno (stûr′nô): a prefix denoting connection with the sternum (breastbone).

sternocleidomastoid artery (stûr′nō-klī′-dô-măs′toid är′tĭr-ē): the artery that supplies blood to the muscles of the neck.

sternocleidomastoideus (stûr′nô-klī′dô-măs-toyd′ê-ûs): a muscle of the neck which depresses and rotates the head.

sternomastoid (stûr-nô-măs′toyd): pertaining to the sternum and the mastoid process.

sternum (stûr′nûm): the flat bone or breastbone that forms the ventral support of the ribs.

steroid (stēr′oid): any of a large group of fat soluble organic compounds, including the sterols and sex hormones.

stigma (stĭg′mă): a mark, spot, scar or other blemish on the skin.

stimulant (stĭm′û-lênt): an agent that arouses organic activity.

stomach (stŭm′ûk): the dilated portion of the alimentary canal, in which one of the processes of digestion takes place.

stopping point (stŏp′ĭng point): in massage, a point on a muscle or over a pressure point where pressing movements are made during the facial or scalp massage.

straight (strāt): extending in one direction without a curve or bend; not curly.

straight elevation (strāt ĕl-ĕ-vā′shûn): in haircutting, a term applied to the method of cutting the hair in a straight sphere or frame.

straightening comb (strāt′ĕn-ĭng kōm): also called a pressing comb; a comb constructed of steel or brass with a wood handle, usually heated electrically; used to remove curl from overcurly hair.

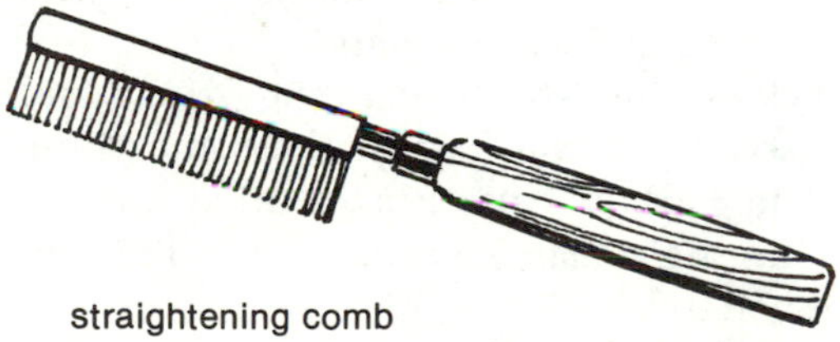

straightening comb

straight permanent wave rod (strāt pûr′-mă-nênt wāv rŏd): a permanent wave rod which is equal in circumference along the entire curling area.

straight profile (strāt prō′fīl): a profile that has evenly balanced facial features; being neither concave nor convex, as seen in profile.

straight wave (strāt wāv): a wave running alongside and parallel to the part.

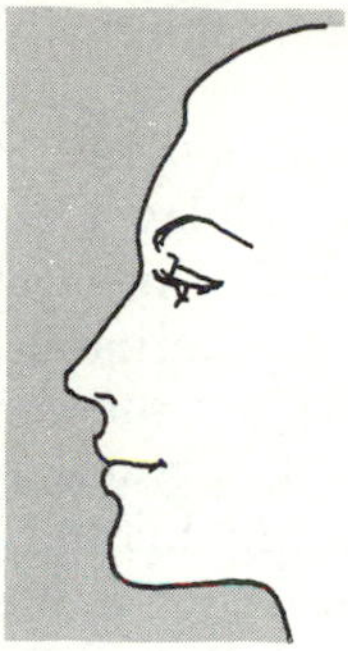

straight profile

strand (strănd): fibers or hairs that form a unit.

strand test (strănd tĕst): a test given before tinting, lightening, permanent waving or hair relaxing to determine the required developing or processing time; a test to determine the degree of porosity and elasticity of the hair, as well as the ability of the hair to withstand the effects of chemicals.

stratum (strā′tûm); pl., **strata** (-ă): a layer, as of tissue.

stratum basale (strā-tŭm bă-sā′lē): basal layer, the cell producing layer of the epidermis.

stratum corneum (strā′tûm kôr′nê-ûm): horny layer of the skin.

stratum germinativum (strāt′tûm jûr-mĭ-nă-tīv′ûm): the deepest layer of the epidermis resting on the corneum.

stratum granulosum (strāt′tûm grăn-û-lō′sûm): granular layer of the skin.

stratum lucidum (strā′tûm lū′sĭ-dûm): the clear, transparent layer of the epidermis under the stratum corneum.

stratum malpighii (strā′tûm mâl-pēg′ē-ī): the germinative or innermost layer of the epidermis including the spinosum or prickle layer.

stratum mucosum (strā′tûm mū-kō′sûm):

S-T

mucous or malpighian layer of the skin.

stratum spinosum (strā′tûm spĭn-ō′sûm): the prickle cell layer of the skin often classified with the stratum germinatum to form the basal layer; prickle-like threads join the cells.

streak (strēk): to lighten a strand of hair to create a highlighted effect.

streaking (strēk′ĭng): lightening thin sections of the hair.

streaking cap (strēk′ĭng kăp): also called frosting cap; a plastic or rubber head covering with punctured holes used to lighten or darken strands of hair.

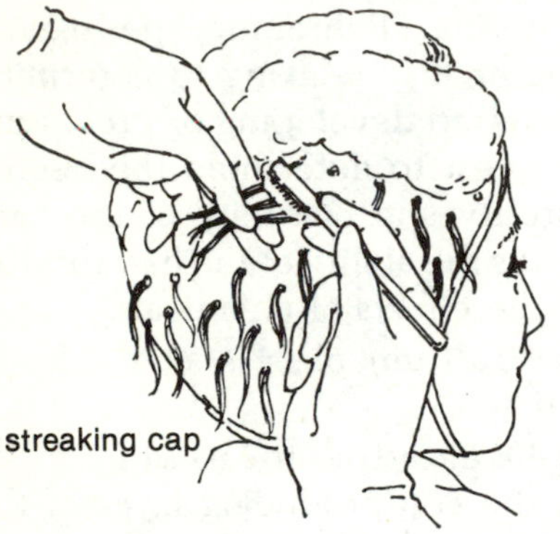

S-T

streptococcus (strĕp-tô-kŏk′ûs); pl., **streptococci** (-kŏk′sī): pus-forming bacteria that arrange in curved lines resembling a string of beads; found in erysipelas and blood poisoning.

stretch wig (strĕch wĭg): a wig which has been constructed with a completely elasticized foundation that will stretch to fit a wide range of head sizes.

striated (strī′āt-ĕd): marked with parallel lines or bands; striped, as voluntary muscle.

stringy hair (strĭng′ē hâr): limp hairs matted together forming a rope-like strand.

stripping (strĭp′ĭng): the removal of color from the hair shaft; bleaching; lightening; strong shampoos or soap removing some of the color from the hair is also known as stripping.

stroking (strōk′ŭng): a gliding movement over a surface; to pass the finger or any instrument gently over a surface; effleurage.

strong hair (strông hâr): hair that is somewhat resistant to treatments, usually coarser than average hair.

strontium sulphide (strŏn′tē-ûm sŭl′fīd): a light gray powder capable of liberating hydrogen sulphide in the presence of water; used as a depilatory.

sty, stye (stī); pl., **sties, styes** (stīz): inflammation of one of the sebaceous glands of the eyelid.

style (stīl): the current, fashionable mode of dress, makeup or hair design; the specific shape, size and placement of curls and waves of a finished hairstyle.

style cut (stīl kŭt): a short hair shaping which has the design and style cut into the top, sides and nape.

style drying (stīl drī′ĭng): the drying and styling of the hair at the same time.

style part (stīl pärt): a planned part in the hair that is visible in the finished hairstyle.

styling chair (stī′lĭng châr): an adjustable chair, usually with a footrest, where the client sits while the hair is being styled.

styling comb (stī′lĭng kōm): a comb designed with one half row of thin, close teeth and the other half with wider spaces between the teeth; used to aid in styling hair.

styling gel (stī′lĭng jĕl): a jelly-like preparation used to aid in styling the hair and add stiffness.

styling iron heater (stī′lĭng ī′ûrn hē′tĕr): an electric apparatus used to heat thermal curling irons.

styling lotion (stī′lĭng lō′shûn): a liquid preparation used to add body and staying power to the finished hairstyle.

styling station (stīl′ĭng stā′shûn): a space or unit in a salon containing the furnishings, implements and products needed to cut and style hair.

stylist (stīl′ĭst): one who develops, designs, advises on, or creates styles.

styptic (stĭp′tĭk): an agent causing contraction of living tissue; used to stop bleeding; an astringent.

styrofoam (stī′rô-fōm): a lightweight plastic foam used for a wig blok, used to keep a styled wig in shape.

sub (sŭb): a prefix denoting under; below.

subclavian (sŭb-klā′vē ûn): lying under the clavicle, as the subclavian artery.

subcutaneous (sŭb-kū-tā′nē-ûs): under the skin.

subcutis (sŭb-kū′tĭs): subdermis; subcutaneous tissue; under or beneath the corium or dermis, the true skin.

subdermis (sŭb-dûr′mĭs): subcutis or subcutaneous tissue of the skin.

subdivide (sŭb′dĭ-vīd): to divide a section into smaller sections.

submental artery (sŭb-mĕn′tâl är′tĭr-ē): artery that supplies blood to the chin and lower lip.

suboccipital nerve (sŭb-ŏk-sĭp′ĭ tâl nûrv): nerve that stimulates the deep muscles of the back of the neck.

subsection (sŭb′sĕk′shûn): dividing a section into smaller parts; the part created by this division.

subsection

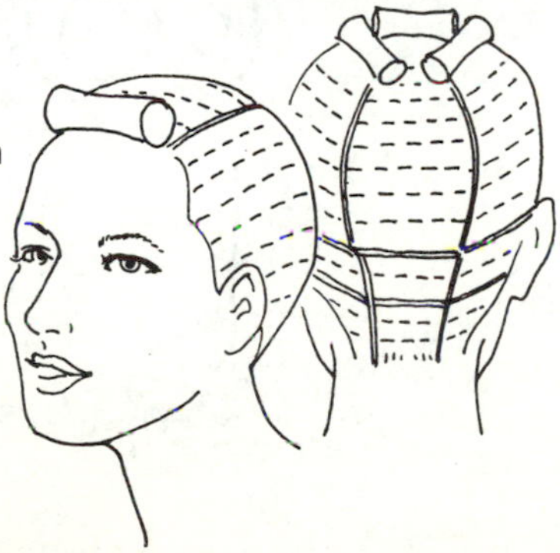

suction machine (sŭk′shûn mă-shēn′): an apparatus used in some facial treatment procedures to dislodge debris from the follicles.

sudamen (sû-dā′mĕn); pl., **sudamina** (sû-dăm′ĭ-nă): a disorder of the sweat glands with obstruction of their ducts.

sudor (sū′dôr): sweat; perspiration.

sudoriferous (sū-dŭr-ĭf′ĕr-ûs): carrying or producing sweat.

sudoriferous ducts (sū-dŭr-ĭf′ĕr-ûs dŭkts): the excretory ducts of the sweat glands.

sudoriferous glands (sū-dŭr-ĭf′ĕr-ûs glăndz): sweat glands of the skin.

sudorific (sū-dŭr-ĭf′ĭk): causing or inducing perspiration.

sulfide (sŭl′fīd): compound of sulfur and an oxide.

sulfite (sŭl′fīt): any salt of sulfurous acid.

sulfonated oil (sŭl′fă-nāt-ĭd oyl): an organic substance prepared by reacting oils with sulphuric acid; used as a base in soapless shampoos and in hair sprays as an emulsifier.

sulfur, sulphur (sŭl′fĕr): a solid, nonmetallic element, usually yellow in color; it is insoluble in water.

sulfur bonds (sŭl′fĕr bŏndz): sulfur cross bonds in the hair, which hold the chains of amino acids together; position determines curl present in the hair.

sulfuric acid (sŭl-fū′rĭk ăs′ĭd): oil of vitriol; colorless and nearly odorless, heavy oily corrosive liquid, employed as a caustic.

sulphide (sŭl′fīd): a compound of sulfur with another element or basic radical.

sunburn (sŭn′bûrn): inflammation of the skin caused by exposure to the sun.

sunburst (sŭn′bûrst): a special form of hair lightening that creates a sun-like effect, usually in the front of the style.

sunflower seed oil (sŭn-flou′ẽr sēd oyl): oil obtained from the seeds of sunflowers; a good source of vitamin E; used in soap manufacturing, salad oil and some food products.

sunlamp (sŭn′lămp): a lamp that radiates ultraviolet rays; used in cosmetic and therapeutic face and body treatments.

sunlighting (sŭn′līt-ĭng): the technique of highlighting the top layer of the hair.

suntan (sŭn′tăn): a brownish coloring of the skin as a result of sun exposure.

super (sū′pẽr): a prefix denoting over; above; beyond.

superciliary (sū-pẽr-sĭl′ê-ẽr-ē): pertaining to or referring to the region of the eyebrow.

supercilium (sū-pẽr-sĭl′ē-ûm); pl., **supercilia** (-ă): the eyebrow.

superficial (sū-pẽr-fĭsh′âl): pertaining to or being on the surface.

superficial cervical (sū-pẽr-fĭsh′âl sûr′vĭ-kâl): a cranial nerve which supplies the muscle and skin of the neck.

superficial fascia (sū-pẽr-fĭsh′âl făsh′ē-ă): a sheet of subcutaneous tissue; tissue that attaches the dermis to underlying structures.

superficial temporal artery (sū-pẽr-fĭsh′âl tĕm′pă-râl är′tĭr-ē): the artery that supplies blood to the muscles of the scalp and head.

superfluous (sū-pẽr′flo͞o-ûs): excessive; more than is wanted or needed.

superfluous hair (sū-pẽr′flo͞o-ûs hâr): unwanted hair.

superior (sū-pĭr′ē-ẽr): higher; upper; better or of more value.

superior auricularis (sū-pĭr′ē-ẽr ô-rĭk-ū-lâr′ĭs): the muscle that draws the ear upward.

superioris (sū-pĭr-ĕ-ŏr′ĭs): a muscle which elevates.

superior labial artery (sū-pĭr′ē-ẽr lā′bē-âl är′tĭr-ē): artery that supplies blood to the upper lip and region of the nose.

superior labial nerve (sū-pĭr′ē-ẽr lā′bē-âl nûrv): nerve that receives stimuli from the skin of the upper lip.

superior maxillary (sū-pĭr′ē-ẽr măk′sĭ-lĕ-rē): the upper jawbone.

superior palpebral nerve (sū-pĭr′ē-ẽr pâl′pĕ-brâl nûrv): nerve that receives stimuli from the upper eyelid.

superior vena cava (sū-pĭr′ē-ẽr vē′nă cā′vă): the large vein that carries blood to the upper right chamber of the heart.

supinate (sū′pĭ-nāt): to turn the forearm and hand so the palmar surface is uppermost.

supinator (sū′pĭ-nāt-ôr): a muscle of the forearm, which rotates the radius outward.

supple hair (sŭp′'l hâr): hair that is easily managed, pliable, and not stiff.

supporting curl (sŭ-pôrt′ĭng kûrl): a pin curl made in the same direction as the first line of curls.

supporting curl

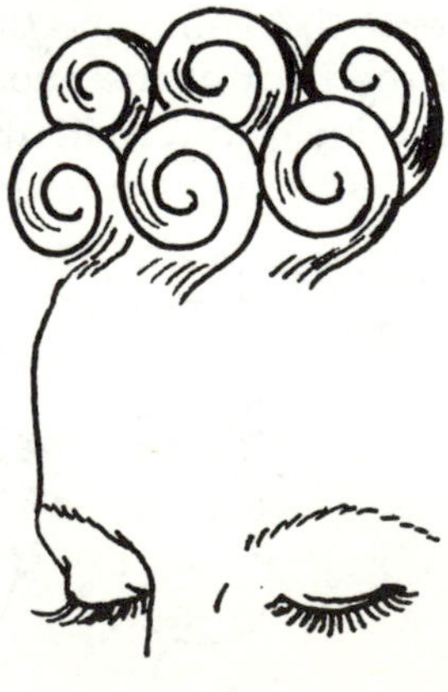

suppuration (sŭp-û-rā′shûn): the formation of pus.

supra (sū′pră): a prefix denoting on top of, above, over, beyond, besides; more than.

supraclavicular (sū′pră-klă-vĭk′ū-lär): above the clavicle.

supraclavicular nerve, intermediate (sū′-pră-klă-vĭk′ū-lär nûrv, ĭn′tĕr-mē′dē-ĭt): nerve that receives stimuli from the lower anterior aspect of the neck and interior chest wall.

supraclavicular nerve, lateral (sū′pră klă-vĭk-ū lär nûrv, lăt′ĕr-ăl): nerve that receives stimuli from the skin of the lateral aspect of the neck and shoulder.

supraorbital (sū-pră-ôr′bĭ-tâl): above the orbit or eye.

supraorbital artery (sū-pră-ôr′bĭ-tâl är′-tĭr-ē): artery that supplies blood to the upper eyelid and forehead.

supraorbital nerve (sū-pră-ôr′bĭ-tâl nûrv): nerve that receives stimuli from the skin of the upper eyelid and the forehead.

suprascapular artery (sū-pră-skăp′ū-lär är′tĭr-ē): the artery that supplies blood to the shoulder joints and muscles surrounding the area.

supratrochlear (sū-pră-trŏk′lē-ĕr): above the trochlea or pulley of the superior oblique muscle.

supratrochlear artery (sū-pră-trŏk′lē-ĕr är-tĭr-ē): artery that supplies blood to the anterior scalp.

supratrochlear nerve (sū-pră-trŏk′lē-ĕr nûrv): nerve that receives stimuli from the skin of the medial aspect of forehead, root of the nose and the upper eyelid.

surface (sûr′fĭs): the outer or topmost boundary of an object; the boundary of any three-dimensional figure.

surface tension (sûrfûs tĕn′shûn): the tension or resistance to rupture possessed by the surface film of a liquid.

surgical glove (sûr′jĭ-kâl glŭv): a thin rubber glove with finger and thumb sections, used to protect the hands from stains and irritants.

suspension (sŭs-pĕn′shûn): a state of matter in which the solid particles are dispersed in or distributed throughout a liquid medium; the particles in the medium are large but not large enough to settle to the bottom under the influence of gravity.

swab (swab): absorbent cotton wrapped around the end of a short, pliable stick; used for the application of solutions and for removing excess makeup.

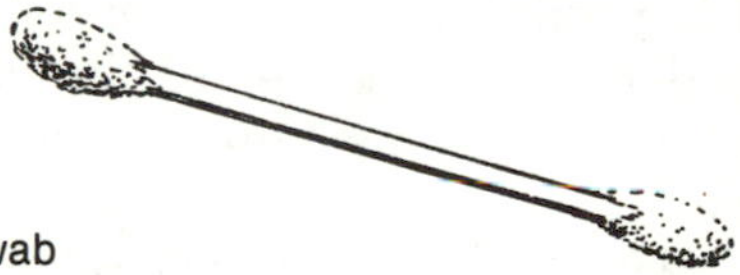

swab

swathe (swäth): knotted or woven hairpiece usually worn at the nape of the neck.

sweat (swĕt): to exude or excrete moisture from the pores of the skin; perspiration.

sweat gland (swĕt glănd): small convoluted tubules that secrete sweat; found in the subcutaneous tissue and ending at the opening of the pores.

Swedish massage (swē′dĭsh mă-säzh′): a system of passive and active exercise movements and techniques for muscles and joints.

Swedish movements (swē′dĭsh mo͞ov′-mêntz): a system of muscular movements employed in massage to treat and develop the body.

sweep (swēp): to brush or comb the hair upward, moving or extending in a wide curve or over a wide area; upsweep.

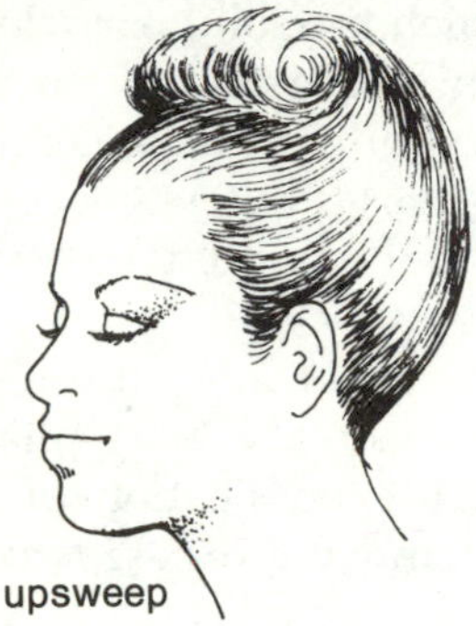

sweep, upsweep

sweet bay oil (swēt bā oyl): an oil produced from the leaves of the laurel; used in soaps, perfumes and emollients.

swirl (swûrl): formation of a wave in a diagonal direction from back to side of head.

switch (swĭch): a long length of wefted hair mounted with a loop on the end; usually constructed with three stem strands to provide flexibility in styling; a separate tress of hair, or of some substitute, worn by women to increase the apparent mass of hair.

swivel clamp (swĭv′âl klămp): a clamp used to secure a wig block or mannikin head to a table top.

sycosis (sī-kō′sĭs): a chronic pustular inflammation of the hair follicles.

sycosis barbae (sī-kō′sĭs bär′bē): a chronic inflammation of the hair follicles of the beard; barber's itch.

sycosis tinea (sī-kō′sĭs tĭn′ē-ă): parasitic ringworm of the beard; barber's itch.

sycosis vulgaris (sī-kō′sĭs vŭl-gâ′rĭs): a pustular, follicular lesion caused by staphylococci; nonparasitic sycosis of the beard.

symbol (sĭm′bâl): conventional abbreviation; a character, sign or mark to represent an object, abstract idea, an element, quantity, etc.

symmetrical (sĭ-mĕt′rĭ-kâl): uniform and balanced in proportion and style.

symmetrical hairstyle (sĭ-mĕt′rĭ-kâl hâr′-stīl): a hairstyle with a similar design on both sides of the face.

symmetrical hairstyle

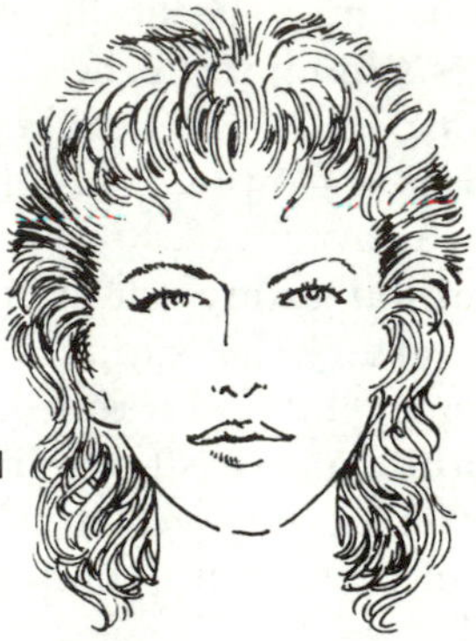

symmetry (sĭ′mĕt-rē): balanced proportions; harmony of line and form.

sympathetic nervous system (sĭm-pă-thĕt′ĭk nûr′vŭs sĭs′tĕm): that part of the autonomic nervous system concerned with mediating involuntary responses of the body such as heart rate, salivary secretion, blood pressure, digestion, etc.

symptomatica alopecia (sĭmp-tûm-ăt′ĭ-kă ăl-ô-pē′shē-ă): loss of hair due to illness.

symptom, objective (sĭmp′tûm, ŏb-jĕk′-tĭv): a symptom that can be seen, as in pimples or pustules.

symptom, subjective (sĭmp′tûm, sŭb-jĕk′-tĭv): a symptom that can be felt but not seen, such as itching.

syn (sĭn): a prefix denoting along with; together; at the same time.

syndactylism (sĭn-dăk′tĭl-ĭz′m): webbed fingers or toes.

synergetic (sĭn′är-jĕt′ĭk): working together; the combined action or effect of two or more organs or agents, or to coordination of muscular or organ functions by the nervous system in such a way that specific movements and actions can be performed.

synovia (sĭ-nō′vē-ă): a transparent viscid lubricating fluid secreted by the lining membranes of joints.

synthetic (sĭn-thĕt′ĭk): produced artificially; not natural.

synthetic hair (sĭn-thĕt′ĭk hâr): a man-made hairlike fiber made from nylon, dynel, rayon, etc., or from any combination of these fibers.

syrian hair (sĭr′ē-ên hâr): a mixture of human hair or animal hair with yak hair.

system (sĭs′tûm): a group of bodily organs acting together to perform one or more of the main bodily functions; an arrangement of objects that complete a unit; a procedure or established way of doing something.

systemic (sĭs-tĕm′ĭk): pertaining to a system or to the body as a whole; affecting the body generally.

T

"T" pin (Tē pĭn): a "T" shaped pin used to attach a hairpiece to a block.

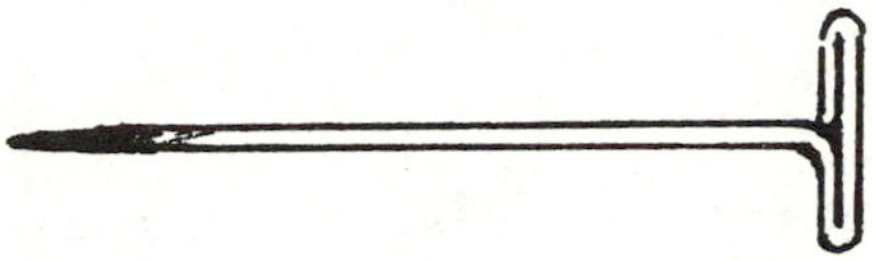

"T" pin

tabes (tā′bēz): wasting away or atrophy due to disease.

tablespoon (tā′b'l spōōn): abbr: tbsp; a large spoon used for serving food and in measuring substances; one tablespoonful equals three teaspoons, or ½ ounce, or 15 milliliters in metric measure.

tache (tăsh): a small, discolored spot on the skin, such as a freckle; a macule.

tactile (tăk′tĭl): pertaining to the sense of touch; capable of being felt.

tactile corpuscle (tăk′tĭl kôr′pŭs'l): small epidermal structures with nerve endings that are sensitive to touch and pressure.

tag (tăg): a small appendage, flap or polyp; skin tag; cutaneous outgrowth of the skin.

tail brush (tāl brŭsh): a small, flat brush with stiff bristles and a long tapering end; used to apply a hair coloring or relaxing product to the hair.

tail comb (tāl kōm): a comb, half of which is shaped into a slender tail-like end; see rat tail comb.

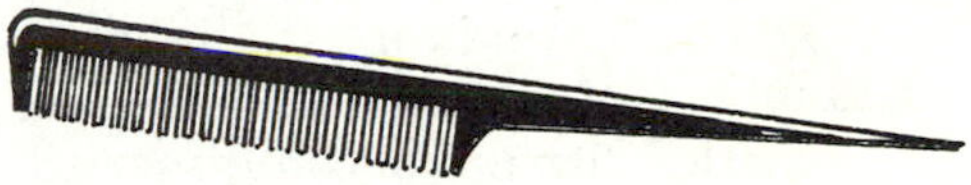

tail comb

tailored neckline (tā′lôrd nĕk′līn): a hair shaping in which the hairline is low and angled in the nape area.

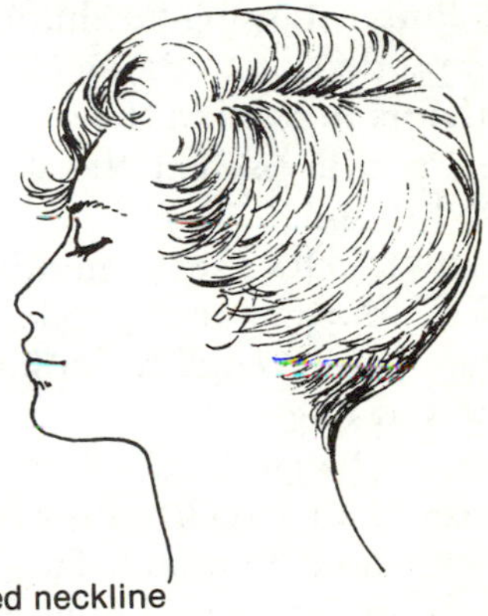

tailored neckline

talc (tâlk): a soft, white hydrous magnesium silicate used in making powder and soaps.

talcum powder (tâl′kûm paủ′dẽr): finely powdered, purified talc used as a face or body powder.

talipes (tâl′ĭ pēz): a deformity of the foot, such as clubfoot.

S-T

talipomanus (tâl-ĭ-pŏm′ă-nûs): a deformity of the hand analogous to clubfoot; clubhand.

talus (tāl′ûs): bone of the ankle that joins the bones of the leg; the ankle.

tan (tăn): sunburn; pigmentation of skin from exposure to the sun.

tan color (tăn kŭl′ẽr): a yellowish-brown color.

tang (tăng): a projection such as the finger rest on scissors.

tangle (tān′g'l): a matted mass of hair; snarled hair; to become snarled.

tangled hair (tān′g'ld hâr): trichonodosis; fraying of the hair resulting in knots, associated with breaking of the hair shaft.

tannic acid (tăn′ĭk ăs′ĭd): tannin; an astringent of plant origin.

tanning lotion (tăn′ĭng lō′shûn): a sunscreen product, containing oil or other ingredients to assist in the sun-tanning process and to protect the skin while exposed to sun.

tap (tăp): to touch or strike gently; to pat the face during the application of makeup; in massage, to strike lightly with flexed fingers.

tape (tāp): in hairstyling, a narrow strip of material to which adhesive is applied and used to attach false hair to the scalp or face, or to hold flat curls or bangs to the face.

taper (tā′pẽr): a gradual decrease in thickness, narrowing to a point; to become progressively narrower at one end.

tapering (tā′pẽr-ĭng): in haircutting, to cut the hair at various lengths; to narrow a strand of hair toward the ends.

tapering shears (tā′pẽr-ĭng shẽrz): scissors designed for thinning hair and shaping blunt ends.

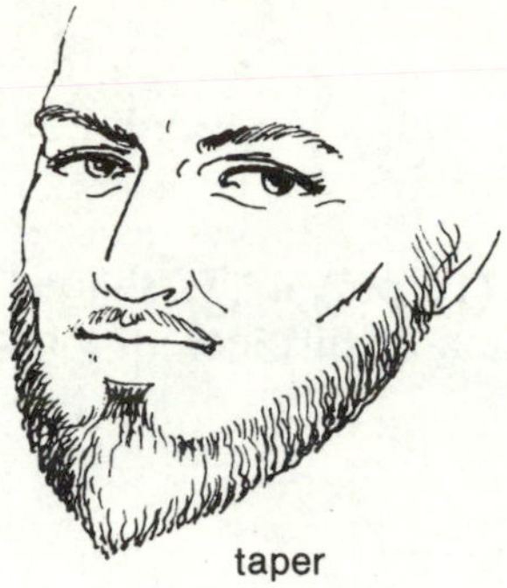

taper

tapotement (tă-pôt-män′): a massage movement using a short, quick slapping or tapping movement.

tapping (tăp′ĭng): a massage movement; striking lightly with the partly flexed fingers.

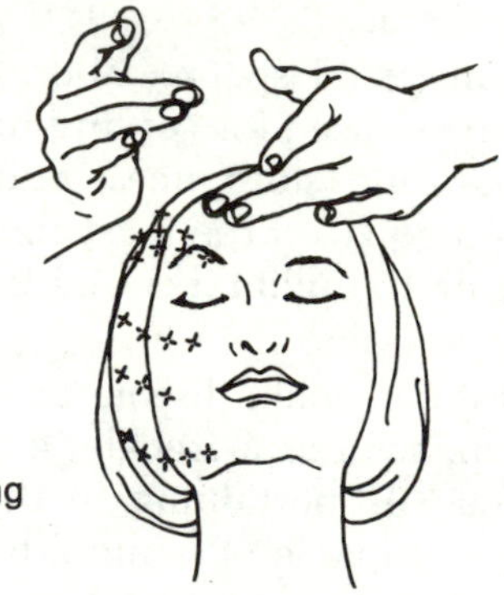

tapping

tar (tär): the thick, semisolid brown or black liquid obtained from various species of pine; used to treat certain skin diseases; pine tar.

tarsal artery (tär′sâl är′tĭr-ē): artery that supplies blood to the foot and tarsal joints.

tarsus (tär′sûs): the root or posterior part of the foot or instep; the seven bones of the instep.

taupe (tōp): the color of moleskin, dark gray with a tinge of brown.

taut (tôt): tightly drawn; firm; not slack.

teal blue (tēl blū): a dull greenish-blue color.

tease (tēz): in hairstyling, to comb small sections of hair from the ends toward the scalp to form a cushion or base; also known as ratting, French lacing or ruffing.

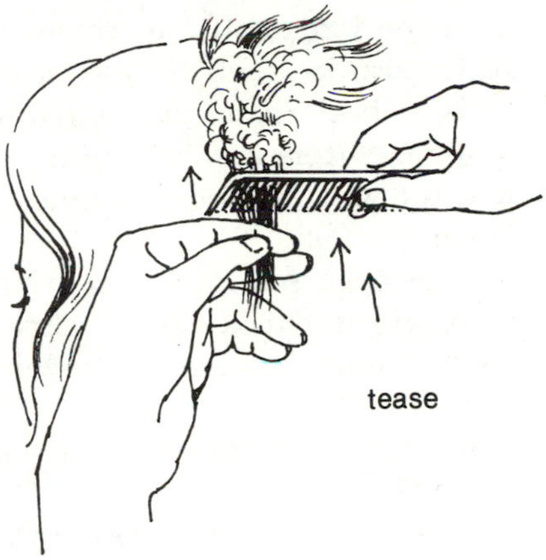

tease

teasing brush (tēz′ĭng brŭsh): a small brush with short, stiff bristles and a long, thin handle; used to brush sections of hair from the ends toward the scalp.

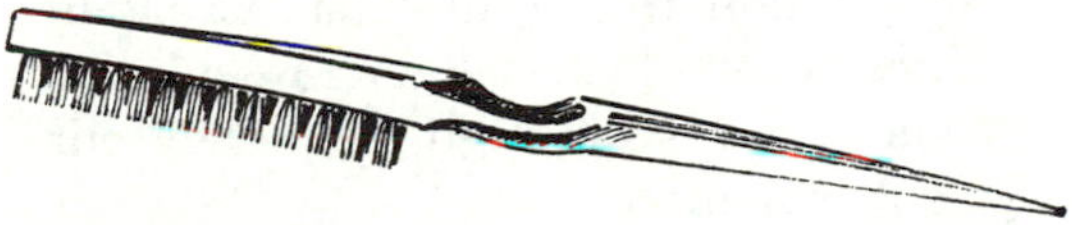

teasing brush

teasing comb (tēz′ĭng kōm): a comb designed with alternating short and long teeth; used to comb sections of hair from the ends toward the scalp.

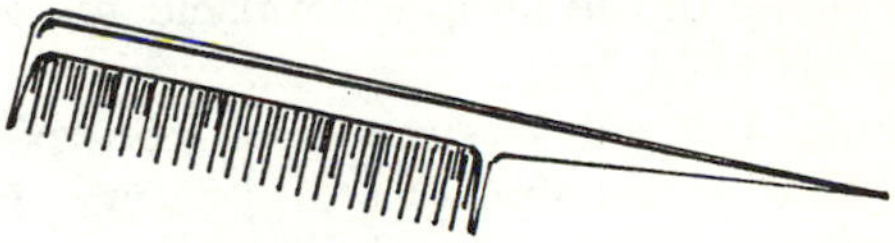

teasing comb

technical (tĕk′nĭ-kâl): relating to a technique; relating to a practical subject organized on scientific principles.

technician (tĕk-nĭ′shûn): an individual trained and expert in a specific skill or subject.

technique (tĕk-nēk): manner of performance; a skill; a process.

tela (tē′lă): a web-like structure.

telangiectasis (tĕl-ăn-jē-ĕk′tă-sĭs): dilation of the capillary vessles and minute arteries, forming a variety of angioma.

telogen effluvin (tĕl′ô jĕn ĕf′lū-vĭn): loss of hair while hair cells are in the resting stage.

telogen phase (tĕl′ô-jĕn fāz): the final resting phase of the hair cycle in a follicle, lasting until the fully grown hair is shed, at which time anogen begins.

telophase (tĕl′ô-fāz): the final stage of cell mitosis in which the chromosomes reorganize to form an interstage nucleus.

temperature (tĕm′pĕr-ă-chĕr): the degree of heat or cold as measured by a thermometer.

temple (tĕm′p'l): the flattened space on the side of the forehead.

temporal (tĕm′pă-râl): of or pertaining to the temple.

temporal artery (tĕm′pă-râl är′tĭr-ē): deep artery that supplies blood to the temporal muscle, the orbit and skull.

temporal artery, medial (tĕm′pă-râl är

S-T

tĭr-ē, mē′dē-âl): artery that supplies blood to the temporal muscle and eyelids.

temporal artery, superficial (tĕm′pâ-râl är′tĭr-ē, soo′pĕr-fĭsh′ăl): artery that supplies blood to the muscles of the head, face and scalp.

temporal bone (tĕm′pă-râl bōn): the bone at the side and base of the skull.

temporalis (tĕm-pă-rā′lĭs): the temporal muscle.

temporal nerve (tĕm′pă-râl nûrv): the nerve that receives stimuli from the temporal muscle at the temple.

temporary (tĕm′pă-rĕ-rē): not permanent; lasting only for a specific time.

temporary color (tĕm′pă-rĕ-rē kŭl′ẽr): a nonpermanent color that may be removed by shampooing.

temporary rinse (tĕm′pă-rĕ-rē rins): a nonpermanent color rinse that is used to color the hair and is easily removed by shampoo.

tendon (tĕn′dôn): fibrous cord or band connecting muscle with bone.

tendril (tĕn′drĭl): a small, wispy curl that appears to be falling downward.

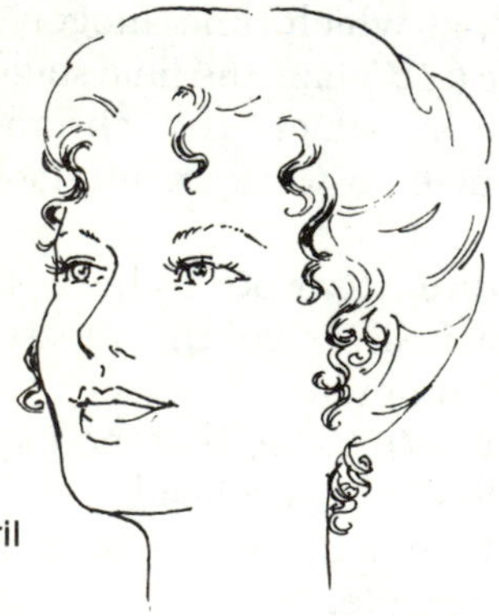

tendril

tensile (tĕn′sĭl): capable of being stretched.

tensile strength (tĕn′sĭl strĕnth): the resistance of a material to the forces of stress.

tension (tĕn′shûn): stress caused by stretching or pulling.

tepid (tĕp′ĭd): neither hot nor cold; lukewarm.

terminal (tûr′mĭ-nâl): of or pertaining to an end or extremity; a part that forms the end.

terminal hair (tûr′mĭ-nâl hâr): tertiary hair; the long, soft hair found on the scalp; also present on legs, arms and body of both males and females.

terminology (tẽr-mĭ-nŏl′ô-jē): the special words or terms used in science, art or business.

terry (tĕr′ē): a pile fabric in which the loops are uncut; a cotton fabric, very water absorbent; used for towels; terry cloth.

tertiary (tûr′shē-ĕ-rē): third in rank, order or formation.

tertiary color (tûr′shē-ĕ-rē kŭl′ẽr): an intermediate color achieved by mixing a secondary color and its neighboring primary color on the color wheel in equal amounts; example: blue mixed with green to produce turquoise.

Tesla current (tĕs′lă kŭr′ênt): commonly called violet ray; a thermal or heat producing current used by cosmetologists for facial and scalp treatments.

Tesla, Nikola (tĕs′lă, nĭ-kō′lă): Croatian-American electrical engineer after whom the Tesla high frequency current is named.

test curls (tĕst kûrlz): a method to predetermine how the client's hair will react to cold waving solution and neutralizer; process of testing the hair to determine curl for motion during the permanent wave.

test strand (tĕst strănd): a small section of hair on which hair color or chemical relaxer is applied to predetermine how the hair will react.

S-T

tetanus (tĕt′nŭs): an infectious disease which causes spasmodic muscle contractions of voluntary muscles; also called lockjaw.

tetter (tĕt′ẽr): any of various skin eruptions such as herpes, eczema and psoriasis.

textometer (tĕks-tŏm′ĕ-tẽr): a device used to measure the elasticity and reaction of the hair to alkaline solutions.

textural combination (tĕks′chẽr-âl käm-bĭ-nā′shûn): a form incorporating two or more of the basic textures.

texture (tĕks′chẽr): the composition or structure of a tissue or organ; the general feel or appearance of a substance.

texture, hair (tĕks′chẽr, hâr): the general quality such as coarse, medium, fine and feel of the hair.

texture, skin (tĕks′chẽr, skĭn): the general feel and appearance of the skin; skin type such as coarse, fine, medium, thin, thick and degree of elasticity.

texturize (teks′chẽr-īz): in hairdressing, to cut for effect within the hair length.

thallium (thă′lĭ-ûm): a bluish-white metallic element, the salts of which have been used for epilation; thallium is highly toxic to humans.

thenar (thē′när): the fleshy prominence of the palm corresponding to the base of the thumb.

theory (thē′ô-rē): an hypothesis; a reasoned and probable explanation.

therapeutic (thĕr-ă-pū′tĭk): pertaining to the treatment of disease by remedial agents or methods.

therapeutic lamp (thĕr-ă-pū′tĭk lămp): an electrical apparatus producing any of the rays of the spectrum; used for skin and scalp treatments.

therapeutics (thĕr-ă-pū′tĭks): branch of medical science concerned with the treatment of disease.

therapeutic treatments (thĕr-ă pū′tĭk trēt′mênts): beneficial treatments for skin, body or scalp.

therapy (thĕr′ă-pē): the science and art of healing.

therm (thûrm): a unit of heat to which equivalents have been given, for example, a small calorie, a kilocalorie.

thermal (thûr′mâl): relating to heat.

thermal curling (thûr′mâl kûrl′ĭng): the process of curling straight or pressed hair with a thermal iron.

thermal hairdressing (thûr′mâl hâr′drĕs-ĭng): the art of dressing or setting hair with dry heat.

thermal irons (thûr′mâl ī′ẽrnz): curling irons.

thermal set (thûr′mâl sĕt): the technique of setting dry hair with a thermal iron or heated hair rollers.

thermal unit (thŭr′mâl ū′nĭt): the amount of heat required to raise the temperature of a pound of water one degree Centigrade or Fahrenheit.

thermo cap (thûr′mō kăp): an insulated cap used in some hair treatments.

thermolysis (thûr-mŏl′ĭ sĭs): the use of high frequency or shortwave current to remove superfluous hair.

thermomassage (thûr′mō-mă-säzh′): massage given with the application of heat.

thermometer (thẽr-mŏm′ĕ-tẽr): any device for measuring temperature.

thermostat (thûr′mô-stăt): an automatic device for regulating temperature.

thiamine (thī′ă-mĭn): a water soluble component of vitamin B complex; primary sources are vegetables, egg yolks, organ meats, and whole grains.

thickening agent (thĭk′ĕn-ĭng ā′gênt): a substance which is employed to thicken watery solutions.

thigh (thī): the part of the lower extremity from the pelvis to the knee.

thighbone (thī′bōn): the long bone of the thigh; femur.

thinner (thĭn′ẽr): a product used to thin nail polish.

thinning, hair (thĭn′ĭng, hâr): decreasing the thickness of the hair where it is too heavy.

thinning scissors (thĭn′ĭng sĭz′ẽrz): also called shears; scissors with single or double notched blades; used to thin hair.

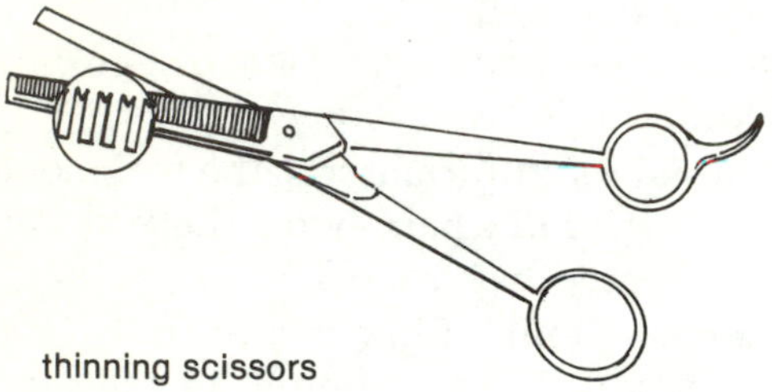

thinning scissors

thio (thī′ō): ammonium thioglycolate and thioglycolic acid; used to break down cross linkages of the hair in chemical straightening or cold waving.

thioglycolic acid (thī-ō-glī′kô-lĭk ăs′ĭd): a colorless liquid or white crystals with a strong unpleasant odor, miscible with water, alcohol or ether; used in permanent wave solutions, hair relaxers and depilatories.

third degree burn (thûrd dĕ-grē′bûrn): a severe burn which destroys the epidermis and underlying tissue, and is more severe than a second degree burn.

third occipital nerve (thûrd ŏk-sĭp′ĭ-tâl nûrv): nerve that receives stimuli from the skin of the posterior aspect of the neck and scalp.

thoracic (thô-răs′ĭk): pertaining to the thorax.

thoracic duct (thô-răs′ĭk dŭkt): the common lymph trunk emptying into the left subclavian vein; the principle duct of the lymphatic system.

thorax (thō′răks): the part of the body between the neck and the abdomen; the chest.

three dimensional (thrē dĭ-mĕn′shûn'l): having length, width, and depth.

three-dimensional shading (thrē dī-mĕn′-shŭn-âl shād′ĭng): a technique in which hair is bleached and toned with two shades of toner, giving a three-dimensional effect.

throat (thrōt): the part of the neck leading from the back of the mouth to the stomach and lungs, including the upper larynx, esophagus and trachea.

thrombocyte (thrŏm′bô-sīt): a blood platelet which aids in clotting.

thumb (thŭm): the short, thick digit next to the forefinger of a human hand.

thumbnail (thŭm′nāl): the nail of the thumb.

thyme (tīm): a shrub plant of the mint family which produces thyme; used in cosmetics and medicinal preparations.

thymol (thī′môl): a compound extracted from the oil of thyme or manufactured synthetically; used in some antiseptics and perfumery.

thymus (thī′mûs): a ductless gland situated in the upper part of the chest; believed to function in the development of the body's immune system.

thyroid cartilage (thī′roid kär′tĭ-lĭg): the largest cartilage of the larynx, composed of two blades which form the Adam's apple.

thyroid gland (thī′roid glănd): a large ductless gland situated in front and on

S-T

either side of the trachea; it produces the hormone thyroxine which regulates the growth and metabolism of the body.

thyroxine (thī răk′sēn): a hormone secreted by the thyroid gland; the gland regulating body metabolism and weight control.

tibia (tĭb′ē-ă): the shinbone; the large bone of the leg below the knee.

tibial arteries (tĭb′ē-âl är′tĭr-ēz): arteries that supply blood to the lower leg and foot.

tibial nerves (tĭb′ē-âl nûrvz): nerves of the leg, sole of the foot, knee and foot joints.

tight scalp (tīt skălp): a scalp that is not easily moved over the underlying structure.

tincture (tĭnk′chēr): an alcoholic solution of a medicinal substance.

tincture of benzoin (tĭnk′chēr of bĕn′zō-ĭn): a protective, antiseptic astringent used in healing skin eruptions.

tincture of capsicum (tĭnk′chēr of kăp′sĭ-kûm): alcoholic solution made from cayenne pepper, which is used in a treatment to stimulate hair growth.

tinea (tĭn′ê-ă): a skin disease, especially ringworm.

tinea barbae (tĭn′ê-ă bär′bē): tinea sycosis.

tinea capitis (tĭn′ê-ă kăp′ĭ-tĭs): tinea tonsurans; ringworm of the scalp.

tinea favosa (tĭn′ê-ă fā-vō′să): favus; honeycomb ringworm.

tinea sycosis (tĭn′ê-ă sī-kō′sĭs): parasitic sycosis; ringworm of the beard; barber's itch.

tinea tonsurans (tĭn′ê-ă tŏn′sū-rănz): tinea capitis; ringworm of the scalp.

tinea unguium (tĭn′ê-ă ŭn′gwē-ŭm): ringworm of the nail.

tinge (tĭnj): to color or tint slightly.

tint (tĭnt): to give coloring; as used in cosmetology, hair tinting; to color the hair by means of a permanent hair tint.

tint back (tĭnt băk): to restore the hair to its original color.

tinting (tĭnt′ĭng): the process of adding artificial color to hair.

tip (tĭp): the narrow end of an object; the end of a hair.

tipping (tĭp′ĭng): similar to frosting, but the darkening or lightening is confined to small strands of hair at the front of the head; lightening the selected ends of the hair.

tipping cap (tĭp′ĭng kăp): a rubber or plastic head covering designed with small holes all over; hair strands are pulled through the holes and the lightening product applied.

Tirrell burner (tĭ-rĕl′bûr′nēr): an apparatus used to burn the hair in ash testing.

tis; sis (tĭs; sĭs): a word termination added to the name of a part to denote inflammation of that part, such a pityriasis, dermatitis.

tissue (tĭsh′û): a collection of similar cells which perform a particular function.

tissue, connective (tĭsh′û, kô-nĕk′tĭv): binding and supporting tissues.

tissue, facial (tĭsh′û, fā′shâl): soft, light absorbent papers, usually of two layers; used as a handkerchief or small towel.

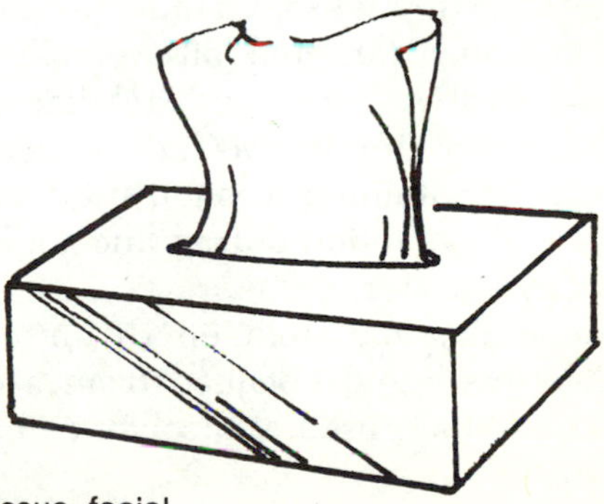

tissue, facial

titanium dioxide (tī-tā′nê-ûm dī-ŏk′sīd): a white, crystalline powder used in the manufacture of some cosmetics for coverage, especially in foundations, cover sticks, mascara, lipstick and nail polish.

titian (tĭsh′ĕn): a reddish, yellow color.

toenail clipper (tō′nāl klĭp′ẽr): also nipper; an instrument designed for clipping toenails.

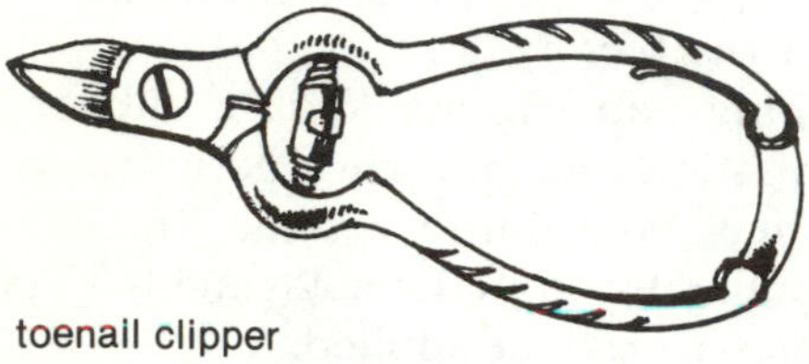

toenail clipper

tocopherol (tō-käf′ă-rôl′): vitamin E; any of a group of four related viscous oils that constitute vitamin E; chief sources are wheat germ and cottonseed oils; used as a dietary supplement, and as an antioxidant in some cosmetic preparations.

S-T

toilet (toy′lĕt): a cloth cover used in shaving or hairdressing; pertaining to one's grooming regimen.

toilet soap (toy′lĕt-sōp): a mild, pure soap containing fats and oils, emollients, preservatives, color and stabilizers.

toilet water (toy′lĕt wô′tẽr): a scented liquid containing alcohol; used as an after shave lotion or fragrance; a light scented water.

toluene diamine (tŏl′ū-ēn dī-ăm′ĭn): a colorless liquid obtained from a coal tar product; used as a solvent in nail polish.

tone (tōn): healthy functioning of the body or its parts; color quality or value.

tone on tone (tōn ŏn tōn): a method of coloring hair in which two sections of hair are lightened and toned into two shades of the same color cast.

toner (tōn′ẽr): an aniline derivative tint; a permanent, penetrating type used primarily on bleached hair to achieve pale, delicate colors.

tonic (tŏn′ĭk): increasing the strength or tone of the bodily system; an agent or drug that increases body tone.

toning (tōn′ĭng): in hair tinting: to tone down; to subdue a color to a softer or less emphatic shade; in facials: to tone up; muscle toning; to strengthen and/or invigorate the muscles of the face.

top coat (tŏp kōt): liquid, colorless nail enamel applied over polish to prevent chipping and to impart a high gloss.

topette (tŏp-ĕt′): a hairpiece such as a wig; wiglet; cascade or fall.

topical (tŏp′ĭ-kâl): pertaining to the surface; limited to a spot or part of the body.

top of the head (tŏp of the hĕd): the uppermost front section of the head.

topper (tŏp′ẽr): a hairpiece, generally made on a round or oval base and designed for use on the top of the head.

topping (tŏp′ĭng): the process of cutting the hair on top of the head.

torsade (tôr-sād′): a woven or foundational hairpiece, dressed into a variation of coils or curls.

tortoise-shelling (tôr′tûs-shĕl′ĭng): the shell of the tortoise (turtle), used for combs and ornaments; in tinting: the use of varying shades of golden blond and platinum on dark and medium dark hair for contrast.

touch up (tŭch ŭp): to brighten or refresh

a recent set; the process of coloring the new growth of tinted or lightened hair.

toupee (tōō-pā′): a small wig used to cover the top or crown of a man's head.

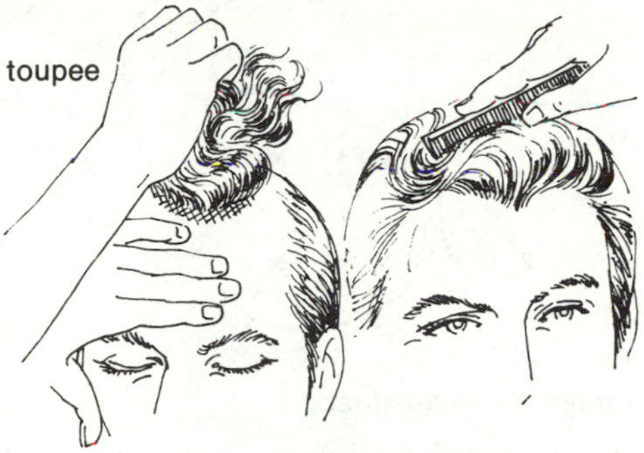

toupee adhesive (tōō-pā′ăd-hē′sĭv): a substance used to adhere the hairpiece to the scalp.

toupet (tōō-pĕt′): a lady's frontal hairpiece, larger than a fringe but not as large as a semitransformation.

towel blot (taù′ĕl blŏt): the technique of gently pressing a towel over the hair to remove excess moisture or lotion.

towel dry (taù′ĕl drī): to remove excess moisture from the hair with a towel.

toxemia (tŏk-sē′mē-ă): form of blood poisoning.

toxic (tŏk′sĭk): due to, or of the nature of poison; poisonous.

toxicoderma (tŏk′sĭ-kō-dûr′mă): disease of the skin due to poison.

toxin (tŏk′sĭn): any of various poisonous substances produced by some microorganisms; many are proteins capable of stimulating the production of antibodies or antitoxins.

"T" pin (tē pĭn): a pin resembling the letter T; used to secure a hairpiece to the block.

trachea (trā′kê-ă): windpipe; air passage from the larynx to the bronchi and the lungs.

trachoma (tră-kō′mă): a contagious disease of the inner eyelids and cornea characterized by scar formation and granulation.

tragacanth (trăg′ă-kănth): a gummy exudation from the stems of Astragalus gummifier; used as a thickener and as an emulsifier.

tranquil (trăn′kwĭl): quiet, calm; free from agitation, as a calm atmosphere.

tranquilizer (trăn′kwĭl-ī-zẽr): any of a class of drugs having the properties of reducing nervous tension and anxiety.

trans (trăns): a prefix used to signify over, across, beyond, through.

transfer rod permanent wave (trăns′fẽr rŏd pûr′mă-nênt wāv): a permanent wave technique in which the hair is rolled on a small rod, transferred to a large rod, and then neutralized.

transformation (trăns-fôr-mā′shûn): a change in the external appearance of an object; an artificial band of hair worn over a person's own hair; a foundational hairpiece completely encircling the hairline.

S-T

transformer (trăns-fôr′mẽr): a device used for increasing or decreasing the voltage of the current used; it can only be used on an alternating current.

translucent (trăns-lū′sênt): somewhat transparent.

translucent powder (trăns-lū′sênt paù′-dẽr): a powder containing the same ingredients as other face powders but to which more titanium dioxide has been added to give the powder an opaque, colorless quality.

transmission (trăns-mĭsh′ûn): passing on of anything; often said of disease.

transmit (trăns-mĭt′): to cause to go across; to send over; dispatch.

transmitter (trăns-mĭt′ẽr): one who or that which transmits.

transparent (trăns-păr′ĕnt): allowing light to pass through; clear.

transplant (trăns′plănt): removal of hair from a part of the body or head by surgical means and affix it to a bald area of the scalp; to transfer tissue or organ from one part of the body to another; graft.

transverse (trăns-vûrs′): lying or being across or crosswise.

transverse facial artery (trăns-vûrs′ fā′shâl är′tĭr-ē): artery supplying the skin, the parotid gland and the masseter muscle.

transverse nerve (trăns-vûrs′ nûrv): nerve that receives stimuli from the skin of the neck.

trapezius (tră-pē′zē-ûs): muscle that draws the head backward and sideways.

trapezoid (trăp′ĕ-zoid): a small bone in the second row of the corpus.

trauma (traů′mă): a wound or injury.

treatment (trēt′mênt): a substance, technique or regimen used in therapeutic practices.

tremble (trĕm′b'l): to shake or quiver involuntarily.

tremor (trĕm′ẽr): an involuntary trembling or quivering.

trend (trĕnd): the general direction, course, or tendency of fashion or style.

tress (trĕs): a lock or ringlet of hair.

tressed (trĕst): hair arranged in braids; long hair.

triangular (trī-ăn′gû-lẽr): having three sides joined at three angles or corners.

triangularis (trī-ăn-gû-lā′rĭs): depressor anguli oris; a muscle that pulls down corners of the mouth.

triangular-shaped face (trī-ăn′gû-lẽr-shāpt fās): a face with a narrow forehead, having the greater width at the jawline.

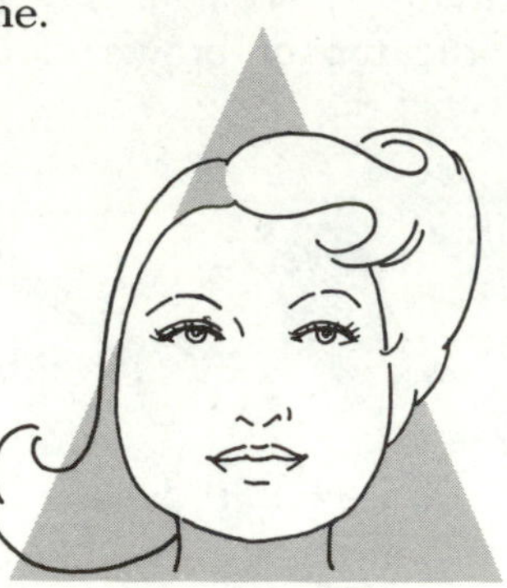

triangular-shaped face

triceps (trī′sĕps): a large muscle at the back of the arm which extends the forearm.

trichiasis (trī-kī′ă-sĭs): a condition in which hairs, especially the eyelashes, turn inward causing irritation of the eyeball.

trichology (trĭ-kŏl′ô-jē): the science dealing with the hair, its diseases and care.

trichomadesis (trĭk-ô-mă-dē′sĭs): abnormal hair loss.

trichonosis (trĭk-ô-nō′sĭs): any disease of the hair.

trichopathy (trĭ-kŏp′ă-thē): pertaining to diseases of the hair.

trichophytina (trĭk-ō-fĭ-tē′nă): a fungus which thrives in the hair follicles, causing tinea.

trichophyton (trī-kŏf′ĭ-tŏn): a fungus that attacks the hair, skin, and nails, causing dermatophytosis.

trichophytosis (trī-kŏf-ĭ-tō′sĭs): ringworm of the skin and scalp due to invasion by fungus.

trichoptilosis (trĭ-kŏp-tĭ-lō′sĭs): a splitting of the hair ends, giving them a feathery appearance.

trichorrhea (trĭk-ô-rē′ă): a rapid loss of hair.

trichorrhexis (trĭk-ô-rĕk′sĭs): brittleness of the hair.

trichorrhexis nodosa (trĭk-ô-rĕk′sĭs nô-dō′să): a hair disease characterized by brittleness and the formation of swellings on the hair shafts.

trichosiderin (trĭ′kô-sĭd′ẽr-ĭn): a pigment containing iron found in human red hair.

trichosis (trĭ-kō′sĭs): any diseased condition of the hair.

trichromat (trī′krō-măt): a person with normal color vision; the ability to distinguish the primary colors: red, yellow and blue.

trichromatic (trī-krō-măt′ĭk): three-colored; having three standard colors.

tricuspid (trī-kŭs′pĭd): having three points, as the right auriculoventricular valve of the heart.

trifacial nerve (trī-fā′shâl nûrv): the fifth cranial nerve; trigeminus nerve; receives stimuli from the face and scalp.

trigeminal (trī-jĕm′ĭ-nâl): relating to the fifth cranial or trigeminus nerve, which divides into three divisions: mandibular, maxillary and ophthalmic.

triglyceride (trī-glĭs′ẽr-īd): a fat found in adipose cells; a compound consisting of three molecules of fatty acid linked to glycerol.

trim (trĭm): a haircut in which the hair is cut without altering the shape of the existing lines; to remove a small amount of hair from the ends.

triolein (trī-ō′lē-ĕn): glyceryl trioleate; an olive oil used in nondrying creams, lotions and other cosmetic preparations.

triphase (trī′fāz): a method of color application; first to the midshaft then to ends of hair and finally to the hair nearest the scalp.

trochlea (trŏk′lê-ă): a pulley-like process; a smooth articular surface of bone upon which another glides.

trochlea muscularis (trŏk′lê-ă mŭs-kū-lâr′ĭs): an attachment which changes the direction of the pull of a muscle.

trochlear nerve (trŏk′lê-ẽr nûrv): the fourth cranial nerve.

trophedema (trō-fĕ-dē′mă): chronic edema of the feet or legs due to damage to nerves or blood-supplying vessels in the area.

trophic (trō′fĭk): pertaining to nutrition and its processes.

trophodynamics (trōf′ô-dī-năm′ĭks): the branch of medical science dealing with the forces governing nutrition.

trophology (trō-fŏl′ă-jē): the science of nutrition.

trophopathy (trŏ-fŏp′ă-thē): a disorder caused by improper or inadequate nutrition, such as a vitamin or mineral deficiency.

trough (trôf): the semicircular area of a wave between two ridges.

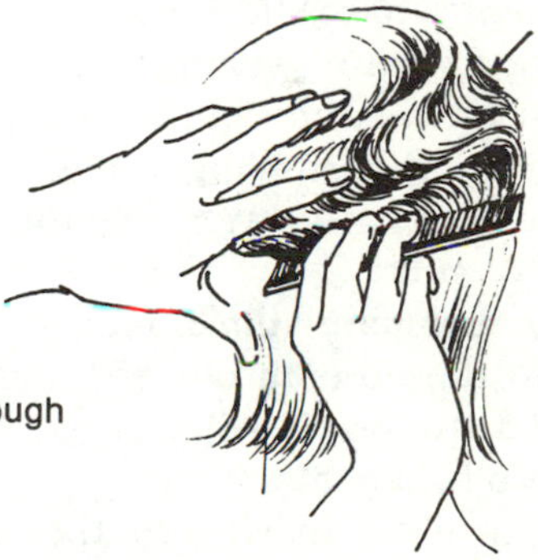

trough

true fixative (trōō fĭk′să-tĭv): substance that makes something permanent; or holds back evaporation of other materials.

true skin (trōō skĭn): the corium; dermis.

S-T

trunk (trŭnk): the human body exclusive of the extremities (arms, legs, neck, head).

trypsin (trĭp′sĭn): an enzyme in the digestive juice secreted by the pancreas; trypsin changes proteins into peptones.

tryptophan (trĭp′tô-făn): an amino acid existing in proteins; essential in human nutrition.

tubercle (tū′bẽr-k'l): an abnormal rounded, solid elevation on the skin, bone or an organ.

tuberculosis (tû-bûr-kū-lō′sĭs): an infectious disease due to a specific bacillus; characterized by the formulation of tubercles, usually in the lungs.

tuberculosis cutis (tû-bûr-kū-lō′sĭs kū′tĭs): tuberculosis of the skin.

tuberose oil (to͞ob′rōz′ oyl): oil obtained from the Mexican plant of the agave family; used in perfumes.

tubular (tūb′û-lẽr): tube shaped; resembling a long, hollow, cylindrical body.

tuck (tŭk): reducing the size of a wig cap by folding the netting into a tuck formation and sewing the fold together.

tumefacient (tū-mă-fā′shênt): swollen; tending to cause swelling.

S-T

tumid (tū′mĭd): swollen; enlarged; puffy.

tumor (tū′mẽr): a swelling; an abnormal mass resulting from excessive multiplication of cells.

turbinal; turbinate (tûr′bĭ-nâl; -nāt): a bone in the nose; turbinated body.

turbinated (tûr′bĭ-nāt-ĕd): shaped like a top; scroll-shaped.

turning (tûrn′ĭng): in wiggery, the procedure by which root ends are arranged to prevent hair from tangling and to assure correct positioning in weaving; to align the roots all on one end.

turpentine gum (tûr′pĕn-tīn gŭm): the brownish-yellow, sticky oleoresin from the terebinth pine and other coniferous trees; used as a solvent in hair preparations and some kinds of soap.

tweezers (twēz′ẽrz): a pair of small forceps to remove hair.

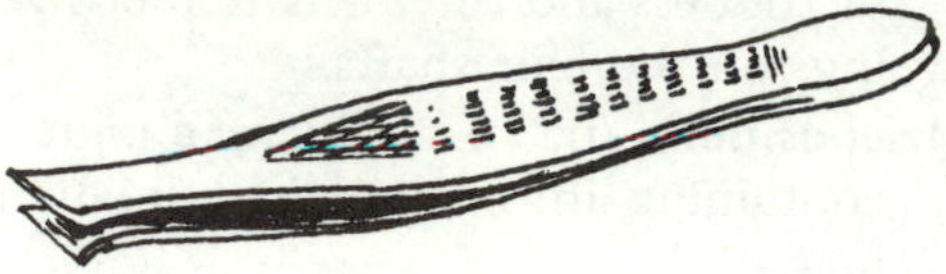

tweezers

tweezing (twēz′ĭng): removing hair with the use of a tweezer.

twice-in-weft (twīs-ĭn-wĕft): a more widely spaced method of weaving than once-in weaving.

twine (twīn): to form a coil of hair; to interlace.

twist (twĭst): in hairdressing, to form the hair into a roll or spiral shape; an overlapping of a section of hair as a French twist or roll.

twist

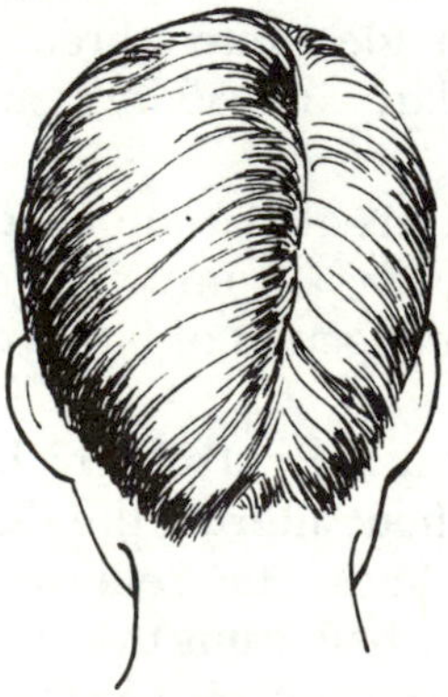

two dimensional (to͞o dĭ-mĕn′shûn'l): having length and width.

two-dimensional shading (to͞o dī-mĕn′-shûn-âl shād′ĭng): a hair coloring effect using two or more colors to add dimension or accentuate a style.

typhoid (tī′foyd): acute, infectious fever with intestinal lesions and an eruption of rose-colored spots on the chest and abdomen.

tyrosine (tī-rō′sĭn): an amino acid widely distributed in proteins, particularly in casein.

U

ulcer (ŭl′sĕr): an open sore on an internal or external part of the body.

ulceroglandular (ŭl′sŭr-ô-glăn′dū-lĕr): pertaining to ulcers involving lymph nodes.

ulna (ŭl′nă): the inner and larger bone of the forearm, attached to the wrist and located on the little finger side.

ulnar (ŭl′nĕr): pertaining to the ulna or to the ulnar, or medial aspect of the arm as compared to the radial (lateral) aspect.

ulnar artery (ŭl′nĕr är′tĭr-ē): artery which supplies blood to the muscle of the little finger side of the arm and the hand.

ulnar nerve (ŭl′nĕr nûrv): the nerve that affects the muscles of the little finger, side of the arm and the hand.

ulodermatitis (ū′lō-dûr′mă-tī′tĭs): inflammation of the skin with formation of cicatrices.

ultra (ŭl′tră): a prefix denoting beyond; on the other side; excessively.

ultramarine blue (ul′tră-mă-rēn′ blū): a blue pigment obtained by grinding lapis lazula or produced synthetically; used in eyeshadows, powders and mascara.

ultraviolet (ŭl′tră-vī′ô-lĕt): invisible rays of the spectrum which are beyond the violet rays; used for germicidal purposes.

un (ŭn): a prefix denoting not; contrary.

unadulterated (ŭn-ă-dŭl′tĕr-āt-ĕd): pure, unmixed.

unciform (ŭn′sĭ-fôrm): hook-shaped; the bone on the inner side of the second row of the carpus.

unctuous (ŭnk′chû-ûs): greasy; oily.

undercut (ŭn′dĕr-kŭt): to cut hair from the underside or the nape area.

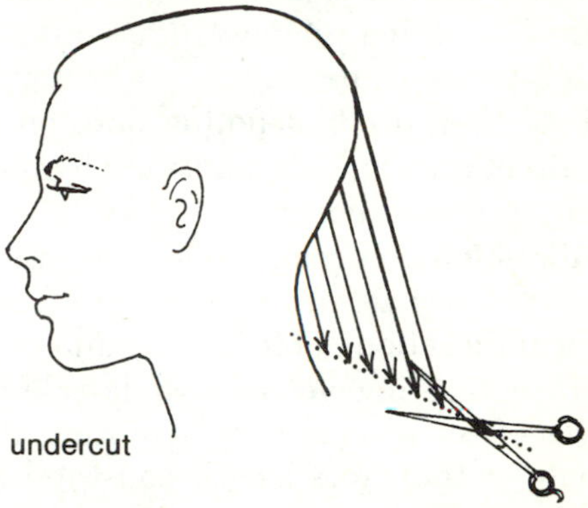

undercut

underdirected (ŭn′dĕr-dĭ-rĕk′tĕd): having less than the usual or normal amount of direction.

underelevation (ŭn′dĕr-ĕl-ĕ-vā′shûn): hair shaping technique in which hair is cut on top of the head, longer at the crown, then progressively shorter to create overlapping.

underknotting (ŭn′dĕr-nŏt′ĭng): fine knotting used under the hairline of foundational hairpieces.

underprocessing (ŭn-dĕr-prŏ′cĕs-ĭng): insufficient exposure of the hair to the chemical action of the waving solution, resulting in little or no change in hair structure and condition of the hair.

undertint (ŭn′dĕr-tĭnt): a subdued tint; not bright.

undertone (ŭn′dĕr-tōn): a subdued shade of a color; a color upon which another color has been imposed and which can be seen through the other color.

undulation (ŭn-dû-lā′shûn): a wave-like movement or shape.

unguent (ŭn′gwĕnt): an ointment or salve.

unguentum (ŭn-gwĕn′tûm); pl., **unguenta** (-ă): a salve or ointment.

unguis (ŭn′gwĭs): the nail of a finger or toe.

unguis incarnatus (ŭn′gwĭs ĭn-kär-nā′-tûs): ingrown fingernails or toenails.

unguium, tinea (ŭn′gwē-ŭm, tĭn′ê-ă): ringworm of the nails.

uni (ūn′ĭ): a prefix denoting one; once.

unidirectional (ūn′ĭ-dī-rĕk′shûn-âl): moving in one direction.

unidirectional current (ūn′ĭ-dī-rĕk′shûn-âl kŭr′ênt): an electric current of uniform direction; a direct current.

uniform layering (yōō′nă-fôrm lā-ẽr′ĭng): the effect produced by sculpting the hair at the same length consistently; using a 90 degree (normal) projection angle.

unipolar (yōō-nĭ-pō′lẽr): having or acting by a single magnetic pole; the application of one electrode of a direct current to the body during a treatment.

unisex (yōō′nĭ-sĕks): cosmetology services suitable for both men and women.

unit (ū′nĭt): a single thing or value.

United States Pharmacopeia (USP) (ū-nīt′ĕd stāts fär-mă-kô-pē′ă): an official book of drug and medicinal standards.

U-V

unprofessional (ŭn-prô-fĕsh′ŭn-âl): in violation of ethical codes or standards of conduct of a profession.

unstable (ŭn-stā′b'l): not firm; not constant; readily decomposing or changing in chemical composition or biological activity.

unwind (ŭn-wīd′): to unwrap hair from a permanent wave or hair setting rod.

upangle cutting (ŭp′ăng′'l kŭt′ĭng): cutting subsections of hair into layers, longer by degrees from the innermost to the outermost layers of hair.

upblending (ŭp-blĕnd′ĭng): blending the hair upward from the nape.

upelevation (ŭp-ĕl-ĕ-vā′shûn): a technique in which hair is cut in graduated lengths, shorter to longer; upangle cutting.

upstroke (ŭp′strōk): stroking upward, as in shaving.

upsweep (ŭp′swēp): a hairstyle combed up from the nape of the neck toward the crown.

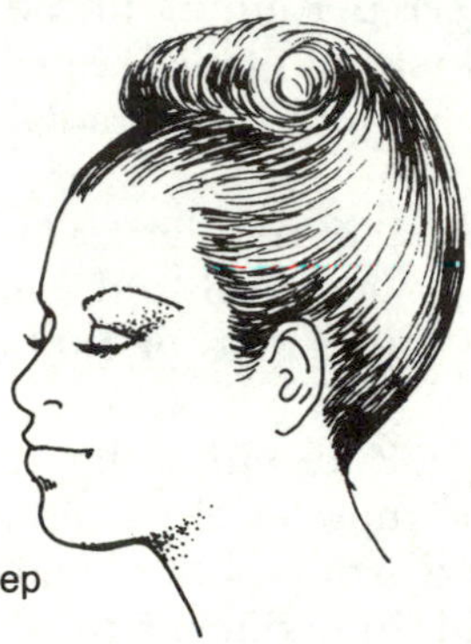

upsweep

urea (ū-rē′ă): a colorless crystalline compound; the chief solid component of urine and an end product of protein metabolism; used in some cosmetic and medicinal products.

urea peroxide (ū-rē′ă pẽr-ŏk′sīd): a combination of urea and peroxide in the form of a cream developer or activator; employed in hair tinting.

uric acid (ū′rĭk ăs′ĭd): a crystalline acid contained in urine; a product of protein metabolism.

uridrosis, urhidrosis (ū-rī-drō′sĭs, ūr-hī-drō′sĭs): the presence of urea in the sweat in excess of normal.

urticaria (ûr-tĭ-kăr-ē-ă): a skin condition characterized by smooth and slightly elevated patches sometimes whiter or redder than the surrounding skin, with severe itching; hives; nettle rash.

urticaria medicamentosa (ûr-tĭ-kăr′ē-ă mĕd′ĭ-kă-mĕn-tō′să): skin eruptions due to the ingestion of a drug to which the individual is allergic.

uticaria papulosa (u-tĭ-kā′rē-ă păp-ū-lō′să): a pruritic skin eruption usually in children, related to insect bites and characterized by papules.

V

vaccination (văc-sĭ-nā′shûn): inoculation; administration of any vaccine.

vaccine (văk′sĭn; -sēn′): any substance used for preventive inoculation.

vacuum (văk′û-ûm): a space entirely devoid of matter; a space from which the air has been exhausted.

vacuum procedure (văk′û-ûm prô-sē′-jẽr): the use of a suction type apparatus to cleanse the pores during a facial treatment.

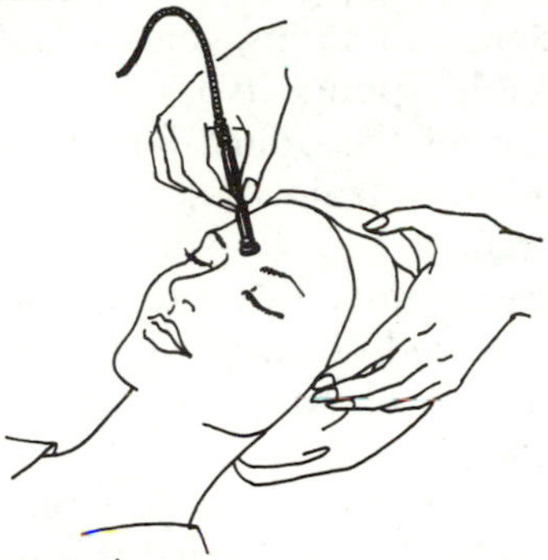

vacuum procedure

vagus (vā′gûs): pneumogastric nerve; tenth cranial nerve.

valence (vā′lĕns): the capacity of an atom to combine with other atoms in definite proportions.

valine (vā′lēn): amino acid essential in human nutrition.

valve (vălv): a structure which temporarily closes a passage or orifice or permits flow in one direction only.

vanishing cream (văn′ĭsh-ĭng krēm): a skin cream formulated to leave no oily residue on the surface of the skin.

vapor (vā′pẽr): a gas; the gaseous form of a substance that at ordinary temperature is a liquid or a solid.

vaporization (vā-pẽr-ĭ-zā′shûn): act or process of converting a solid or liquid into a vapor.

vaporizer (vā′pẽr-ī-zẽr): an apparatus designed to turn water or other substance into vapor; used in hair and skin treatments; a vaporizing machine.

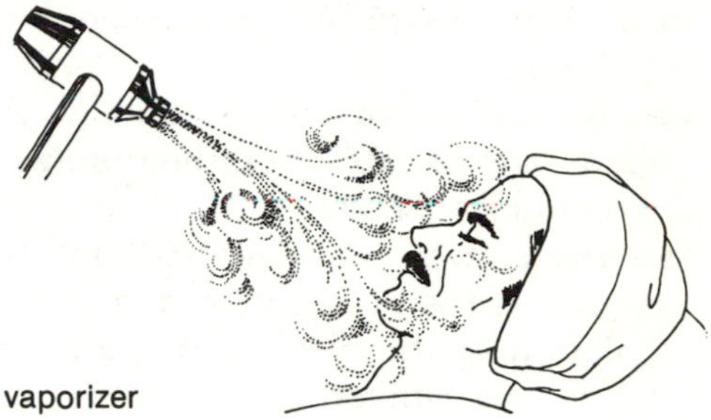

vaporizer

variable (văr′ē-ă-b'l): changeable; subject to variations or changes.

variation (văr-ē-ā′shûn): changes or differences, as in procedures or styles.

varicolored (văr′ē-kŭl-ẽrd): having various or several colors.

varicophlebitis (văr′ĭ-kō-flĕ-bī′tĭs): inflammation of a varicose vein or veins.

varicose veins (văr′ĭ-kōs vānz): swollen or knotted veins.

varicosis (văr-ĭ-kō′sĭs): a dilated or varicose state of a vein or veins.

variegating (văr′ē-ă-gāt′ĭng): lightening small sections or strands of hair throughout the head; also known as frosting.

varnish (vär′nĭsh): a product used to give the nails a smooth, glossy appearance; nail polish.

vasa lymphatica profunda (vā′să lĭm-

U-V

făt′ĭk-ă prō-fŭn′dă): the deep lymphatic vessels.

vasa lymphatica superficialia (vā′să lĭm-făt′ĭk-ă sū-pĕr-fĭsh-ē-ā′lē ă): the superficial lymphatic vessels.

vascular (văs′kû-lẽr): supplied with small blood vessels; pertaining to a vessel for the conveyance of a fluid, such as blood or lymph.

vascular bed (văs′kū-lẽr bĕd): the total blood supply system of an organ or region of the body: arteries, capillaries, veins.

vascularity (văs-kû-lăr′ĭ-tē): the condition of being vascular.

vascularization (văs-kî-lăr-ĭ-zā′shûn): the formation of capillaries; the process of becoming vascular.

vascular system (văs′kû-lẽr sĭs′têm): the organs of the body involved in the circulation of the blood: heart, arteries, veins and capillaries.

vasoconstrictor (vāz′ô-kôn-strĭk′tẽr): a nerve or agent that causes narrowing of blood vessels.

vasodilator (văs′ô-dĭ-lā′tẽr): a nerve or agent that causes expansion of the blood vessels.

vegetable dye (vĕj′tă-b'l dī): a natural organic coloring obtained from the leaves or bark of plants; examples are henna and camomile which are used to tint hair.

U-V

vegetable facial mask (vĕj-ĕ-tă-b'l fā′shâl măsk): a mask made of fresh vegetables such as cucumber or avocado; used on the face for their beneficial enzyme action.

vegetable oil (vĕg′tă-b'l oyl): any of various liquid fats obtained from seeds of certain plants; examples are peanut, olive and sesame seed oil; used in hypoallergenic and a wide variety of other cosmetics including baby preparations, creams, lotions, powders and hair grooming products.

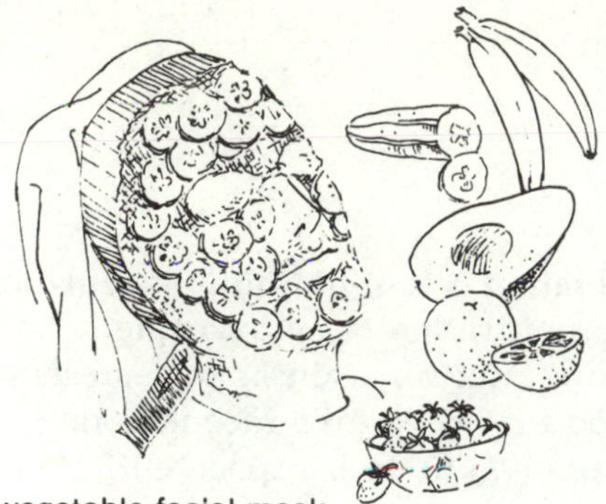

vegetable facial mask

vegetable peel (vĕj′ĕ-tă-b'l pēl): a mild skin peeling process using creams or lotions containing vegetable enzymes.

vegetable sponge (vĕj′ĕ-tă-b'l spŭnj): a genes of the gourd family producing a fibrous fruit used as a sponge; a loofah.

vegetable tints (vĕj′ĕ-tă-b'l tĭnts): tints comprised of Egyptian henna, indigo, or camomile; used as hair tints or hair rinses.

vein; vena (vān; vē′nă): a blood vessel carrying blood toward the heart.

vellus (vĕl′ûs): the fine, downy hair that appears on the body, with the exception of the palms of the hands and soles of the feet.

vena cava (vē′nă kă′vă): one of the two large veins which carry the blood to the right auricle of the heart.

vena cutanea (vē′nă kū-tā′nē-ă): a cutaneous vein.

venenata, dermatitis (vĕn-ĕn-ā′tă dûr-mă-tī′tĭs): inflammation produced by local action of irritating substances.

venous (vē′nûs): pertaining to or marked with veins.

ventilate (vĕn′tĭ-lāt): to renew the air in a place; to oxygenate the blood in the capillaries of the lungs.

ventilated (vĕn′tĭ-lāt-ĕd): describes a method of knotting single strand groups of hair individually to the net foundation of a wig.

ventilating needle (vĕn′tĭ-lāt-ĭng nē′d'l): a miniature crocheting needle, made of spring steel; used in attaching hair to a foundation.

ventricle (vĕn′trĭ-k'l): a small cavity, particularly in the brain or heart; one of the two lower chambers of the heart.

venule (vĕn′ūl): a small vein or smallest branch of a vein.

vermillion (vẽr-mĭl′yĕn): a bright orange red color; also called Chinese red and cinnabar.

verruca (vĕ-ro͞o′kă): a wart; a circumscribed hypertrophy of the papillae and epidermis.

verrucose; verrucous (vĕr′o͝o-kōs, vĕr-o͝o′-kōs, -kûs): warty; presenting wart-like elevations.

versicolor (vûr′sĭ-kŭl-ẽr): having a variety of colors; iridescent; changing color under different light.

vertebra (vûr′tĕ-bră); pl., **vertebrae** (-brē): a bony segment of the spinal column.

vertebral artery (vûr′tĕ-brâl är′tĭr-ē): artery that supplies blood to the muscles of the neck.

vertex (vûr′tĕks): the crown or top of the head; top; highest point.

vertical (vûr′tĭ-kâl): in an upright position; usually described in terms of up and down as opposed to left and right.

vertical base (vûr′tĭ-k'l bās): a vertical section of a hair form used in practical exercises.

vesicant (vĕs′ĭ-kănt): an agent which produces blisters on the skin.

vesicle (vĕs′ĭ-k'l): a small blister or sac; a small elevation on the skin.

vesicle bulla (vęb′ĭ-k'l bo͞ol′ă): a large vesicle; blister.

vesicular (vê-sĭk′û-lẽr): relating to or containing vesicles.

vesiculopapular (vĕ-sĭk′û-lō-păp′ū lẽr): consisting of both vesicles and papules.

vesiculopustular (vĕ-sĭk′û-lō-pŭs′tū-lẽr): consisting of both vesicles and pustules.

vessel (vĕs′'l): tube or canal in which blood, lymph, or other fluid is contained and conveyed or circulated.

vibex (vī′bĕks); pl., **vibices** (vī′bĭ-sēz): a narrow linear mark on the skin; stretchmark; a condition generally caused by pregnancy or rapid weight gain.

vibrate (vī′brāt): to swing; to mark or to measure by oscillation.

vibration (vī-brā′shûn): shaking; a to and fro movement.

vibration, massage movement (vī-brā′shûn mă-säzh′ mo͞ov-mênt): also called shaking movement; consists of pressing fingertips to the point of application and shaking the arms to produce a stimulating effect on tissues.

vibration treatment (vī′brā-shûn trēt′-mênt): massage by rapid shaking of the body part; given by hand, machine or oscillator.

vibrator (vī′brā-tẽr): an electrically driven apparatus used in some massage procedures.

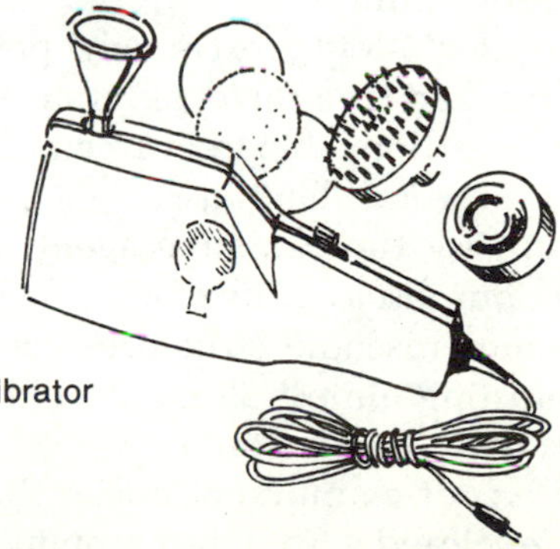

vibrator

vibrator scalp treatment (vī′brā-tẽr skălp trēt′mênt): massage for the scalp given with the aid of a hand vibrator.

vibratory (vī′bră-tô-rē): vibrations or light, rapid percussion used in massage, and given by hand or an electrical apparatus.

vibrissa (vī-brĭs′ă); pl., **vibrissae** (vī-brĭs′ē): stiff hairs in the nostrils.

vibroid (vī′broyd): a vibratory movement in massage.

villus (vĭl′ûs); pl., **villi** (-ī): minute finger-like processes covering the surface of the mucous membrane of the small intestine.

vinegar (vĭn′ĕ-gẽr): a sour liquid used as a condiment or as a preservative, formed by fermentation of dilute alcoholic liquids as wine, cider, etc.; it contains acetic acid.

violet (vī′ô-lĕt): a bluish-red color; bluish-purple hue.

violet-ray (vī′ô-lĕt-rā): high frequency; an electric current of medium voltage and medium amperage; also called Tesla current.

virgin bleaching (vûr′jĭn blēch′ĭng): first bleaching (lightening) of the hair.

virgin hair (vûr′jĭn hâr): normal hair which has had no previous bleaching or tinting treatments.

U-V

virgin tint (vûr′jĭn tĭnt): first time the hair has been tinted.

virulent (vĭr′ū-lênt): extremely poisonous; marked by a rapid, severe course, as an infection; able to overcome bodily defense mechanisms.

virus (vī′rûs): the causative agent of an infectious disease; any of a large group of submicroscopic structures capable of infesting almost all plants and animals, including bacteria.

viscera (vĭs′ẽr-ă): plural of viscus; the organs enclosed within the cranium, thorax, abdomen or pelvis, especially the organs within the abdominal cavity.

visceral (vĭs′ẽr-âl): pertaining to viscera.

visceral cranium (vĭs′ẽr-âl krā-nē-ûm): the part of the skull that forms the face and jaws.

viscid (vĭs′ĭd): sticky or adhesive; glutinous.

viscosity (vĭs-kŏs′ĭ-tē): the degree of density, thickness, stickiness and adhesiveness of a substance.

viscous (vĭs′kûs): sticky or gummy.

vicus (vĭs′kûs); pl., **viscera** (vĭs′ẽr-ă): an internal organ located in the cavity of the trunk or in the thorax, cranium or pelvis.

visible rays (vĭs′ĭ-b'l rāz): light rays which can be seen.

vital (vī′tâl): relating to life; concerned with or necessary to the maintenance of life.

vitality (vī-tăl′ĭ-tē): vigor; to grow, develop, and perform the functions of a living body.

vitamin (vī′tă-mĭn): one of a group of organic substances present in a very small quantity in natural food stuffs, which are essential to normal metabolism and the lack of which causes deficiency diseases.

vitamin chart (vī′tă-mĭn chärt): a chart showing the essential vitamins and minerals, their sources and benefits.

vitiligines (vĭt-ĭ-lĭ′jĭ-nēz): depigmented areas of the skin.

vitiligo (vĭt-ĭ-lī′gō): milky-white spots of the skin.

volatile (vŏl′ă-tĭl): easily evaporating; diffusing freely; explosive.

volt (vōlt): the unit of electromotive force; the electromotive force that, steadily applied to a conductor whose resistance is one ohm, will produce a current of one ampere.

voltage (vōl′tĭj): electrical potential difference expressed in volts.

voltage drop (vōl′tĭj drŏp): the decrease in the potential energy in an electric circuit due to the resistance of the conductor.

voltaic cell (vŏl-tā′ĭk sĕl): a receptacle for producing direct electric current by chemical action.

voltaic current (vŏl-tā′ĭk kŭr′ênt): galvanic current.

voltaic electricity (vŏl-tā′ĭk ê-lĕk-trĭs′ĭ-tē): galvanic electricity.

voltmeter (vōlt′mē-tẽr): an instrument used for measuring (in volts) the differences of potential between different points of an electrical circuit.

volume (vŏl′ūm): amount (bulk or mass); quantity; space occupied, as measured in cubic units; the lift, elevation and height created by the formation of curls or waves in the hair; measure of potential oxidation of varying strengths of hydrogen peroxide.

volume curl (vŏl′ūm kûrl): a pincurl with the stem moving upward from the scalp to create fullness.

volume of peroxide (vŏl′ūm of pẽr-ŏk′-sīd): the concentration of hydrogen peroxide in water solution; as 20 volume peroxide.

voluntary (vŏl′ûn-tẽr′ē): under the control of the will; being done by choice.

voluntary muscle (vŏl′ûn-tẽr′ē mŭs′′l): striated muscle under the control of the will.

vomer (vō′mẽr): the thin plate of bone between the nostrils.

vortices pilorum (vôr′tī-sēz pī-lō′rûm): hair whorls; commonly called a cowlick.

vulgaris, acne (vŭl-gā′rĭs, ăk′nē): common pimple condition.

W

wall plate (wôl plāt): an apparatus equipped with indicators and controlling devices to produce various currents.

wall socket (wôl sŏk′ĕt): a wall receptacle into which may be fitted the plug of an electrical appliance.

walnut (wôl′nŭt): a warm, reddish brown color.

walnut stain (wôl′nŭt stān): one of the wood extracts historically used as a hair coloring.

warm (wôrm): having the color or tone of something that imparts heat, as in the range of colors from yellow or gold through orange and red.

wart (wôrt): verruca; a circumscribed hypertrophy of the papillae of the corium, usually of the hand, covered by thickened epidermis.

water blister (wô′tẽr blĭs′tẽr): a blister with watery contents.

water, hard (wô′tẽr, härd): water containing certain minerals; does not lather with soap.

water, soft (wô′tẽr, sŏft): water which lathers easily with soap and is relatively free of minerals.

water softener (wô′tẽr sŏf′′n-ẽr): certain chemicals, such as the carbonate or phosphate of sodium, used to soften hard water to permit the lathering of soap.

water soluble (wô′tẽr sŏl′ū-b'l): able to dissolve in water.

water vapor (wô′tẽr vā′pẽr): water diffused in a vaporous form; used in some facial treatments.

water wrapped perm (wô′tẽr răpt pûrm): a permanent wave wrapped with water and the waving lotion applied after the entire head is wrapped; this is done to control timing during the process.

watt (wŏt): the electrical unit of energy; the power required to cause a current of one ampere to flow between points differing in potential by one volt.

wattage (wŏt′ĭj): amount of electric power expressed in watts.

watt hour (wôt aůr): one watt of power expended for one hour.

wave (wāv): two connecting c-shapings placed in alternating directions.

wave clip (wāv klĭp): a clamp-like device with rows of small teeth used to hold a wave in place while the hair dries.

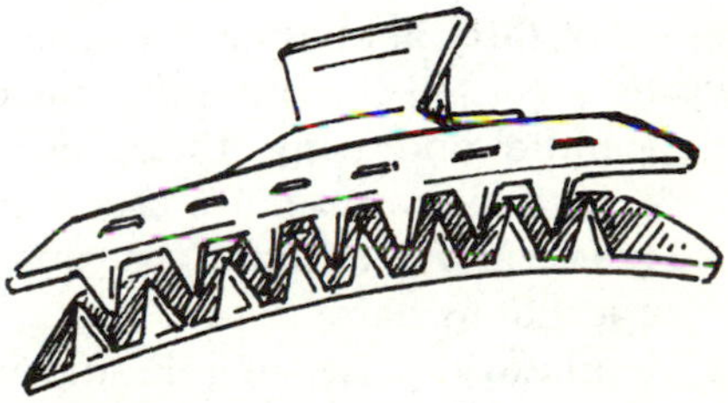

wave clip

wave, cold (wāv, kōld): a method of permanent waving using chemicals instead of heat.

wave, croquignole marcel (wāv, krō′kwĭ-nōl mär-sĕl): a wave produced with the marcel iron, using the croquignole winding.

wave, marcel (wāv, mär-sĕl′): a wave that resembles a perfect natural wave; produced by means of heated irons.

W-X

waves (wāvz): hair formation resulting in a side by side series of S-like movements or half-circles going in opposite directions.

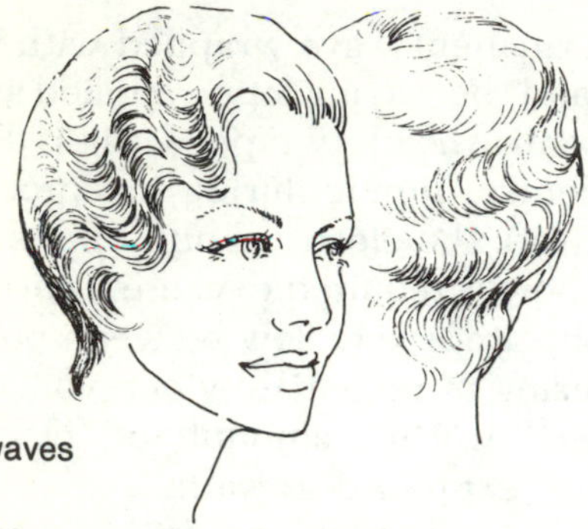

waves

wave, shadow (wāv, shă′dō): a wave with low ridges and shallow waves.

wax (wăks): a substance insoluble in water but soluble in most organic solvents; derived from animal sources such as beeswax, stearic acid and Chinese wax; vegetable sources such as carnauba, bayberry, etc.; mostly composed of fatty acid esters and alcohol; waxes are used in cosmetics, packaging, candles and many other products; in cosmetology, waxes are used for facial masks and as an aid to the removal of superfluous hair.

wax depilatory (wăks dē-pĭl′ă-tô-rē): a soft wax applied to remove superfluous hair.

wax heater (wăks hēt′ẽr): a thermostatically controlled heating pot used to warm wax to be used for a facial or depilatory treatment.

wax mask (wăks măsk): a special mixture of oils and waxes used to form a facial mask for facial treatments; these waxes may be combinations of beeswax, mineral oil and similar oils and waxes.

weave (wēv): a technique in hair styling accomplished by interlacing strands of hair to form intricate patterns.

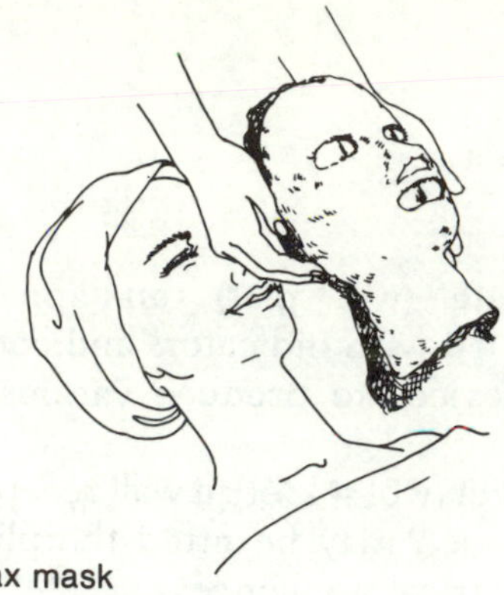

wax mask

weaving, hair (wēv′ĭng, hâr): a special technique of sewing or weaving, wefts of matched hair into a net-shaped base, of nylon thread, which had previously been tied into the remaining hair on the head.

weaving silk (wēv′ĭng sĭlk): a strong, fine silk used on weaving sticks when weaving hair into a weft.

wedged parting (wĕj′'d pärt′ĭng): a triangular sectioning pattern used as a base for a standup curl.

wedged parting

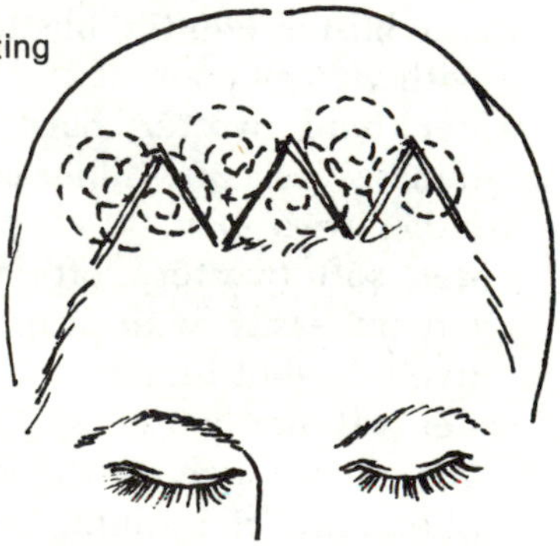

weft (wĕft): an artificial section of woven hair used for practice work or as a substitute for natural hair.

weft wig (wĕft wĭg): a wig made of wefts of hair sewn into a wig base; a machine-made wig.

weight (wāt): mass in form and space; the length concentration in a hair design.

weight line (wāt līn): the line of maximum length within the weight area.

welt (wĕlt): a ridge or lump usually caused by a blow.

wen (wĕn): a sebaceous cyst, usually on the scalp.

wet pack (wĕt păk): packing the body or a part in towels that have been saturated in water or other fluids for therapeutic purposes.

wet sanitizer (wĕt săn′ĭ-tī-zẽr): a container filled with a germicidal solution into which implements are placed for sanitizing.

wetting agent (wĕt′ĭng ā′jênt): a substance that causes a liquid to spread more readily on a solid surface, chiefly through a reduction of surface tension.

wheal (hwēl): a raised ridge on the skin, usually caused by a blow, a bite of an insect, uticaria, or a sting of a nettle.

wheat germ oil (hwēt jûrm oyl): the oil of the wheat embryo used in oils, fats, food and cosmetic products as a stabilizer.

white (hwīt): the color produced by reflection of all the light rays in the spectrum; the absence of pigment; having light colored skin; having the color of milk or new snow.

white corpuscle (hwit kôr′pus'l): leukocyte; cell in the blood whose function is to destroy disease germs.

whitehead (hwīt′hĕd): milium.

whiten (hwīt′'n): to make white or lighter as in the use of a white lead to whiten tips of the fingernails.

whorl (whûrl; whôrl): hair which forms in a swirl effect, as on the crown.

widow's peak (wĭd′ōz pēk): a "V" shaped growth of hair at the center of the forehead; see peak.

wig (wĭg): an artificial covering for the head consisting of a network of interwoven hair.

wig bar (wĭg bär): a showcase or counter for the sale of ready-to-wear wigs and hairpieces.

wig block (wĭg blŏk): a head-shaped block (which may be constructed of wood, cork-filled cloth, plastic or other materials) on which hairpieces and wigs are formed or dressed.

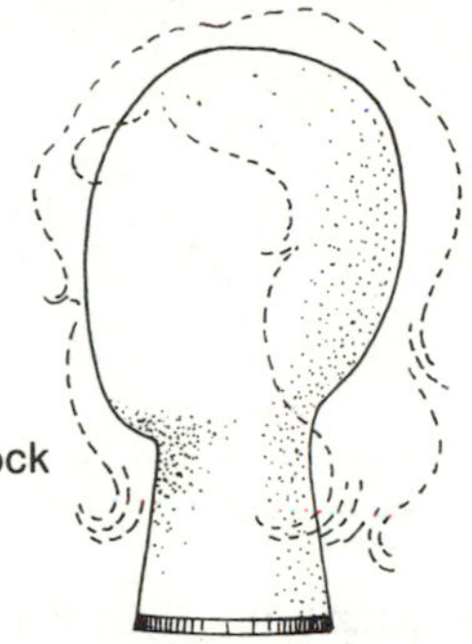

wig brush (wĭg brŭsh): a brush with semistiff bristles used to comb and disentangle a wig after cleaning.

wig cap (wĭg kăp): the foundation to which the hair or fiber of a wig is attached.

wig cleaner (wĭg klēn′ẽr): any type of dry cleaning fluid which may be used to clean wigs and hairpieces.

wig conditioner (wĭg kôn-dĭ′shûn-ẽr): a product, in cream, lotion or spray form, which is used to restore life and add luster to wigs or hairpieces.

wiglet (wĭg′lĕt): a hairpiece with a flat base which is used in special areas of the head.

wig net (wĭg nĕt): a soft, narrow-meshed net of silk, cotton, linen or nylon, used in the base of a wig or hairpiece.

wig pin (wĭg pĭn): a steel pin about two inches in length with a "T" shaped head, used to secure a wig to a canvas headblock while combing and styling.

wig spray (wĭg sprā): a hair spray used to hold coiffures set in wigs.

wig spring (wĭg sprĭng): a small spring inserted into a wig or hairpiece to hold it to the head.

wig stand (wĭg stănd): a head-shaped stand designed for keeping wigs in the proper shape when not being worn.

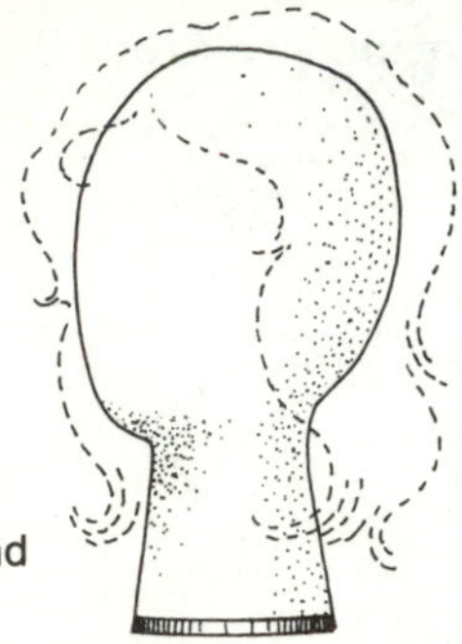

wig stand

winding, croquignole (wĭnd′ĭng, krō′-kwĭ-nōl): winding the hair from the hair ends towards the scalp.

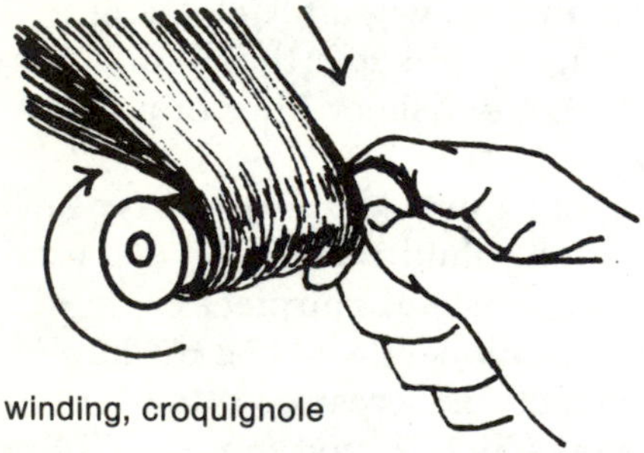

winding, croquignole

windpipe (wĭnd′pīp): the trachea.

wine color (wīn kûl′ĕr): the color of red wine; dark purplish red, similar to burgandy wine.

wintergreen oil (wĭn′tĕr-grēn oyl): an oil made from the leaves of the wintergreen shrub or bark of sweet birch; used in flavorings, mouthwashes, toothpastes and some medicinal products.

wire mesh roller (wīr mĕsh rō′lĕr): a hair roller made of wire open-work mesh to allow for faster drying of the hair.

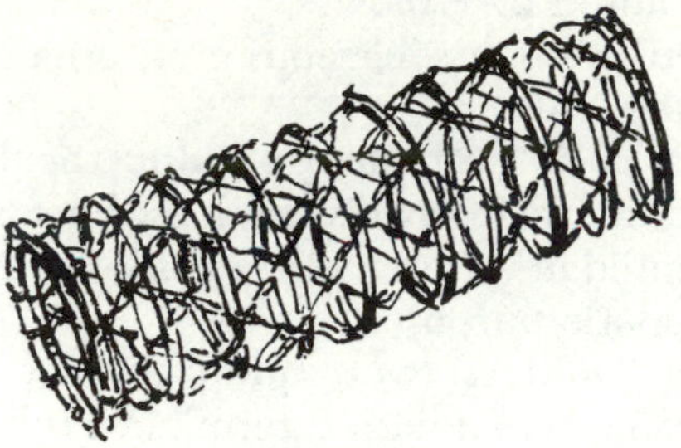

wire mesh roller

wiry hair (wīr′ēhâr): a hair fiber that is strong and resilient, difficult to form into a curl formation, and having a smooth, hard, glossy surface.

wisp (wĭsp): a small, lightweight, thin strand of hair; light, fluffy curls.

witch hazel (wĭch hā′z'l): an extract of the bark of the hamamelis shrub; soothing and mildly astringent; used as a lotion and mild medication.

wood's lamp (wo͞odz lămp): a light used to study and analyze skin conditions.

wool crepe (wo͞ol krāp): a material used to keep hair ends smooth when winding in permanent waving.

wooly hair (wo͞ol′ē hâr): short, overcurly hair.

wrap (răp): to wind the hair on permanent wave rods.

wrapping (răp′ĭng): winding hair on rollers or rods in order to form curls.

wring (rĭng): to squeeze or compress by twisting.

wrinkle (rĭnk′'l): a small ridge or furrow on the skin.

wrinkle remover (rĭn′k'l rĭ-mo͞o′vĕr): a cream or lotion claimed to be formulated to puff up and fill out lines in the face; there is no scientific evidence to support claims that such products actually remove wrinkles from the skin.

wrist (rĭst): the joint between the hand and arm.

wrist electrode (rĭst ê-lĕk′trōd): an electrode for high frequency current attached to the wrist to produce mild current during a phase of a facial treatment.

X

xanthochroid (zăn′thō-kroyd): characterized by a light yellow or fair complexion.

xanthochromia (zăn-thō-krō′mē-ă): a yellowish discoloration of the skin or cerebrospinal fluid.

xanthoma (zăn-thō′mă): a skin disease characterized by the presence of yellow nodules or slightly raised plates in the subcutaneous tissue, often around tendons.

xanthoma palpebrarum (zăn-thō′mă păl-pĕ-brā′rûm): yellowish, raised patches occurring around the eyelids resulting from lipid filled cells in the dermis.

xanthosis (zăn-thō′sĭs): a discoloration of the skin caused by eating an overabundance of carotene-producing foods, such as squash, carrots, etc.; the condition is reversible.

xanthous (zăn′thûs): having yellowish skin tone.

xerasia (zĕ-rā′zē-ă, zĕ-rā′zhă): a disease of the hair marked by cessation of growth, dryness and general lifeless appearance.

xeroderma (zē-rō-dûr′mă): a condition of excessively dry skin; a mild form of ichthyosis marked by a dry, discolored, rough condition of the skin.

xerosis (zē-rō′sĭs): a condition of abnormal dryness of tissue such as the eyes, skin, or mucous membranes.

x rays (ĕks′ rāz): Roentgen rays; electromagnetic radiations of very short wave length; rays used in some medical therapy procedures.

xyrospasm (zī′rō-spăz'm): a spasm of the wrist and forearm muscles; an occupational condition which may affect cosmetologists, estheticians and barbers.

Y

yak (yăk): the long-haired ox of Tibet and central Asia; hair used for making wigs.

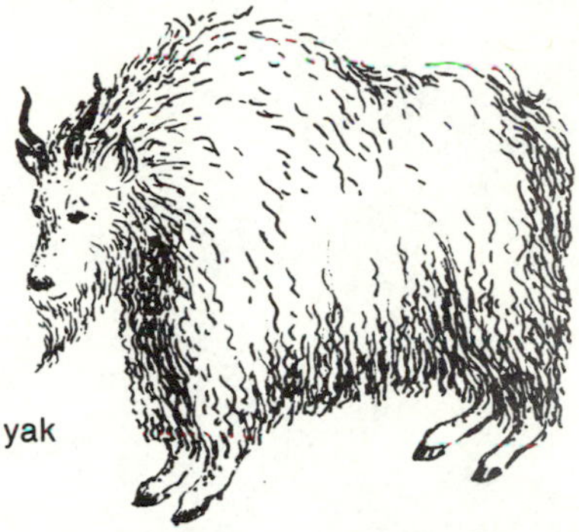

yak

yak hair (yăk hâr): hair from the yak; this long, coarse, curly hair is used in the manufacture of inexpensive wigs and hairpieces; it is often mixed with the soft hair from the Angora sheep to add body and strength to Angora hair.

yang and yin (yän and yĭn): a Chinese philosophy often applied to personality and fashion theories; yang is active, positive, masculine, and a source of heat and light, contrasted with and complimentary to yin; yin is the passive, negative, feminine force, and source of heat and light, contrasted with and complimentary to yang.

yard (yärd): a standard English-American measure of length equal to 3 feet or 36 inches.

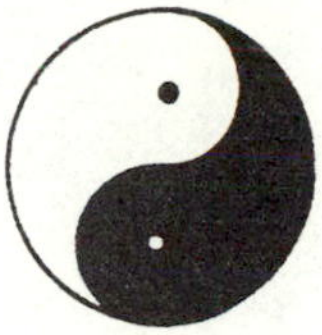

yin and yang

yeast (yēst): a substance consisting of minute cells of fungi; used to promote fermentation; a high source of vitamin B.

yellow (yĕl′ō): one of the three primary colors; having the color of ripe lemons.

yin (yīn): Pertaining to the Chinese philosophy and art of Yin and Yang.

ylang ylang (ē′lŏng ē′lŏng): an Asiatic tree producing greenish yellow flowers from which a perfume oil is produced.

yoga (yō′gă): A Hindu system of philosophy that involves physical and mental disciplines; a system of exercise.

yogurt (yō′gōōrt) A thick, curdled milk regarded as a nutritious and beneficial food; sometimes used as a facial mask.

Z

zeis's glands (tsĭce glăndz): the sebaceous glands associated with the cilia.

zeolite (zē′ō-līt): a chemical mixture of natural or synthesized silicates used to soften hard water.

zero projection (zē′rō prô-jĕk′shûn): in haircutting, no elevation or projection; hair held as close to the scalp as possible.

zigzag (zĭg′zăg): pertaining to short, sharp angled partings used during some roller settings to prevent separation of strands during comb-out.

zinc (zĭnk): a white crystalline metallic element; used in some cosmetics such as powders and ointments; salts of zinc are used in some antiseptics and astringents.

zinc ointment (zĭngk oynt′mênt): a medicated ointment containing zinc oxide and petrolatum, used for skin disorders.

zinc oxide (zĭngk ŏk′sīd): a fine, white compound used as a mild antiseptic and astringent.

zinc sulphate (zĭnk sŭl′fāt): a salt often employed as an astringent, both in lotions and creams.

zinc sulphocarbonate (zĭngk sŭl-fô-kär′-bôn-āt): a fine white powder having the odor of carbolic acid; used as an antiseptic and astringent in deodorant preparations.

zoodermic (zō′ō-dûr′mĭk): pertaining to skin graft done with the grafts from the tissue or skin of an animal.

zoster herpes (zŏs′tẽr hûr′pēz): an acute viral infectious disease affecting the skin and mucous membranes.

zygoma (zī-gō′mă): a bone of the skull which extends along the front or side of the face, below the eye; the molar or cheekbone.

zygomatic (zī-gô-măt′ĭk): pertaining to the zygoma (the molar or cheekbone).

zygomatic artery (zī-gô-măt′ĭk är′tĭr-ē): superficial temporal artery supplying blood to the orbit and orbicularis.

zygomatic bone (zī-gô-măt′ĭk bōn): the cheekbone.

zygomatic nerve (zī-gô-măt′ĭk nûrv): temporal nerve that supplies stimuli to the skin of the temple area.

zygomatic process (zī-gô-măt′ĭk prŏ′sĕs): the process of the temporal bone that helps to form the zygoma.

zygomaticus (zī-gô-măt′ĭ-kûs): a muscle that draws the upper lip upward and outward.

zymosis (zī-mō′sĭs): fermentation; any infectious or contagious disease; the development or spread of an infectious disease.

ANATOMY TABLE I

The Skeletal System—Anterior View

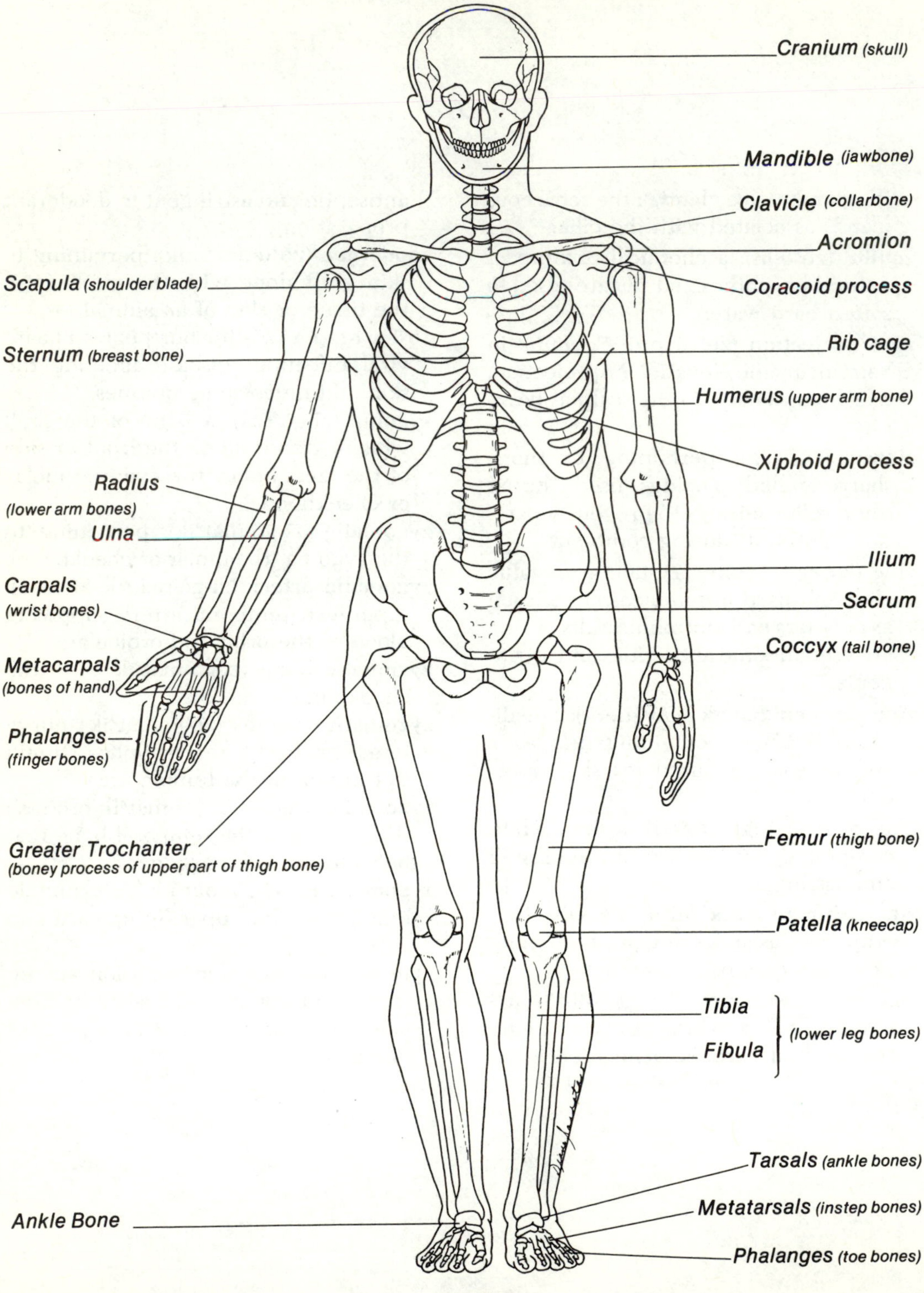
Cranium (skull)
Mandible (jawbone)
Clavicle (collarbone)
Acromion
Scapula (shoulder blade)
Coracoid process
Sternum (breast bone)
Rib cage
Humerus (upper arm bone)
Xiphoid process
Radius
(lower arm bones)
Ulna
Ilium
Carpals
(wrist bones)
Sacrum
Coccyx (tail bone)
Metacarpals
(bones of hand)
Phalanges
(finger bones)
Greater Trochanter
(boney process of upper part of thigh bone)
Femur (thigh bone)
Patella (kneecap)
Tibia
Fibula
(lower leg bones)
Tarsals (ankle bones)
Metatarsals (instep bones)
Ankle Bone
Phalanges (toe bones)

ANATOMY TABLE II
Posterior View of the Skeletal System

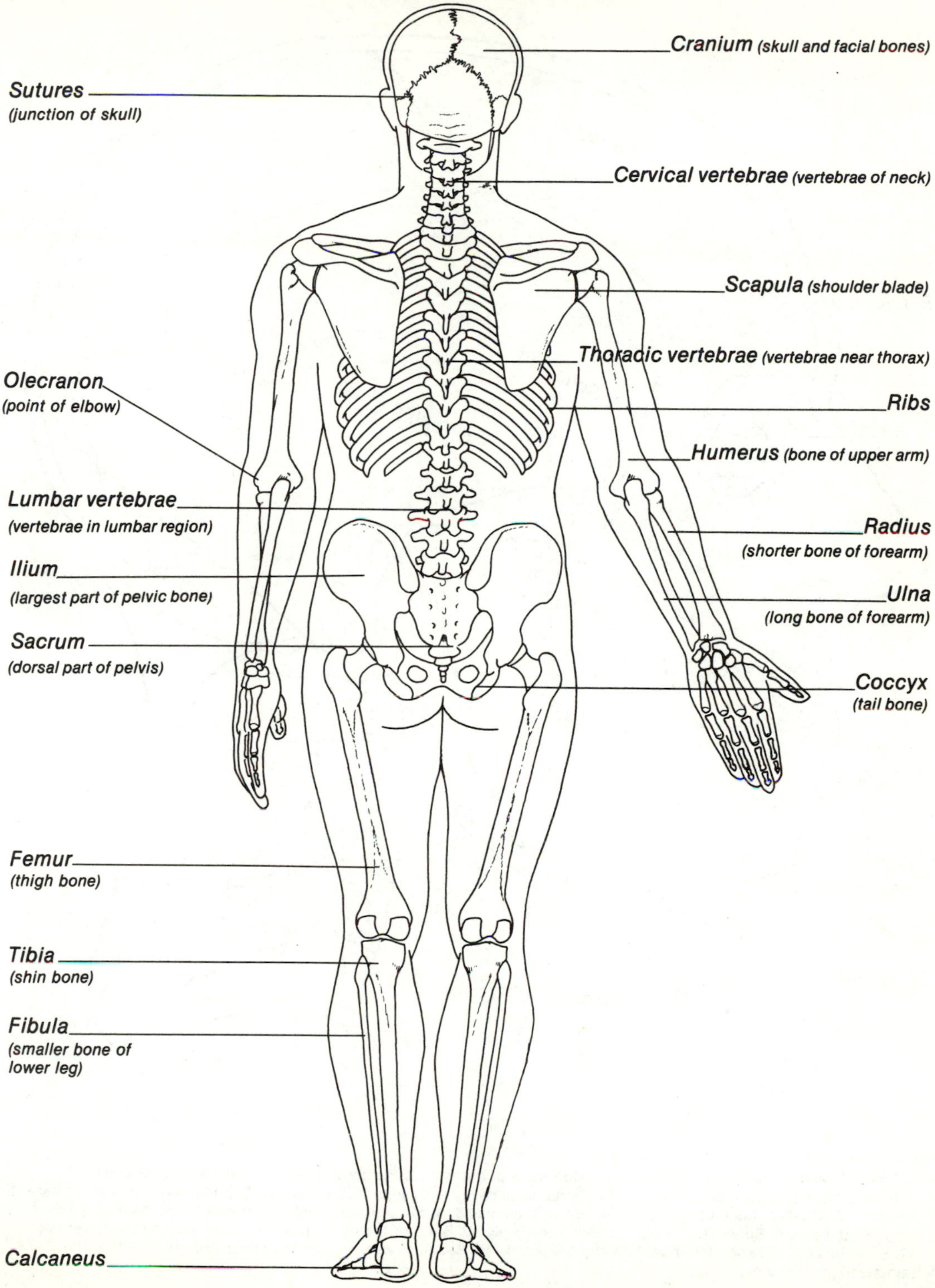

ANATOMY TABLE III
Cranium, Face and Neck Bones

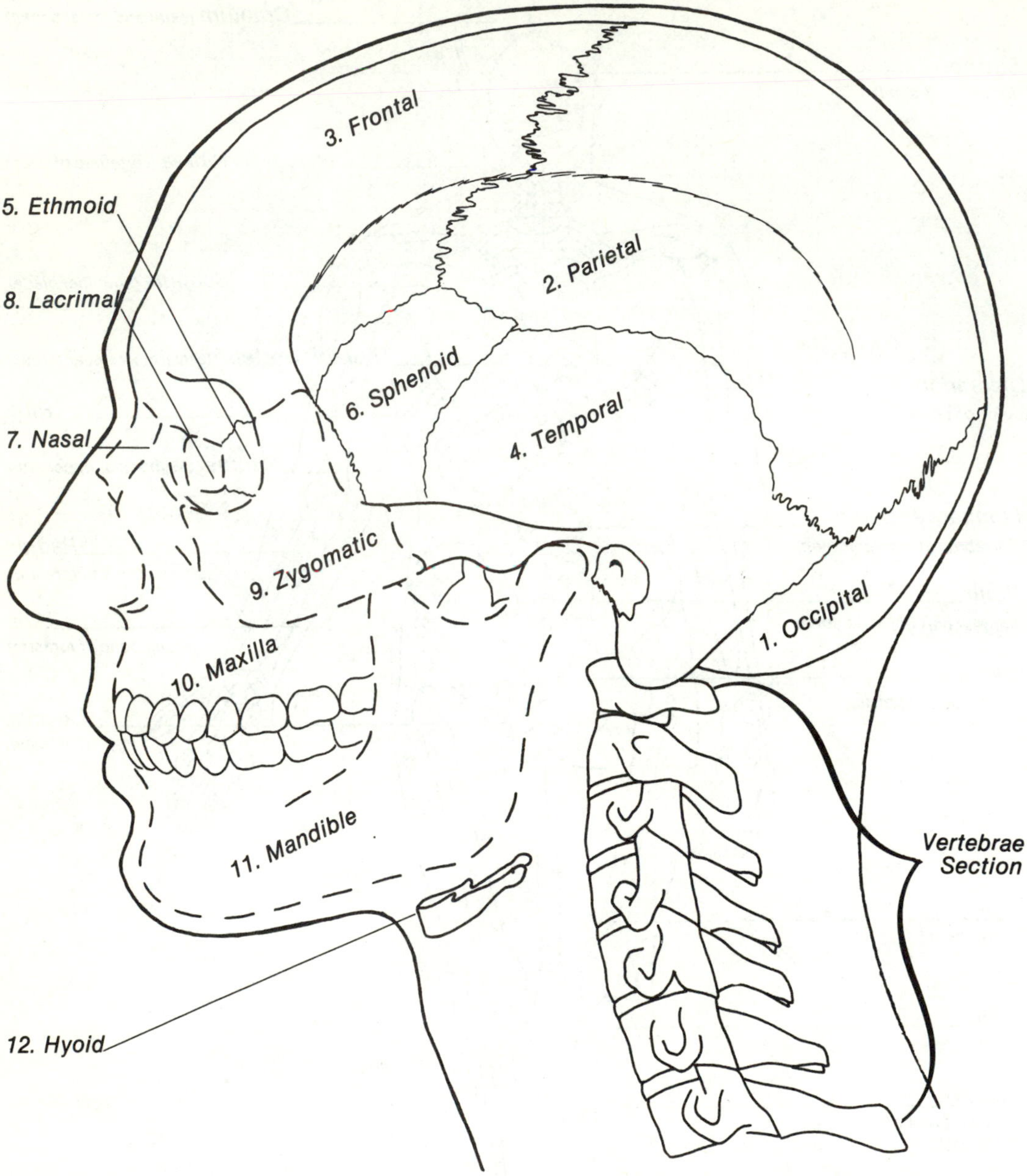

1. Base of skull. **2.** Large part of upper and side walls of cranium. **3.** Forms forehead, nasal cavity and orbits. **4.** Forms sides and base of cranium. **5.** Supports nasal cavity and helps to form orbits. **6.** Forms anterior part of base of cranium. **7.** A pair of bones forming the bridge of the nose. **8.** A pair of bones making up part of the orbit at the inner angle of the eye. **9.** Bone which helps to form the cheek. **10.** Bone of the upper jaw. **11.** Bone forming the lower jaw. **12.** Bone located between the mandible and the larynx. **13.** Smallest vertebrae of the spinal column; forming the framework of the neck.

ANATOMY TABLE IV
The Muscular System—Anterior View

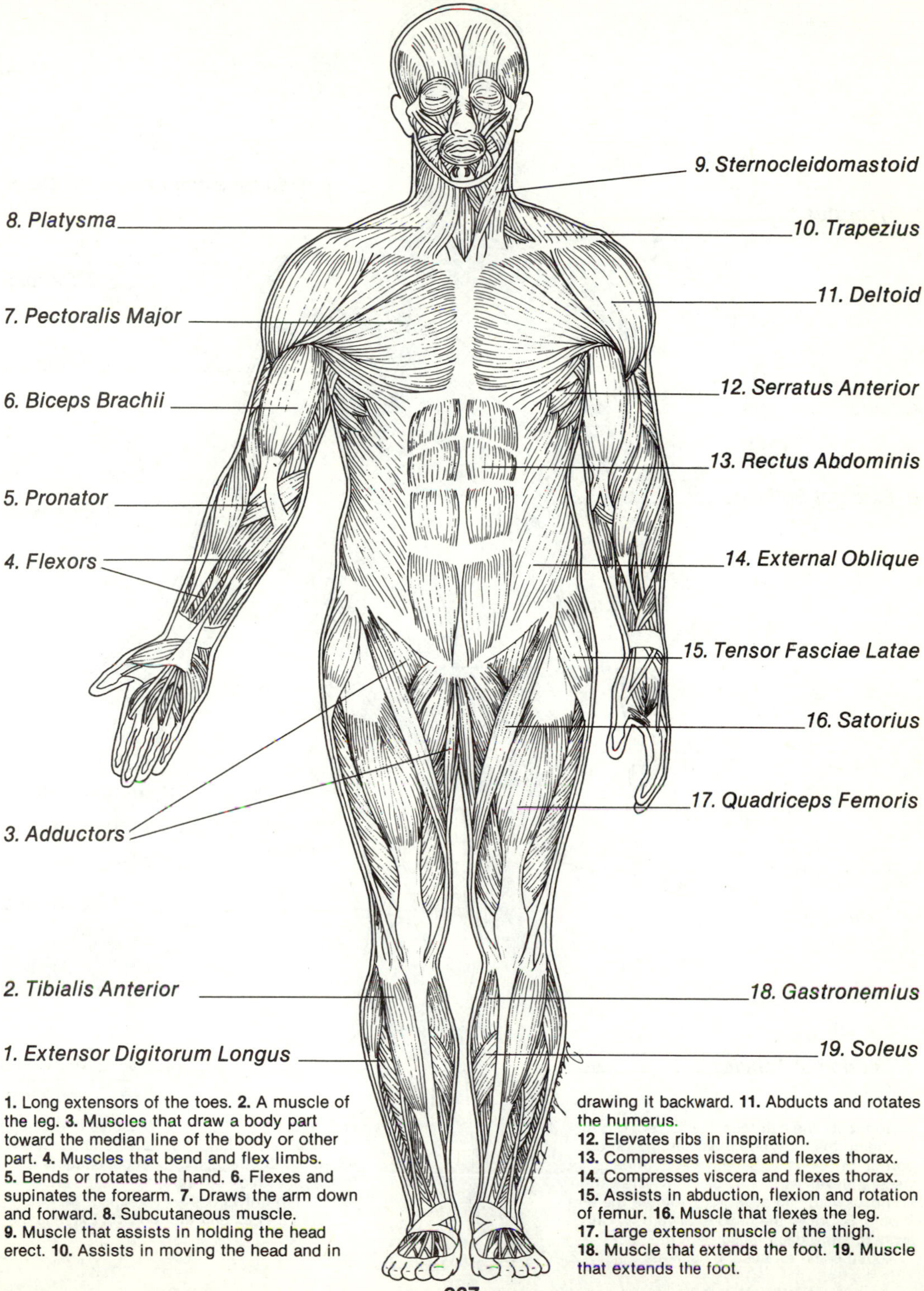

1. Long extensors of the toes. **2.** A muscle of the leg. **3.** Muscles that draw a body part toward the median line of the body or other part. **4.** Muscles that bend and flex limbs. **5.** Bends or rotates the hand. **6.** Flexes and supinates the forearm. **7.** Draws the arm down and forward. **8.** Subcutaneous muscle. **9.** Muscle that assists in holding the head erect. **10.** Assists in moving the head and in drawing it backward. **11.** Abducts and rotates the humerus.
12. Elevates ribs in inspiration.
13. Compresses viscera and flexes thorax.
14. Compresses viscera and flexes thorax.
15. Assists in abduction, flexion and rotation of femur. **16.** Muscle that flexes the leg.
17. Large extensor muscle of the thigh.
18. Muscle that extends the foot. **19.** Muscle that extends the foot.

ANATOMY TABLE V

The Muscular System—Posterior View

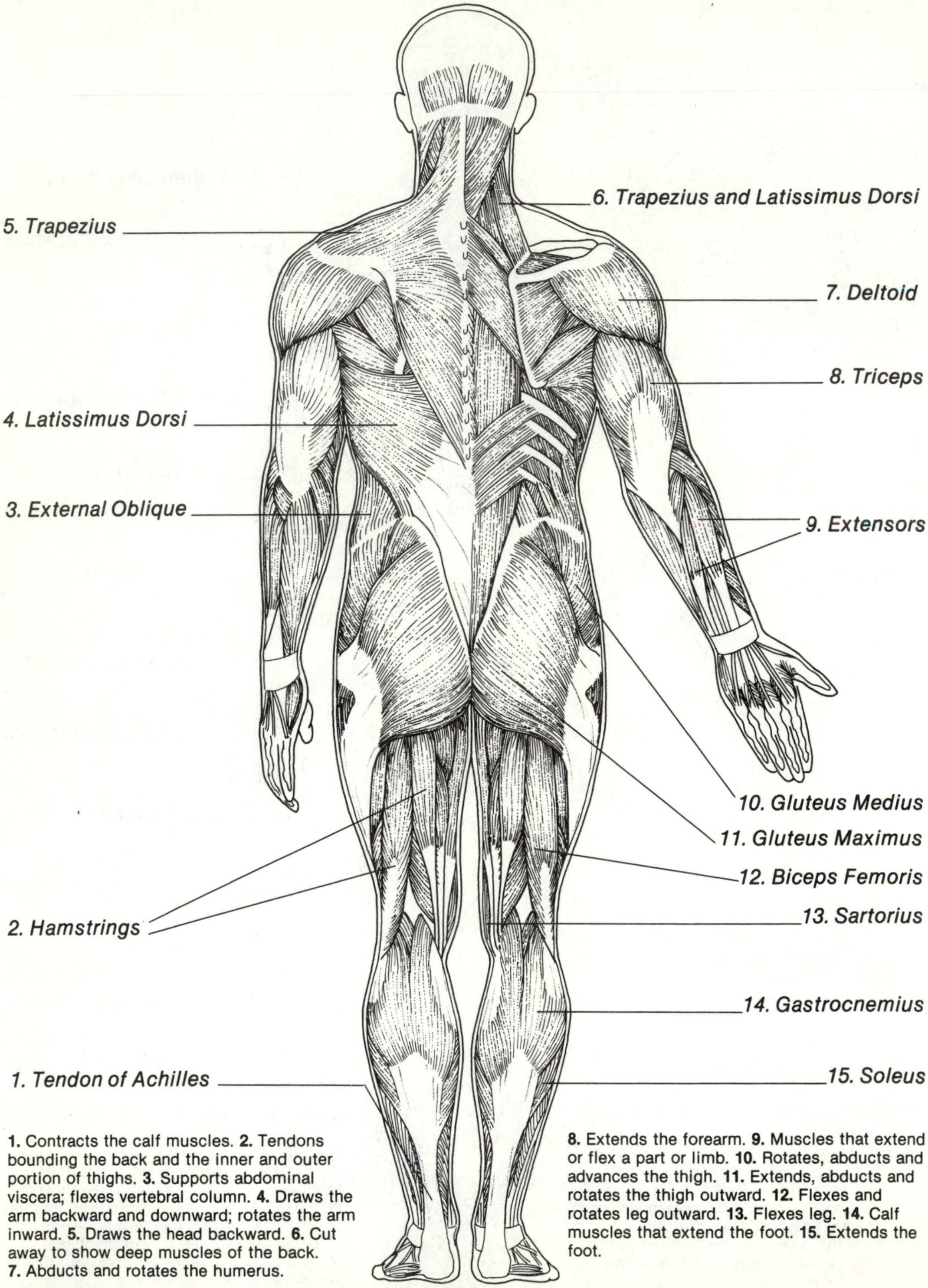

1. Contracts the calf muscles. **2.** Tendons bounding the back and the inner and outer portion of thighs. **3.** Supports abdominal viscera; flexes vertebral column. **4.** Draws the arm backward and downward; rotates the arm inward. **5.** Draws the head backward. **6.** Cut away to show deep muscles of the back. **7.** Abducts and rotates the humerus.

8. Extends the forearm. **9.** Muscles that extend or flex a part or limb. **10.** Rotates, abducts and advances the thigh. **11.** Extends, abducts and rotates the thigh outward. **12.** Flexes and rotates leg outward. **13.** Flexes leg. **14.** Calf muscles that extend the foot. **15.** Extends the foot.

ANATOMY TABLE VI
Muscles of the Head, Face and Neck

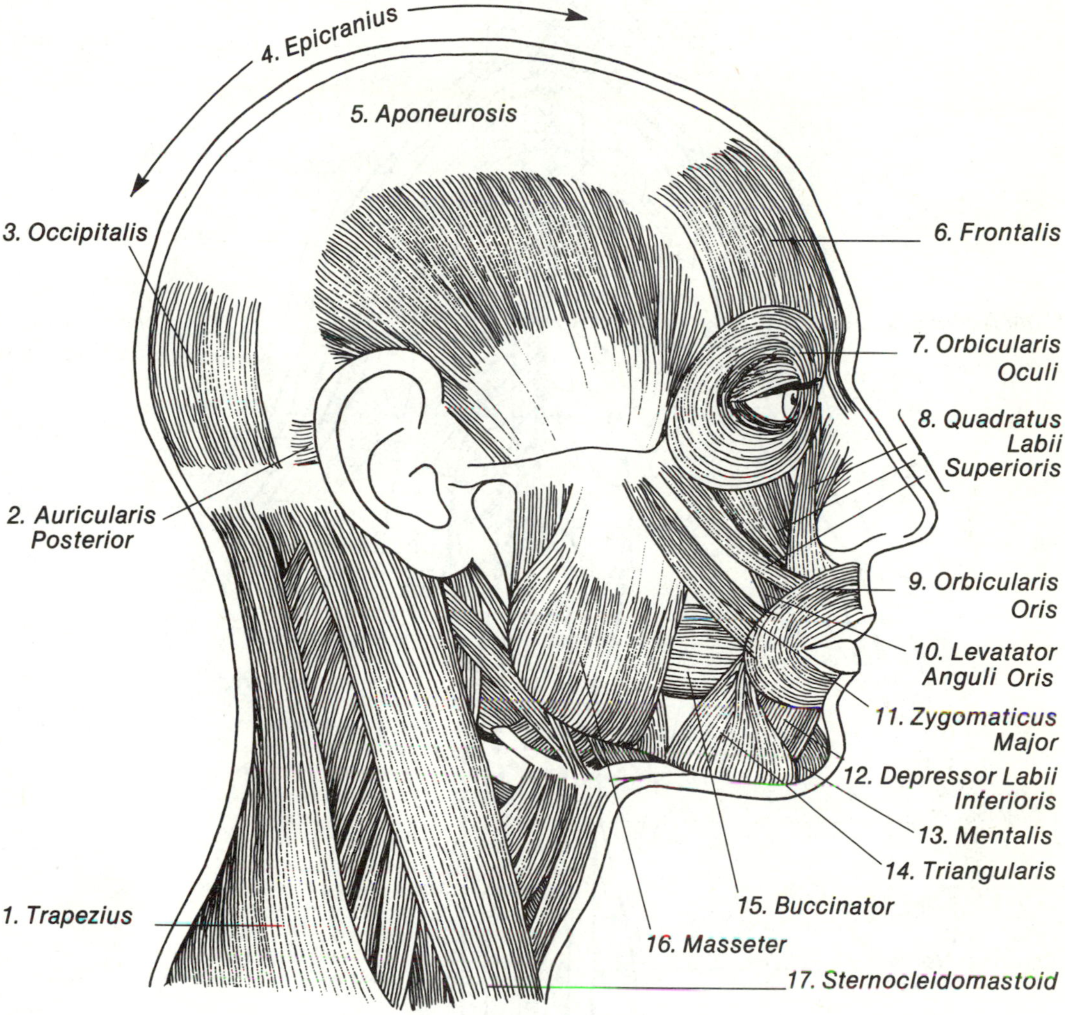

1. Allows movement of shoulders. **2.** Moves auricle, the external part of the ear. **3.** Posterior part of the epicranius muscle. **4.** Draws scalp backward. **5.** Fibrous or membranous sheet to which flat muscles are attached at origin of insertion. **6.** Elevates eyebrows and wrinkles skin of forehead. **7.** The ring muscle of the eye. **8.** A muscle of facial expression with insertion in skin of upper lip. **9.** Muscle of expression, especially smile; opens and closes lips; ring muscle of the mouth. **10.** Muscle of facial expression at the angle of the mouth. **11.** Muscle which pulls the mouth upward and back when laughing. **12.** Muscle of facial expression; everts and draws the lower lip downward. **13.** Muscle which raises and protrudes lower lip. **14.** Muscle of facial expression at angle of mouth. **15.** Largest muscle of facial expression; purses the lips. **16.** Muscle which closes the jaw. **17.** Muscle which helps to hold the head erect.

ANATOMY TABLE VII
The Nervous System:
The Brain, Spinal Cord and Main Nerves of the Body

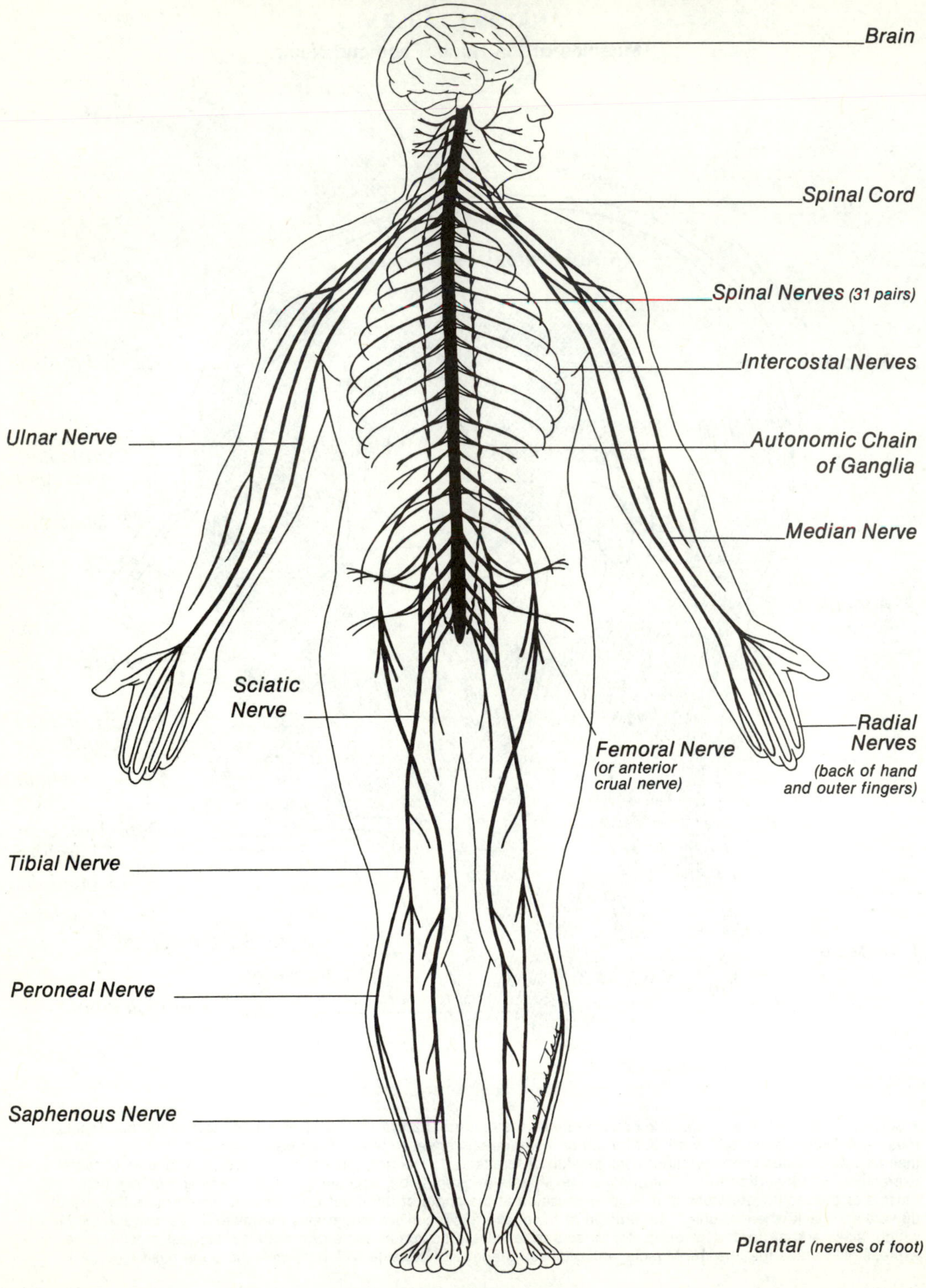

ANATOMY TABLE VIII
Nerves of the Head, Face and Neck

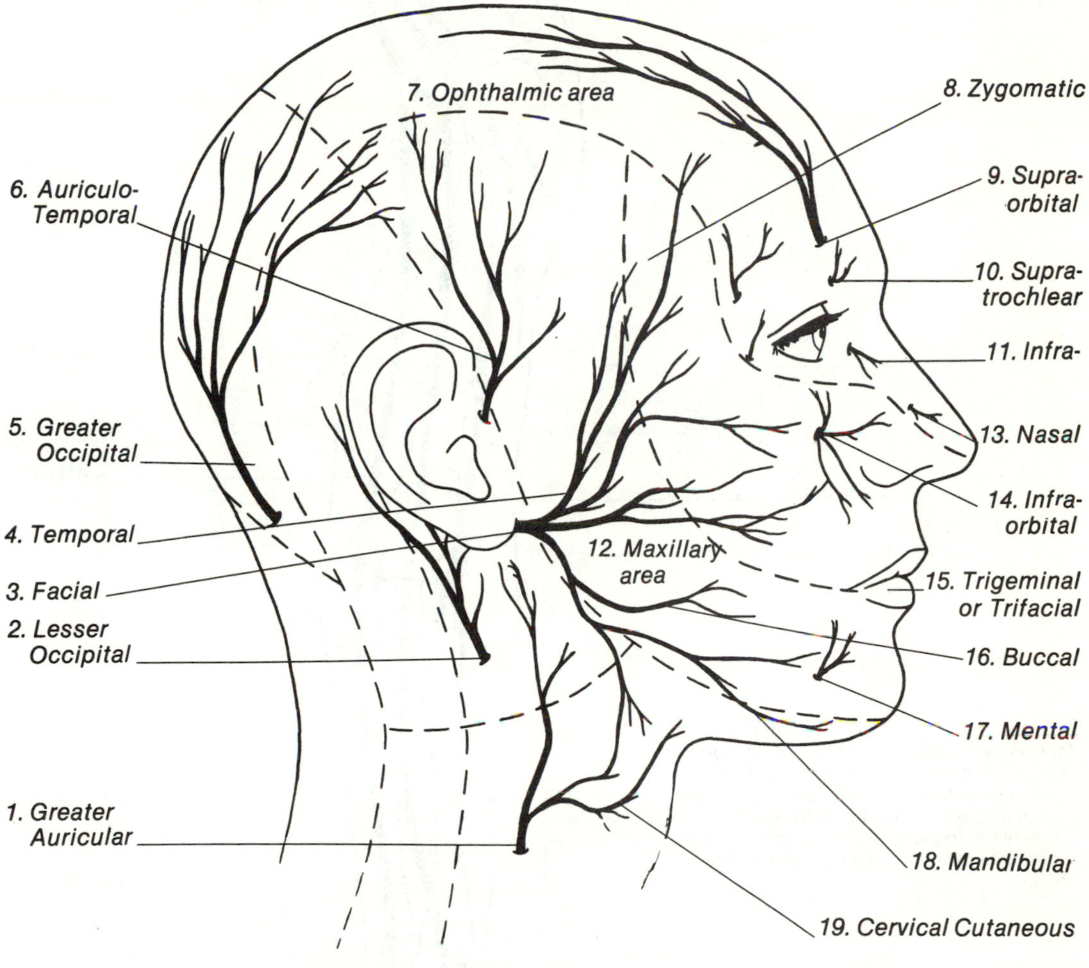

1. Nerves of the side of the neck and ear. **2.** Nerves of skin behind the ear and back of scalp. **3.** Nerves of muscles of expression. **4.** Nerves of the temporal muscle. **5.** Nerves of skin over back part of the head. **6.** Nerves of the side of the scalp. **7.** Nerves of tear glands, eye membrane, skin of forehead and nose. **8.** Zygomatic sensory nerve, a branch of the maxillary nerve which innervates the skin in the temple area, side of forehead and upper part of cheek. **9.** Nerves of the skin of the forehead. **10.** Nerves of the skin of upper eyelids and root of the nose. **11.** Nerves of skin of lower eyelids and sides of nose. **12.** Nerves of the nasal pharynx, teeth of the upper jaw and skin of the cheek. **13.** Nerves of skin and mucous membrane of the nose. **14.** Nerves of the skin of the cheek and lower eyelid. **15.** Nerves of skin of face, tongue, teeth and muscles of mastication. **16.** Nerves of buccinator and orbicularis oris. **17.** Nerves of lower lip and chin. **18.** Nerves of teeth and lower jaws and cheek area. **19.** Nerves which supply the skin of the jaw back of ear, lateral and anterior sides of neck and skin of upper anterior thorax.

ANATOMY TABLE IX
Nerves of the Arm and Hand

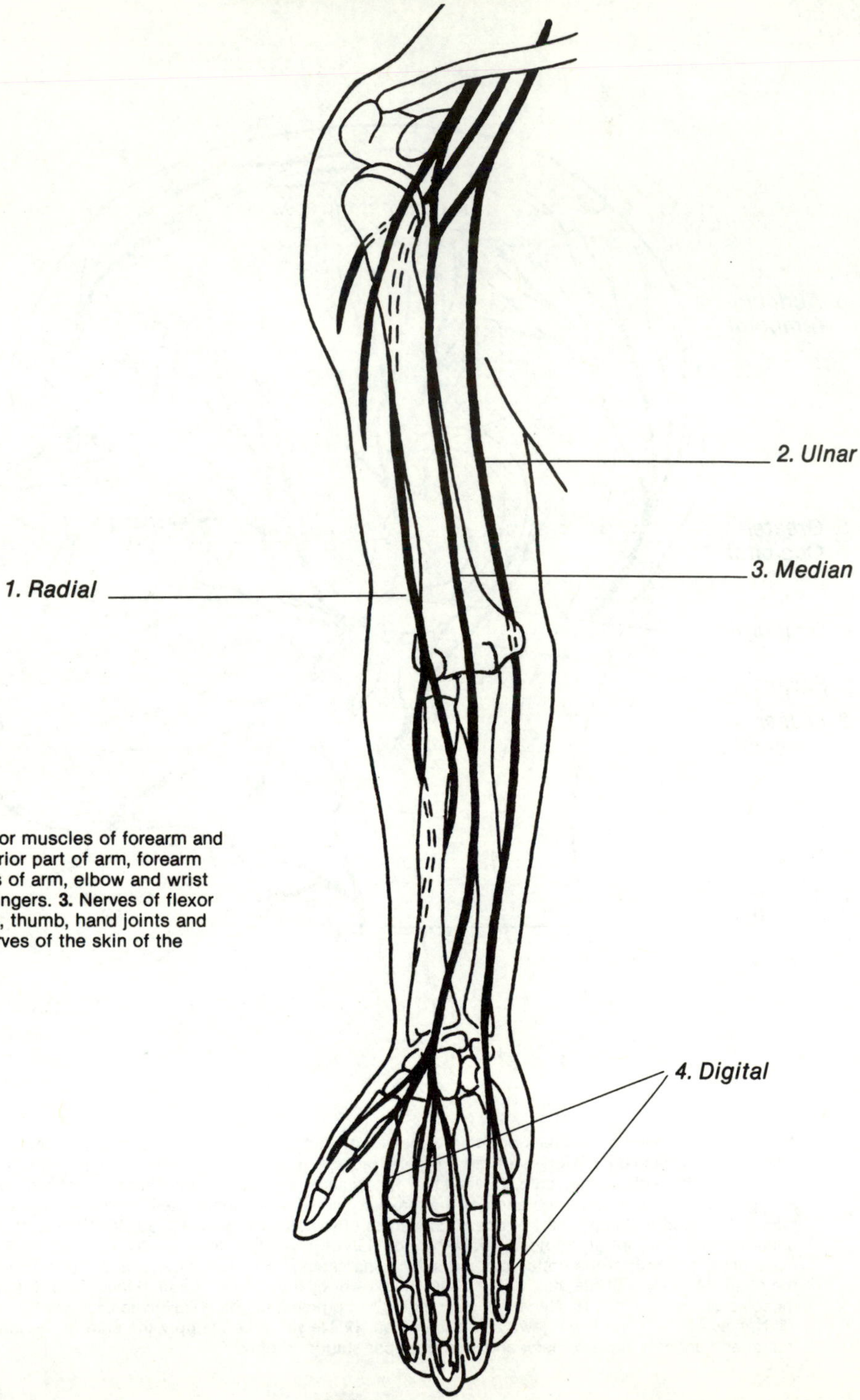

1. Nerves of extensor muscles of forearm and hand, skin of posterior part of arm, forearm and wrist. **2.** Nerves of arm, elbow and wrist joints and skin of fingers. **3.** Nerves of flexor muscles of forearm, thumb, hand joints and skin of hand. **4.** Nerves of the skin of the fingers.

ANATOMY TABLE X

Motor Nerve Points of the Face and Neck

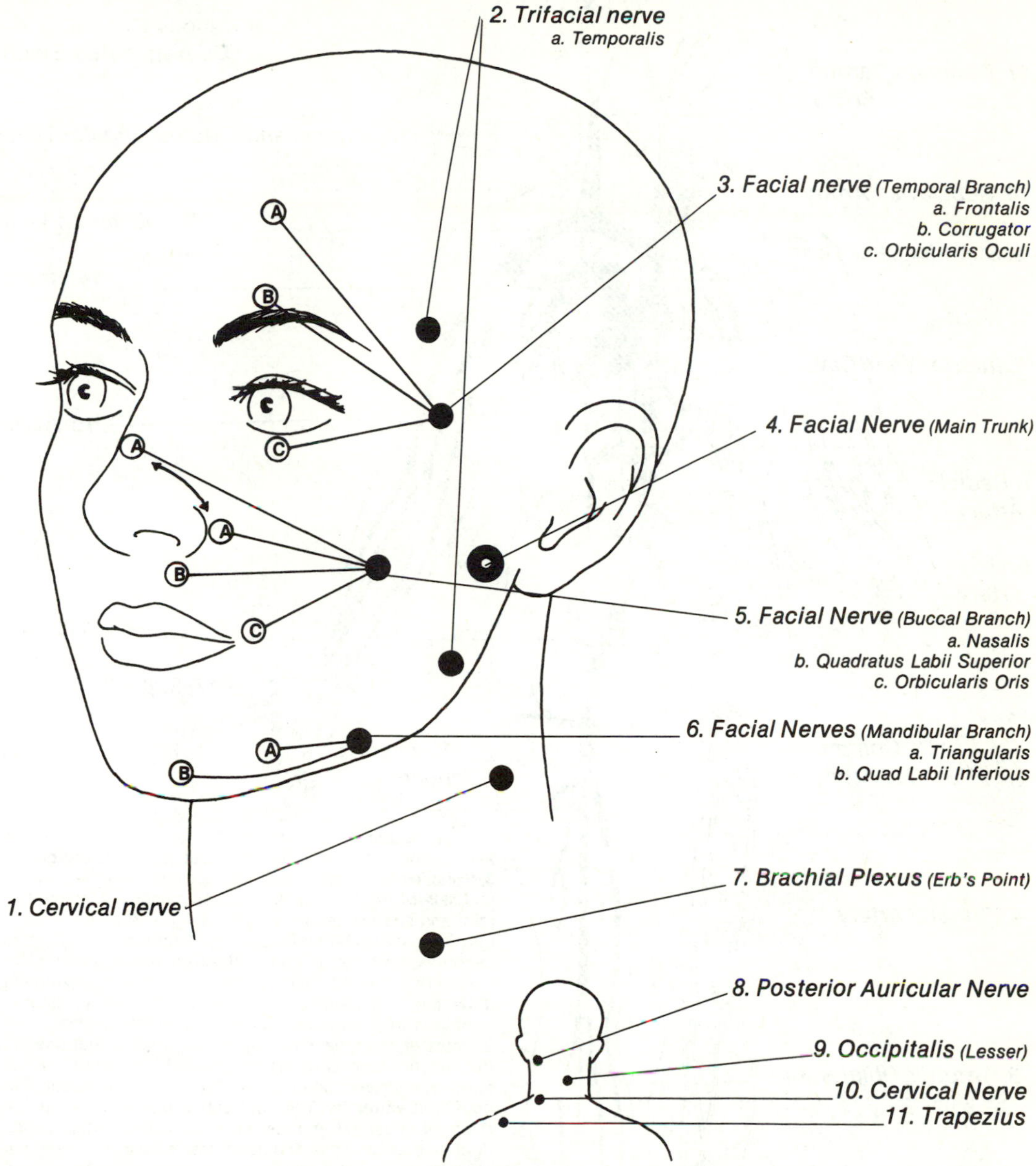

1. Nerve serving the skin of jaw, back of ear, lateral and posterior sides of the neck, and skin of upper anterior thorax. **2.** Nerves of skin of face, tongue, teeth and muscles of mastication. **2a.** Nerves of the temporal muscle. **3a.** Nerve serving skin of forehead. **3b.** Nerve serving the muscle that draws eyebrows downward and inward. **3c.** Nerves of muscle surrounding the orbit. **4.** Controls facial muscles of expression. **5a.** Serves skin and mucous membrane of the nose. **5b.** Nerves that raise lip and dilate nostrils. **5c.** Muscles ringing the mouth that function in pursing of the lips. **6a.** Nerves serving the triangularis muscle. **6b.** Nerves of the lower lip. **7.** Nerves located in the neck and axilla. **8.** Nerve of epicranius and auricular muscle. **9.** Nerve of skin behind the ear and on back of scalp. **10.** Nerve serving the skin of back of neck. **11.** Nerve serving the trapezius muscles that draw the head sideward and backward.

ANATOMY TABLE XI
The Circulatory System

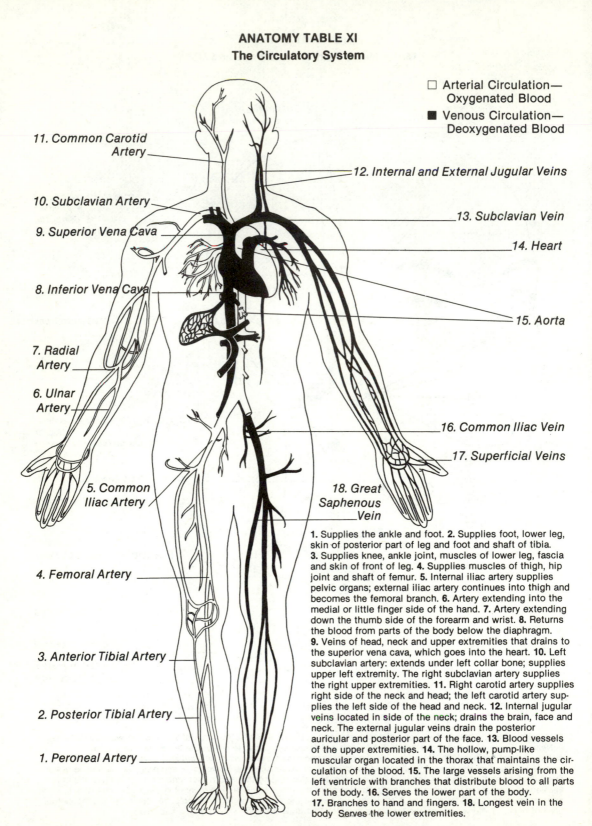

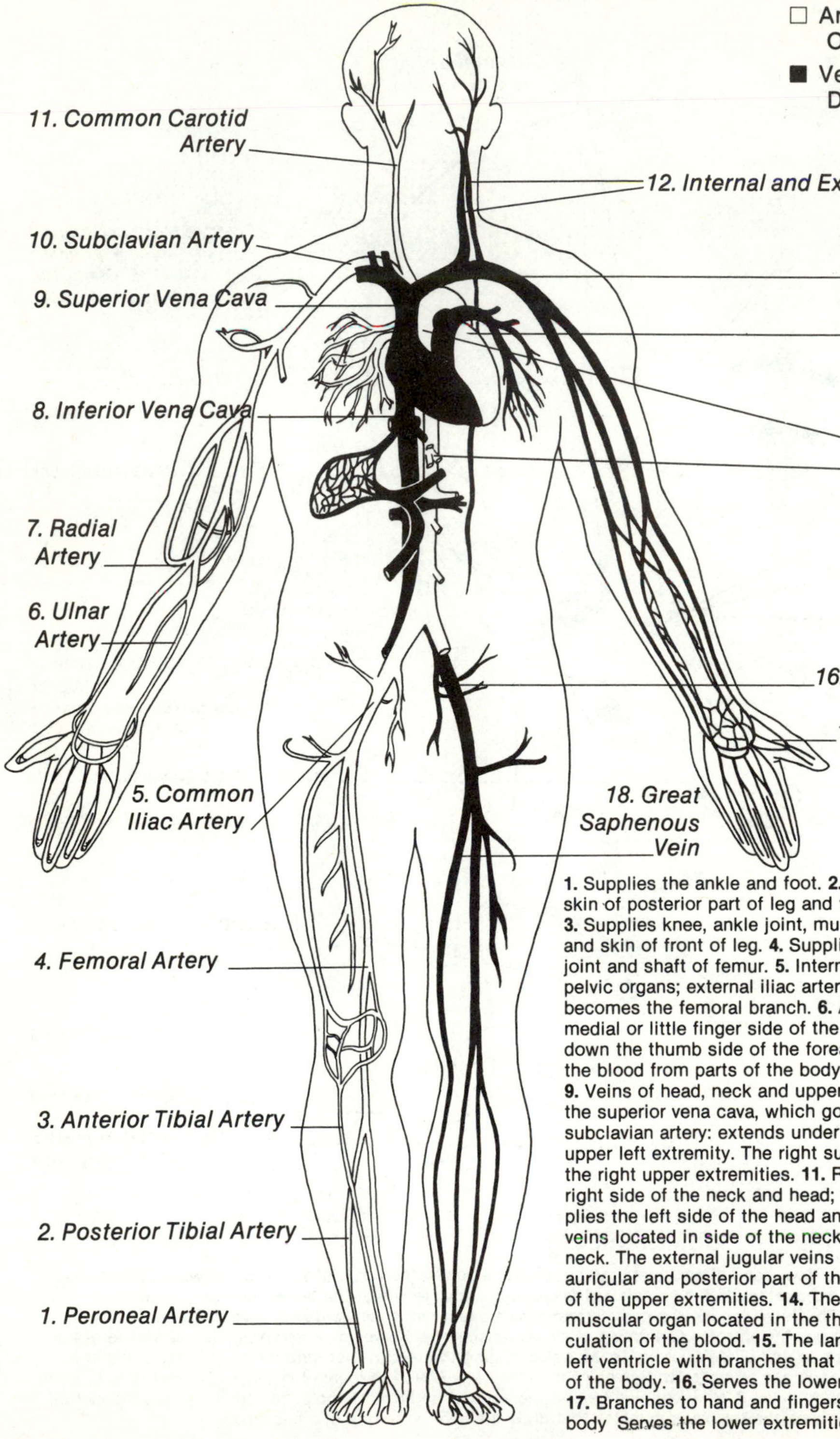

1. Supplies the ankle and foot. **2.** Supplies foot, lower leg, skin of posterior part of leg and foot and shaft of tibia. **3.** Supplies knee, ankle joint, muscles of lower leg, fascia and skin of front of leg. **4.** Supplies muscles of thigh, hip joint and shaft of femur. **5.** Internal iliac artery supplies pelvic organs; external iliac artery continues into thigh and becomes the femoral branch. **6.** Artery extending into the medial or little finger side of the hand. **7.** Artery extending down the thumb side of the forearm and wrist. **8.** Returns the blood from parts of the body below the diaphragm. **9.** Veins of head, neck and upper extremities that drains to the superior vena cava, which goes into the heart. **10.** Left subclavian artery: extends under left collar bone; supplies upper left extremity. The right subclavian artery supplies the right upper extremities. **11.** Right carotid artery supplies right side of the neck and head; the left carotid artery supplies the left side of the head and neck. **12.** Internal jugular veins located in side of the neck; drains the brain, face and neck. The external jugular veins drain the posterior auricular and posterior part of the face. **13.** Blood vessels of the upper extremities. **14.** The hollow, pump-like muscular organ located in the thorax that maintains the circulation of the blood. **15.** The large vessels arising from the left ventricle with branches that distribute blood to all parts of the body. **16.** Serves the lower part of the body. **17.** Branches to hand and fingers. **18.** Longest vein in the body Serves the lower extremities.

ANATOMY TABLE XII
Arteries of the Head, Face and Neck

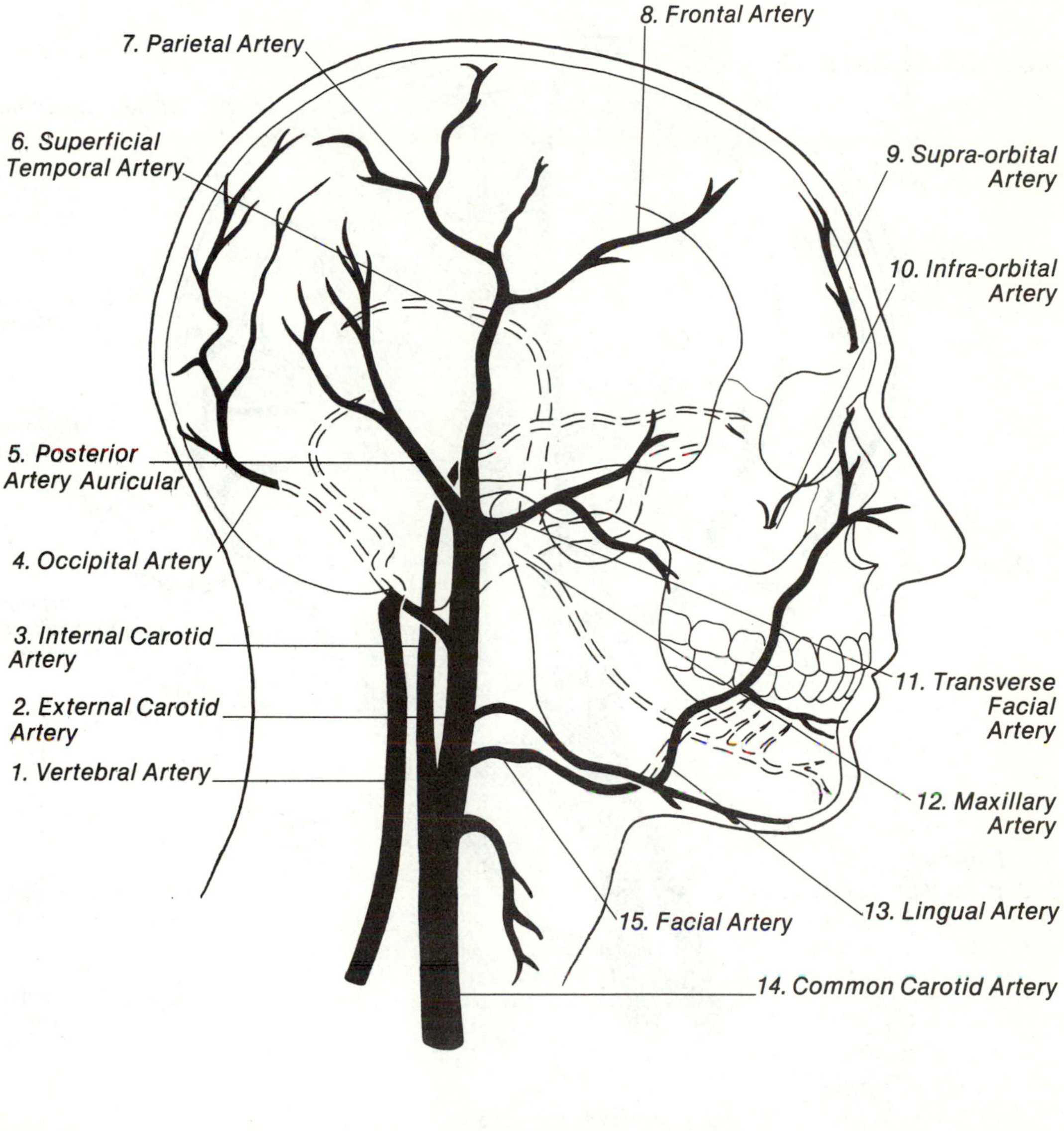

1. Supplies muscles of neck, posterior fossa of skull. **2.** Supplies face, tonsils, root of tongue and submandibular gland. **3.** Supplies brain, sinuses, parts of the head. **4.** Supplies muscles of neck, ear area and scalp. **5.** Supplies area of ear, scalp and parotid gland. **6.** Supplies the masseter muscle. **7.** Located in the parietal bone of the skull. **8.** Supplies frontal bone, upper eyelid. **9.** Supplies root of orbit, frontal bone, upper eyelid. **10.** Supplies muscle of eye and upper lip. **11.** Supplies masseter muscle, parotid gland, skin of face. **12.** Supplies jaws, ear and deep structure of face.
13. Supplies membrane of tongue and mouth, gums, tonsils, soft palate, epiglottis. **14.** Right side supplies right side of head and face, left side supplies the left side of the head and face. **15.** Supplies face, root of tongue, submandibular gland.

ANATOMY TABLE XIII
Veins of the Head, Face and Neck

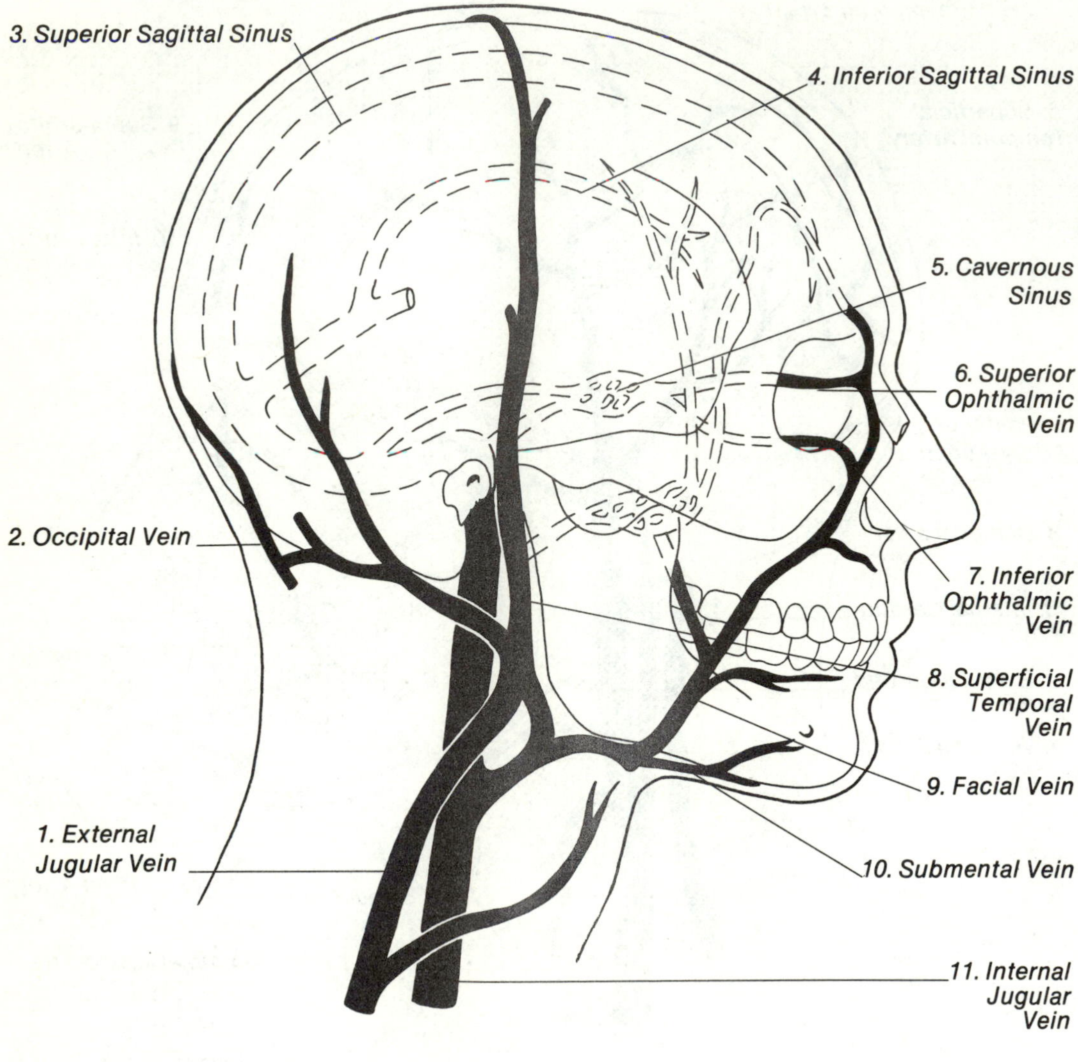

1. Vein located in side of the neck that drains the posterior part of the face area supplied by carotid arteries.
2. Drains into confluence of sinuses. **3.** A single long space located in midline above the brain. Ends in an enlargement called the confluence of sinuses. **4.** A small venous sinus of the dura mater, situated in the posterior half of the lower concave border of the cerebral falx. **5.** Situated behind the eyeball and drains the ophthalmic veins of the eye.
6. Drains veins of the eye. **7.** Veins supplying the eye area. **8.** Vein serving the temple region of the head on either side.
9. Vein supplying the anterior side of the face. **10.** A vein situated below the chin that follows the submental artery and opens into the facial vein. **11.** Vein located in side of the neck and drains the brain, face, neck and transverse sinus.

ANATOMY TABLE XIV

Blood Supply for the Arm and Hand

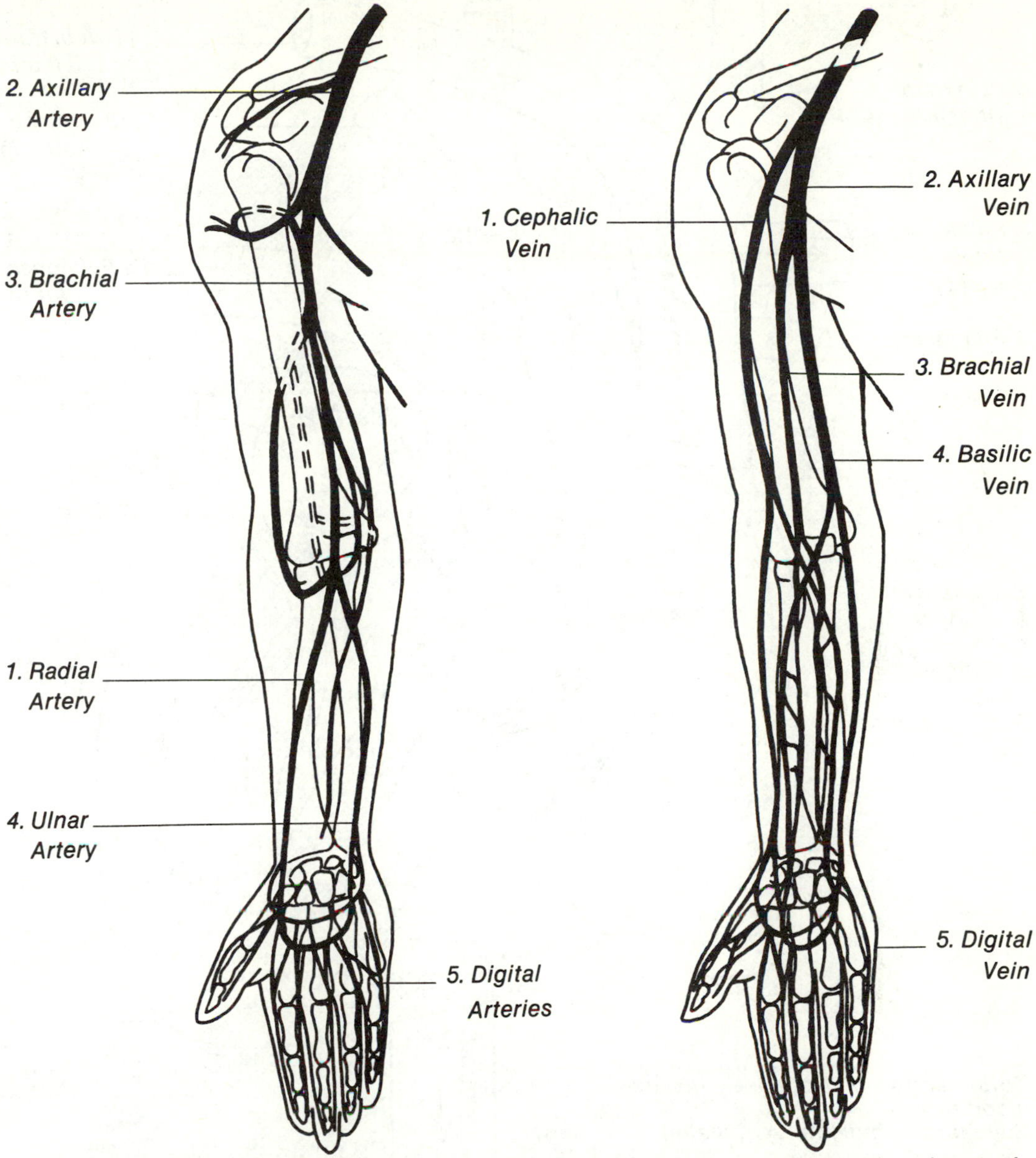

I. Arteries: Large thick-walled tubes comprising a system that carries blood directly from the heart to the main parts of the body. **1.** Principal artery of thumb and deep palmar arch. **2.** A continuation of the subclavian extending from the outer border of the first rib to the tendon of the teres major muscle where it becomes the brachial. **3.** Distributes blood to various muscles of the arm, the humerus, elbow joint, forearm and hand. **4.** Artery which supplies muscles of the forearm, shafts of radius and ulna, ulnal half of the hand and skin of these areas. **5.** Arteries serving the dorsal areas of the fingers.

II. Veins: Blood vessels that carry blood from parts of the body back toward the heart. **1.** The superficial vein rising from the radial side of the arm which supplies the biceps and deltoid muscles. **2.** A continuation of the basilic ending in the outer border of the first rib in the subclavian vein. **3.** Deep veins of the forearm and arm. **4.** Veins beginning in the ulnar part of the dorsal network and extending to join the accessory cephalic vein. **5.** Veins of the fingers.

ANATOMY TABLE XV

Anatomy of the Heart

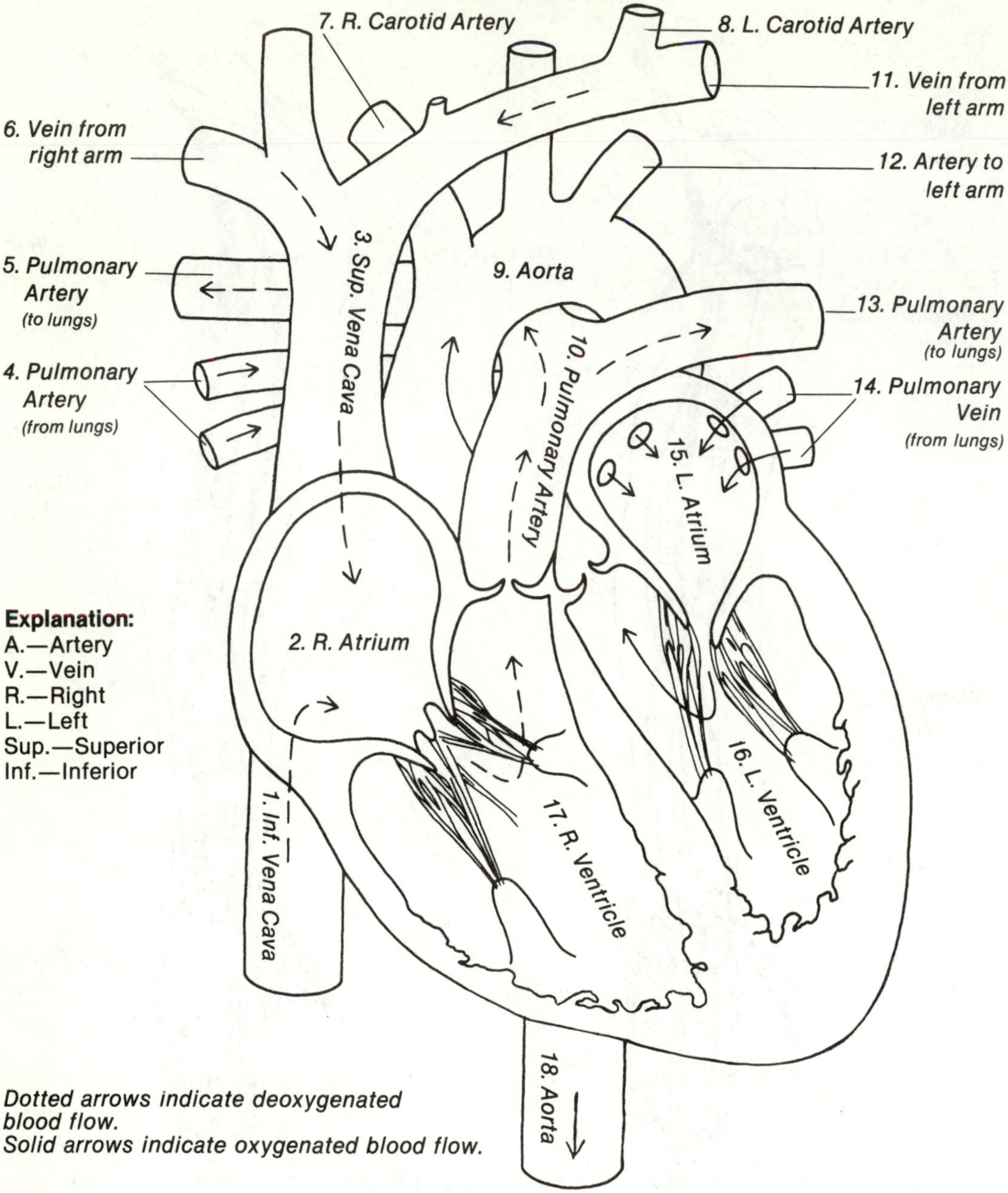

Explanation:
A.—Artery
V.—Vein
R.—Right
L.—Left
Sup.—Superior
Inf.—Inferior

Dotted arrows indicate deoxygenated blood flow.
Solid arrows indicate oxygenated blood flow.

1. Veins of abdomen, pelvis and lower extremities empty into this vein. **2.** Receives impure blood from the vena cava. **3.** Veins of the head, neck, thorax and upper extremities empty into this vein. **4.** Conveys oxygenated blood from the lungs to the left atrium. **5.** Conveys venous blood from the right ventricle to the lungs. **7.** The principal large artery on the right side of the neck. **8.** The principal large artery on the left side of the neck. **9.** Main artery of the body; carries blood from the left ventricle to all arteries of the body. **10.** Divides into left and right branches and takes blood into the lungs. **15.** Receives purified blood through the pulmonary vein. **16.** From the left ventricle the aorta sends blood to all parts of the body except the lungs. **17.** Venous blood is carried through the pulmonary artery up to the lungs to be oxygenated and purified. **18.** A large vessel arising from the left ventricle which, by way of its branches, distributes arterial blood to all parts of the body.

ANATOMY TABLE XVI
The Digestive System

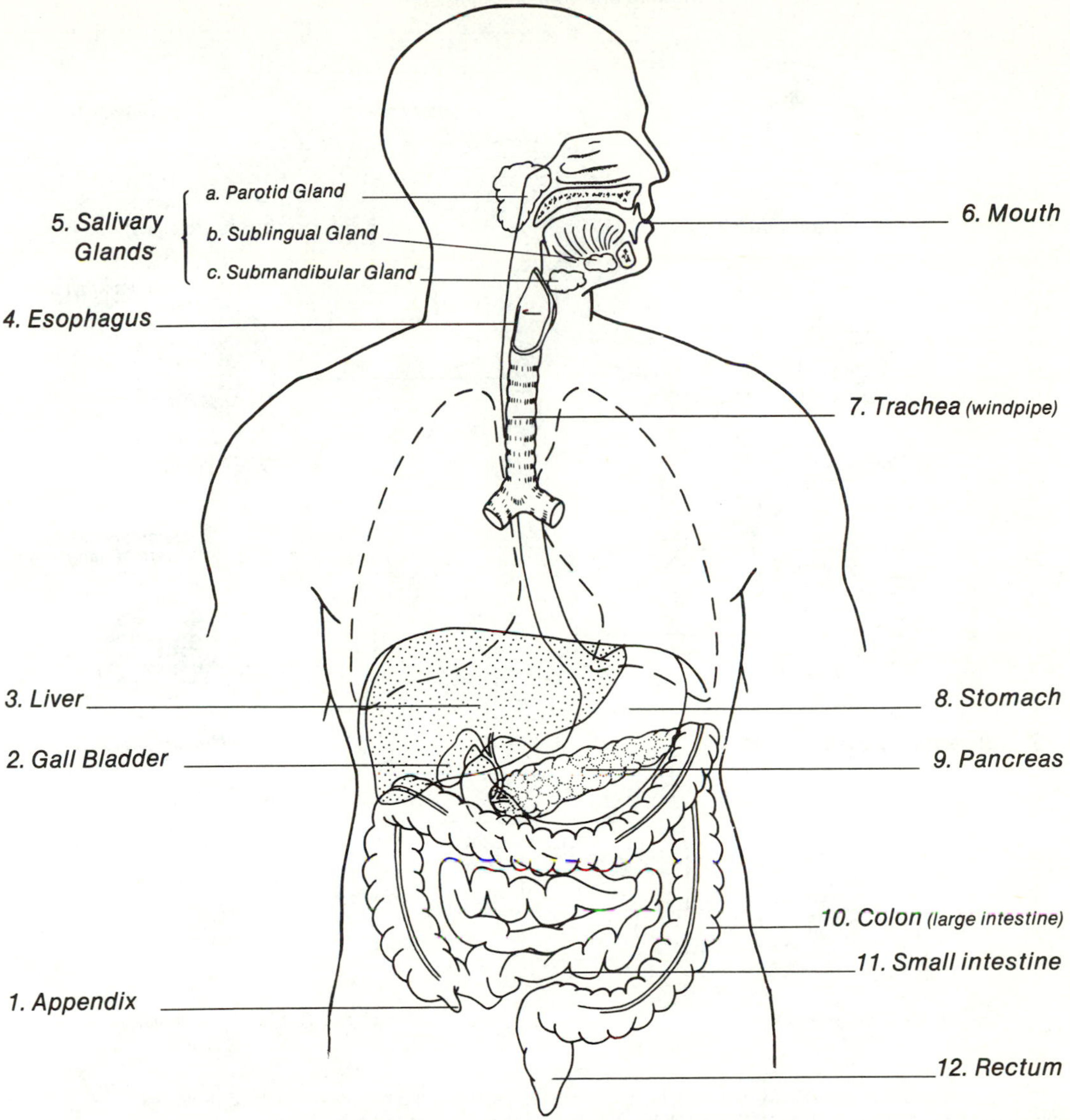

1. A narrow tube attached to the cecum, a part of the colon. **2.** The gall bladder is located on the underside of the liver. It receives bile from liver and expels the bile (as needed) into the duodenum. **3.** Produces bile, which acts as fat solvent. The largest gland of the body, the liver functions to maintain and regulate homeostasis of body fluids and help to control body processes. **4.** Moves food to the stomach.
5. Buccal glands. **5a.** Located under and in front of ear. **5b.** Located below the jaw and under the tongue. **5c.** Located in floor of mouth beneath the tongue. **6.** Principal functions of mouth and salivary glands are mastication and changing starch to sugar. **7.** Windpipe (respiratory tract). **8.** Serves as a receptacle for food; manufactures gastric juice during digestion. **9.** Lies behind the stomach and produces enzymes which act on fat, proteins, starch and carbohydrates to complete the digestive process. Aids in regulation of glucose metabolism.
10. Responsible for absorption and elimination of foodstuffs. **11.** Serves in the absorption and elimination of foodstuffs.
12. Serves to eliminate waste.

ANATOMY TABLE XVII

The Endocrine System

(Both male and female glands are shown)

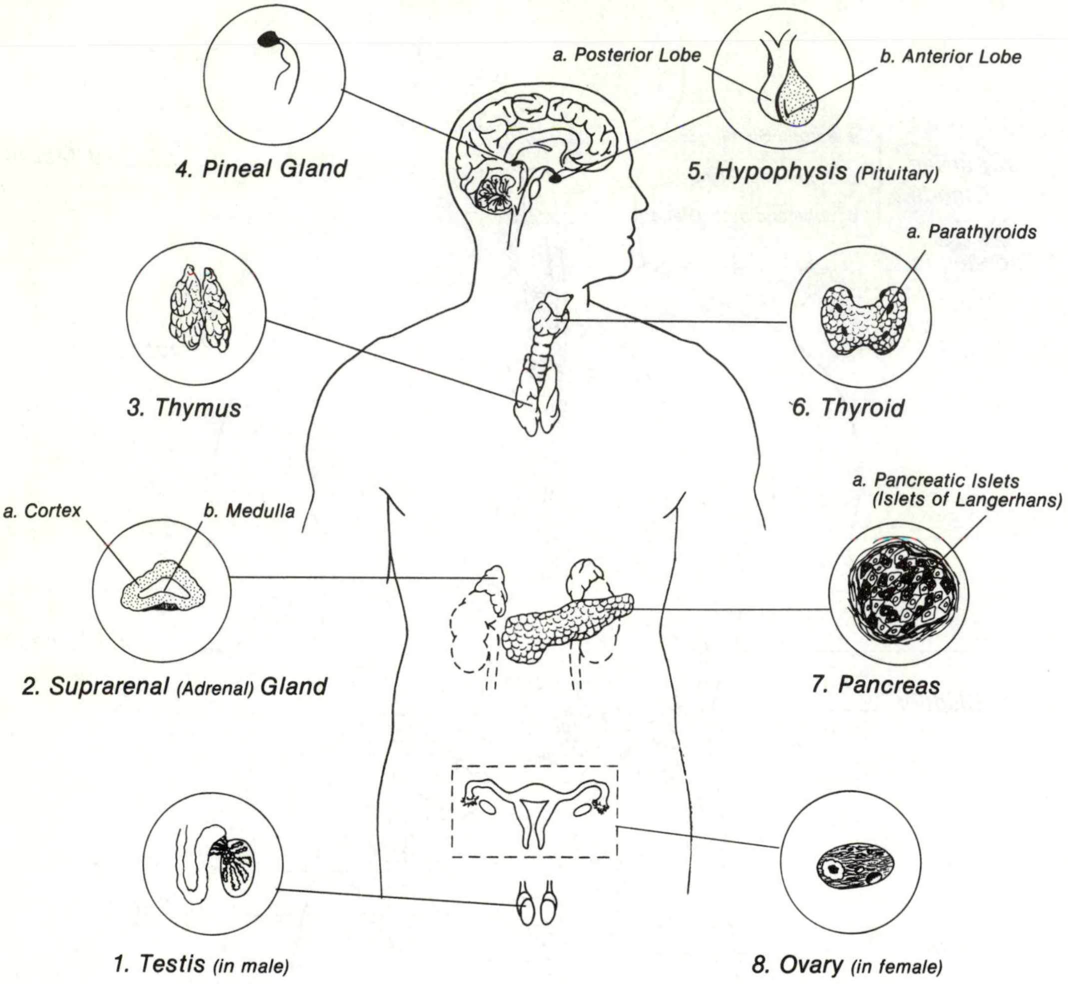

1. Two glandular male reproductive organs which produce testosterone, the hormone which controls sex characteristics in males. **2.** Two small glands located above the upper end of each kidney.
2a. External tissue. **2b.** Chromaphil tissue. **3.** The thymus is part of the lymphatic system located in the upper chest cavity along the trachea. Necessary in early life for development and maturation of immunological functions. **4.** A gland attached to the roof of the third ventricle of the brain. Function is stimulation of adrenal cortex.
5. Called the master or dominating gland. Controls skeletal growth, thyroid secretion and other metabolic processes. **5a.** Affects blood pressure, heartbeat, constriction and contraction of some muscles.
5b. Affects thyroid secretions. **6.** Gland that influences growth and development. Located in front of trachea below thyroid cartilage. **6a.** Four glands arranged in pairs that play a part in maintaining the normal calcium level of the blood, regulate phosphorus metabolism and play a part in the functioning of the nervous system and muscles. **7.** Located between the first and second lumbar vertebrae behind the stomach. Aids in the synthesis of sugar to glycogen, storage of glycogen, and conversion of glycogen to glucose in the liver.
7a. A special group of cells that secrete insulin, which is essential for normal glucose metabolism.
8. Two almond shaped bodies located on each side of the uterus that produce estrogen and progesterone and are essential in the development of female characteristics.

ANATOMY TABLE XVIII
The Respiratory System

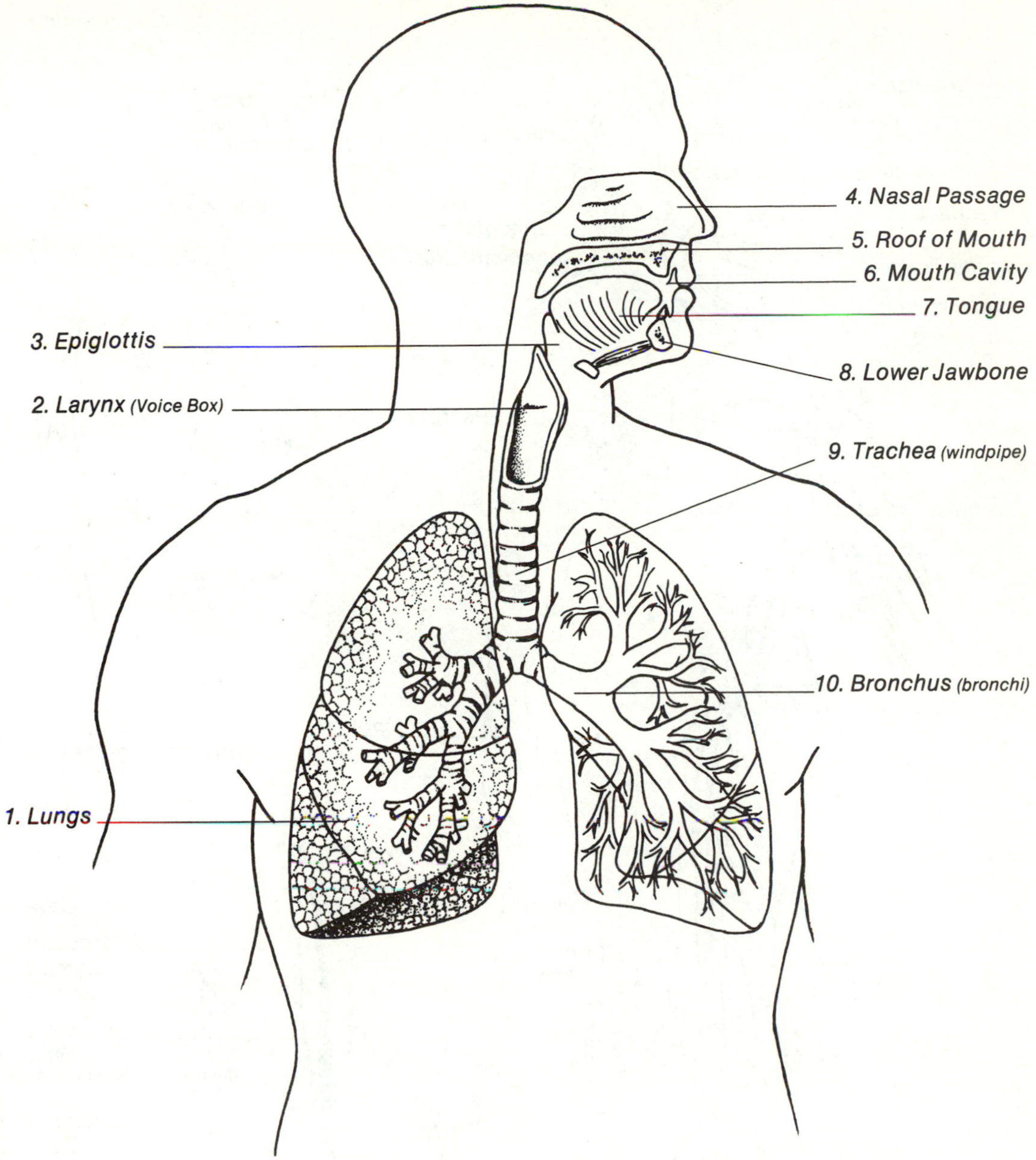

1. Organs of external respiration located in lateral chambers of the thoracic cavity and consisting of three right and two left lobes. **2.** Situated between the tongue and trachea. Functions in production of vocal sounds. **3.** Forms part of larynx and assists in swallowing. **4.**Air passage extending from nostrils to pharynx. **9.** Located in front of esophagus. **10.** Air tubes entering the lungs.

ANATOMY TABLE XIX
The Lymphatic System

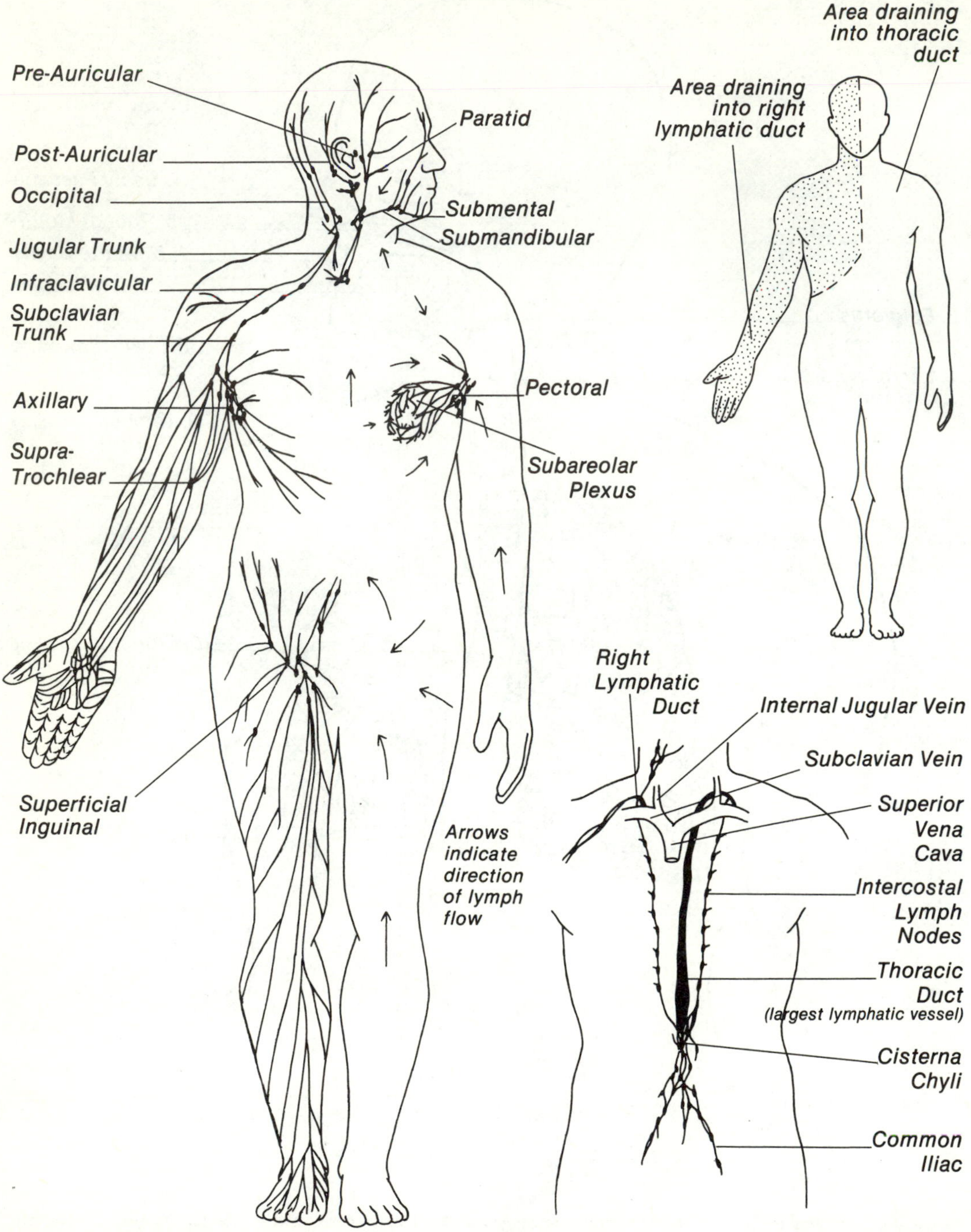

- *Major locations of lymph nodes*
- *Lymphatic vessels are named according to their location*

ANATOMY TABLE XX

The Integumentary Svstem
(showing the skin and hair)

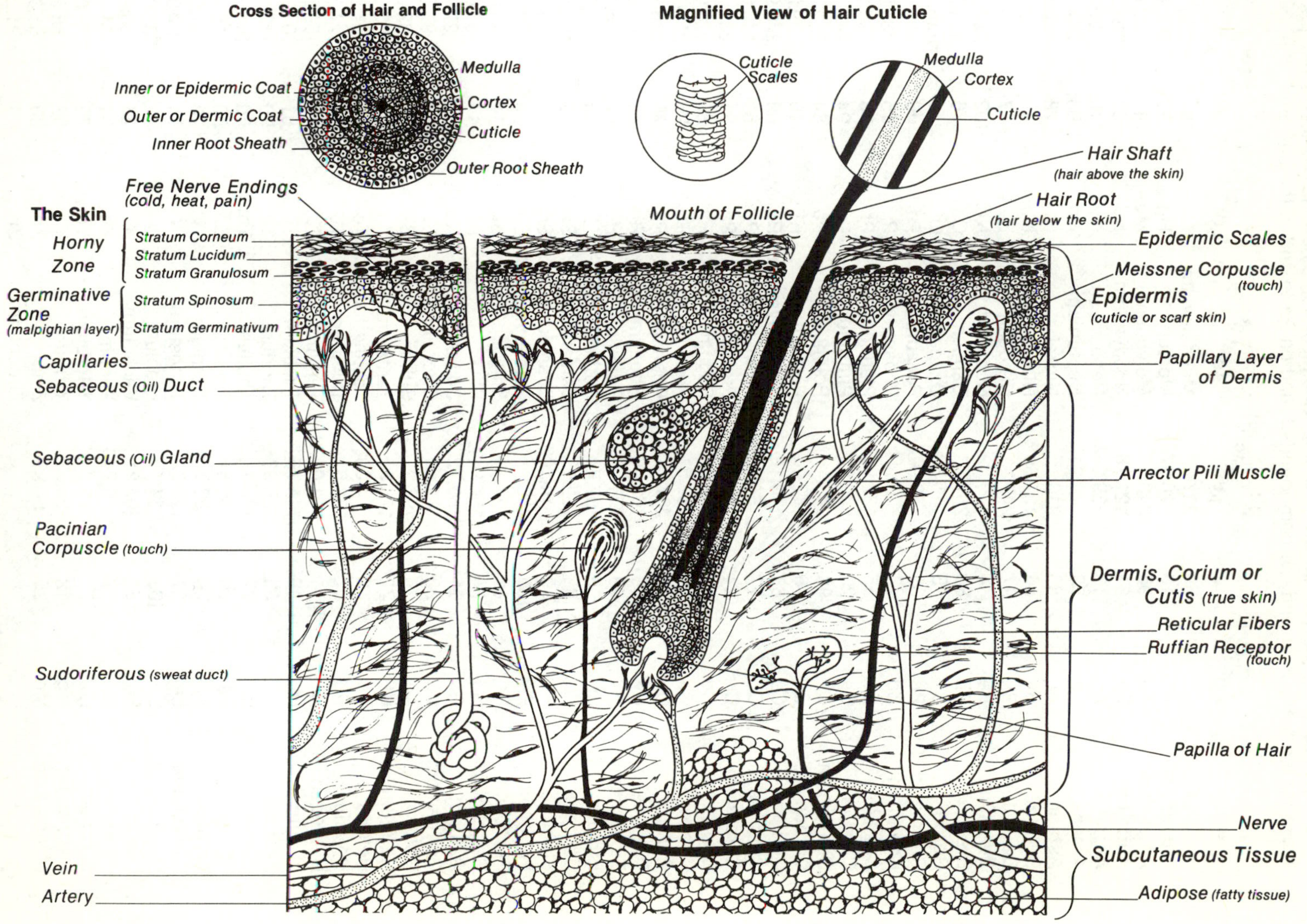
Cross Section of Hair and Follicle
Medulla
Inner or Epidermic Coat
Cortex
Outer or Dermic Coat
Cuticle
Inner Root Sheath
Outer Root Sheath
Magnified View of Hair Cuticle
Cuticle Scales
Medulla
Cortex
Cuticle
Hair Shaft
(hair above the skin)
Hair Root
(hair below the skin)
Free Nerve Endings
(cold, heat, pain)
Mouth of Follicle
The Skin
Horny Zone
Stratum Corneum
Stratum Lucidum
Stratum Granulosum
Germinative Zone
(malpighian layer)
Stratum Spinosum
Stratum Germinativum
Epidermic Scales
Meissner Corpuscle
(touch)
Epidermis
(cuticle or scarf skin)
Capillaries
Papillary Layer of Dermis
Sebaceous (Oil) Duct
Sebaceous (Oil) Gland
Arrector Pili Muscle
Pacinian Corpuscle (touch)
Dermis, Corium or Cutis (true skin)
Reticular Fibers
Ruffian Receptor
(touch)
Sudoriferous (sweat duct)
Papilla of Hair
Nerve
Subcutaneous Tissue
Vein
Artery
Adipose (fatty tissue)

TABLE OF ELEMENTS

This table identifies the 103 known elements. Chemical combinations of these elements make up the many thousands of compounds found on Earth and in the universe.

Element	Symbol	Atomic No.	Atomic Wt.	Element	Symbol	Atomic No.	Atomic Wt.
Actinium	Ac	89	227	Mendelevium	Mv	101	256
Aluminum	Al	13	26.97	Mercury	Hg	80	200.61
Americium	Am	95	243	Molybdenum	Mo	42	96.0
Antimony	Sb	51	121.76	Neodymium	Nd	60	144.27
Argon	A	18	39.944	Neon	Ne	10	20.183
Arsenic	As	33	74.91	Neptunium	Np	93	237
Astatine	At	85	210	Nickel	Ni	28	58.69
Barium	Ba	56	137.36	Niobium	Nb	41	92.91
Berkelium	Bk	97	247	Nitrogen	N	7	14.008
Beryllium	Be	4	9.02	Nobelium	No	102	254
Bismuth	Bi	83	209	Osmium	Os	76	191.5
Boron	B	5	10.82	Oxygen	O	8	16.000
Bromine	Br	35	79.916	Palladium	Pd	46	106.7
Cadmium	Cd	48	112.41	Phosphorus	P	15	31.02
Cesium	Cs	55	132.91	Platinum	Pt	78	195.23
Calcium	Ca	20	40.08	Plutonium	Pu	94	242
Californium	Cf	98	249	Polonium	Po	84	210
Carbon	C	6	12.01	Potassium	K	19	39.096
Cerium	Ce	58	140.13	Praseodymium	Pr	59	140.92
Chlorine	Cl	17	35.457	Prometheum	Pm	61	146.0?
Chromium	Cr	24	52.01	Protactinium	Pa	91	231
Cobalt	Co	27	58.94	Radium	Ra	88	226.05
Copper	Cu	29	63.57	Radon	Rn	86	222
Curium	Cm	96	247	Rhenium	Re	75	186.31
Dysprosium	Dy	66	162.46	Rhodium	Rh	45	102.91
Einsteinium	E	99	254	Rubidium	Rb	37	85.48
Erbium	Er	68	167.64	Ruthenium	Ru	44	101.7
Europium	Eu	63	152.0	Samarium	Sm	62	150.43
Fluorine	F	9	19.000	Scandium	Sc	21	45.10
Fermium	Fm	100	253	Selenium	Se	34	78.96
Francium	Fr	87	223	Silicon	Si	14	28.06
Gadolinium	Gd	64	156.9	Silver	Ag	47	107.88
Gallium	Ga	31	69.72	Sodium	Na	11	22.997
Germanium	Ge	32	72.60	Strontium	Sr	38	87.63
Gold	Au	79	197.2	Sulfur	S	16	32.06
Hafnium	Hf	72	178.6	Tantalum	Ta	73	180.88
Helium	He	2	4.002	Technetium	Tc	43	97.8
Holmium	Ho	67	163.5	Tellurium	Te	52	127.61
Hydrogen	H	1	1.0078	Terbium	Tb	65	159.2
Indium	In	49	114.76	Thallium	Tl	81	204.39
Iodine	I	53	126.92	Thorium	Th	90	232.12
Iridium	Ir	77	193.1	Thulium	Tm	69	169.4
Iron	Fe	26	55.84	Tin	Sn	50	118.70
Krypton	Kr	36	83.7	Titanium	Ti	22	47.90
Lanthanum	La	57	138.92	Tungsten	W	74	184.0
Lawrencium	Lw	103	257	Uranium	U	92	238.07
Lead	Pb	82	207.21	Vanadium	V	23	50.95
Lithium	Li	3	6.940	Xenon	Xe	54	131.3
Lutetium	Lu	71	175.0	Ytterbium	Yb	70	173.04
Magnesium	Mg	12	24.32	Yttrium	Y	39	88.92
Manganese	Mn	25	54.93	Zinc	Zn	30	65.38
				Zirconium	Zr	40	91.22

THE pH SCALE

The symbol pH is used to express the hydrogen-ion concentration of a solution, which determines the relative degree of its acidity or alkalinity. The pH scale ranges from 0 to 14. A pH of 7 represents neutrality; numbers less than 7, down to 0, represent increasing acidity, and numbers greater than 7, up to 14, represent increasing alkalinity.

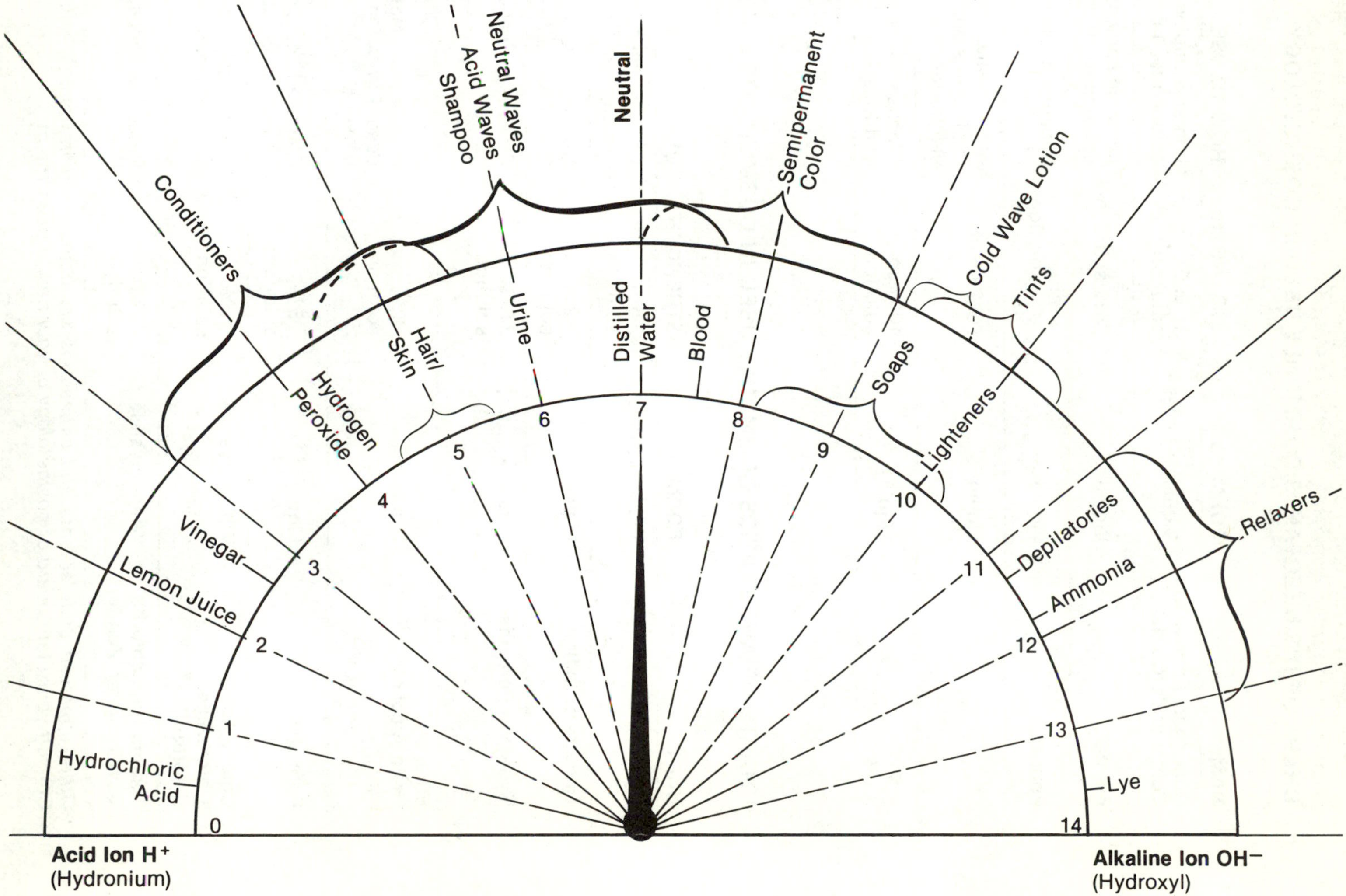

CHART OF DISINFECTANTS COMMONLY USED IN COSMETOLOGY

NAME	FORM	STRENGTH	HOW TO USE
Quaternary Ammonium Compounds (Quats)	Liquid or tablet	1:1000 solution	Immerse implements in solution for 1-5 minutes.
Formalin	Liquid	25% solution	Immerse implements in solution for 10 minutes.
Formalin	Liquid	10% solution	Immerse implements in solution for 20 minutes.
Ethyl or Grain Alcohol	Liquid	70% solution	Sanitize sharp cutting implements and electrodes.
Cresol (Lysol)	Liquid	10% soap solution	Cleanse floors, sinks, and toilets.

CHARTS OF ANTISEPTICS COMMONLY USED IN COSMETOLOGY

NAME	FORM	STRENGTH	USE
Boric Acid	White crystals	2-5% solution	Cleanse the eyes.
Tincture of Iodine	Liquid	2% solution	Cleanse cuts and wounds.
Hydrogen Peroxide	Liquid	3-5% solution	Cleanse skin and minor cuts.
Ethyl or Grain Alcohol	Liquid	60% solution	Cleanse hands, skin, and minute cuts. Not to be used if irritation is present.
Formalin	Liquid	5% solution	Cleanse hands, shampoo bowl, cabinet, etc.
Chloramine-T (Chlorazene; Chlorozol)	White crystals	½% solution	Cleanse skin and hands, and for general use.
Sodium Hypochlorite (Javelle water; Zonite)	White crystals	½% solution	Rinse the hands.

Other approved disinfectants and antiseptics are being used in schools and salons. Consult your state board of cosmetology or your health department.

WEIGHTS AND MEASURES WITH METRIC EQUIVALENTS

Approximate Metric Equivalents

1 decimeter	4 inches
1 liter	1.06 quarts liquid, 0.9 qt. dry
1 meter	1.1 yards
1 kilometer	⅝ of a mile
1 hektoliter	2⅝ bushels
1 hectare	2½ acres
1 kilogram	2⅕ pounds
1 stere, or cubic meter	¼ of a cord
1 metric ton	2,200 pounds

Linear Measure

1 centimeter	0.3937 inches
1 inch	2.54 centimeters
1 decimeter	3.937 in. . . . 0.328 foot
1 foot	3.048 decimeters
1 meter	39.37 inches . . . 1.0936 yds.
1 yard	0.9144 meter
1 dekameter	1.9884 rods
1 rod	0.5029 dekameter
1 kilometer	0.62137 mile
1 mile	1.6093 kilometers

Square Measure

1 square centimeter	0.1550 sq. inches
1 square inch	6.452 square centimeters
1 square decimeter	0.1076 square foot
1 square foot	9.2903 sq. dec.
1 square meter	1.196 sq. yds.
1 square yard	0.8361 square meter
1 acre	160 square rods
1 square rod	0.00625 acre
1 hectare	2.47 acres
1 acre	0.4047 hectare
1 square kilometer	0.386 sq. mile
1 square mile	2.59 sq. kilometers

Measure of Volume

1 cubic centimeter	0.061 cu. inch
1 cubic inch	16.39 cubic centimeters
1 cubic decimeter	0.0353 cubic foot
1 cubic foot	28.317 cubic decimeters
1 cubic yard	0.7646 cubic meter
1 stere	0.2759 cord
1 cord	3.624 steres
1 liter	0.908 qt. dry . . . 1.0567 qts. liq.
1 quart dry	1.101 liters
1 quart liquid	0.9463 liter
1 dekaliter	2.6417 gals. . . . 1.135 pecks
1 gallon	0.3785 dekaliter
1 peck	0.881 dekaliter
1 hektoliter	2.8375 bushels
1 bushel	0.3524 hektoliter

Weights

1 gram	0.03527 ounce
1 ounce	28.35 grams
1 kilogram	2.2046 pounds
1 pound	0.4536 kilogram
1 metric ton	0.98421 English ton
1 English ton	1.016 metric ton

METRIC CONVERSION FACTORS

Approximate Conversions to Metric Measures

Symbol	When You Know	Multiply by	To Find	Symbol
LENGTH (speed)				
in	inches	2.5	centimeters	cm
ft	feet	30	centimeters	cm
yd	yards	0.9	meters	m
mi	miles	1.6	kilometers	km
AREA				
in^2	square inches	6.5	square centimeters	cm^2
ft^2	square feet	0.09	square meters	m^2
yd^2	square yards	0.8	square meters	m^2
mi^2	square miles	2.6	square kilometers	km^2
a	acres	0.4	hectares	ha
MASS (weight)				
oz	ounces	28	grams	g
lb	pounds	0.45	kilograms	kg
	short tons (2000 lb)	0.9	tonnes	t
VOLUME				
tsp	teaspoon	5	milliliters	ml
tbsp	tablespoon	15	milliliters	ml
fl oz	fluid ounces	30	milliliters	ml
c	cups	0.24	liters	l
pt	pints	0.47	liters	l
qt	quarts	0.95	liters	l
gal	gallons	3.8	liters	l
ft^3	cubic feet	0.03	cubic meters	m^3
yd^3	cubic yards	0.76	cubic meters	m^3
TEMPERATURE (exact)				
^0F	Fahrenheit temperature	5/9 after subtracting 32)	Celsius temperature	^0C

EVERYDAY METRIC-AID

The following conversions have been made strictly in accordance with conversion tables and information supplied by the U.S. Department of Commerce.

Spoonfuls

¼ tsp.	1.25 milliliters
½ tsp.	2.5 milliliters
¾ tsp.	3.75 milliliters
1 tsp.	5 milliliters
¼ tbls.	3.75 milliliters
½ tbls.	7.5 milliliters
¾ tbls.	11.25 milliliters
1 tbls.	15 milliliters

Fluid Ounces

¼ oz.	7.5 milliliters
½ oz.	15 milliliters
¾ oz.	22.5 milliliters
1 oz.	30 milliliters

Cups

¼ cup	59 milliliters
⅓ cup	78 milliliters
½ cup	118 milliliters
⅔ cup	157 milliliters
¾ cup	177 milliliters
1 cup	236 milliliters

Pints-Quarts-Gallons

½ pint	236 milliliters
1 pint	473 milliliters
1 quart	946.3 milliliters
1 gallon	3785 milliliters

Aditional Information About Teaspoon and Tablespoon Measurements

60 drops = 1 teaspoon (5 ml)*
3 teaspoons = 1 tablespoon (15 ml)
2 tablespoons = 1 fluid ounce (30 ml)
8 fluid ounces = 1 cup = 16 tablespoons (0.24 l)*
2 cups = 1 pint = 16 fluid ounces (0.47 l)
2 pints = 1 quart = 32 fluid ounces (0.95 l)

1/8 cup = 2 tablespoons = 1 fluid ounce
= 6 teaspoons (30 ml)
1/4 cup = 4 tablespoons = 2 fluid ounces (30 ml)
3/8 cup = 6 tablespoons = 3 fluid ounces (90 ml)
1/2 cup = 8 tablespoons = 4 fluid ounces (120 ml)
3/5 cup = 10 tablespoons = 5 fluid ounces (150 ml)
3/4 cup = 12 tablespoons = 6 fluid ounces (180 ml)
7/8 cup = 14 tablespoons = 7 fluid ounces (210 ml)
1 cup = 16 tablespoons = 8 fluid ounces (0.24 l)

*l = liters; ml = milliliters

Weight in Ounces

¼ oz.	7.1 grams
½ oz.	14.17 grams
¾ oz.	21.27 grams
1 oz.	28.35 grams

Pounds

¼ lb.	.113 kilograms
½ lb.	.227 kilograms
¾ lb.	.340 kilograms
1 lb.	.454 kilograms
2.205 lbs.	1 kilogram

Length

1 inch	2.544 centimeters
1 foot	30.48 centimeters
1 yard	91.44 centimeters
100 ft.	30.48 meters
1 mile	1.609 kilometers
50 mph	80.45 kilometers/hr.

Temperature

32° F.	0° Celsius
68° F.	20° Celsius
212° F.	100° Celsius

Square Measure

1 sq. in.	6.452 sq. cm.
1 sq. ft.	929 sq. cm.
1 sq. yd.	.8361 sq. meters
1 acre	4047 sq. meters

Volume

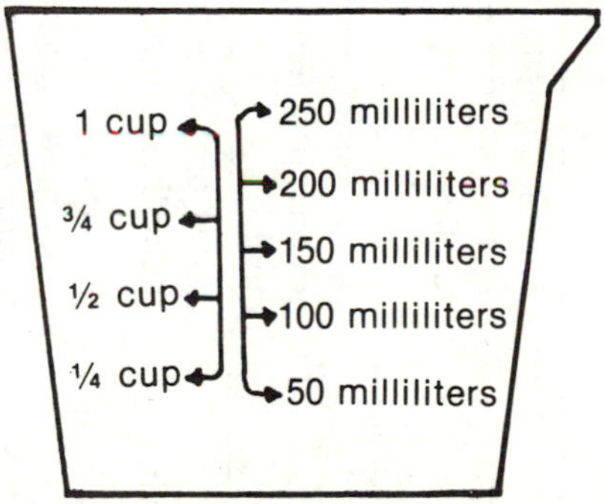

VITAMIN AND MINERAL INFORMATION CHART*

Vitamin; RDA*	Best Sources	Functions	Deficiency Symptoms
A Carotene 5,000 IU	Liver, eggs, yellow & green fruits & vegetables, milk & dairy products, fish liver oil	Growth & repair of body tissues, bone & tooth formation, visual purple formation (necessary for night vision)	Night blindness, dry scaly skin, loss of smell & appetite, susceptibility to infection, frequent fatigue, tooth decay
B1 Thiamin 1.0-1.4 mg	Wheat germ, yeast, liver, whole grains, nuts, fish, poultry, beans, meat	Necessary for metabolism, appetite maintenance, nerve function, growth & muscle tone	Heart irregularity, nerve disorders, fatigue, loss of appetite, forgetfulness
B2 Riboflavin 1.6 mg	Whole grains, green leafy vegetables, organ meats	Necessary for metabolism, cell respiration, formation of antibodies & red blood cells	Eye problems, cracks in corners of mouth, digestive disturbances
B6 Pyridoxine 1.5-1.8 mg	Leafy green vegetables, yeast, organ meats, bananas, whole grains	Necessary for metabolism, formation of antibodies, sodium/potassium balance	Nervousness, dermatitis, blood disorders, muscular weakness, insulin sensitivity, skin cracks, anemia
B12 Cobalamin 3 mcg	Organ meats, eggs, milk, fish, cheese	Necessary for metabolism, maintains healthy nervous system, blood cell formation	Pernicious anemia, nervousness, neuritis, fatigue
Biotin 150-300 mcg	Yeast, organ meats, legumes, eggs, grains	Metabolism, formation of fatty acids	Dry, grayish skin, depression, muscle pain, fatigue, poor appetite
Choline (No RDA)	Organ meats, lecithin, soybeans, fish, wheat germ, egg yolk	Nerve transmission, metabolism, regulates liver & gall bladder	High blood pressure, bleeding, stomach ulcers, liver & kidney problems
Folic Acid Folacin 400 mcg	Green leafy vegetables, organ meats, yeast, milk products	Red blood cell formation, metabolism, growth & cell division	Anemia, gastrointestinal troubles, poor growth
Inositol (No RDA)	Whole grains, citrus fruits, yeast, molasses, milk	Vital for hair growth, metabolism, lecithin formation	High cholesterol, hair loss, skin problems, constipation, eye abnormalities
Niacin 13-18 mg.	Yeast, meat, poultry, fish, milk products, peanuts	Metabolism, health of skin, tongue and digestive system, blood circulation	General fatigue, indigestion, irritability, loss of appetite, skin disorders

*RDA = recommended dietary allowances; IU = international unit; mg = milligram; mcg = microgram.

Vitamin; RDA*	Best Sources	Functions	Deficiency Symptoms
PABA (No RDA)	Liver, yeast, wheat germ, molasses	Metabolism, red blood cell formation, healthy intestines, hair coloring, sunscreen	Digestive disorders, fatigue, depression, nervousness, irritability, constipation
Pangamic Acid B15 (No RDA)	Yeast, brown rice, whole grains, pumpkin and sesame seeds	Metabolism, stimulates nerve and glandular systems, cell respiration	Heart disease, glandular and nervous disorders, impaired circulation
Pantothenic Acid 5-10 mg	Organ meats, yeast, egg yolks, whole grain cereals, legumes	Converts nutrients into energy, formation of some fats, vitamin utilization	Vomiting, stomach stress, restlessness, infections, muscle cramps
C Ascorbic Acid 45 mg	Citrus fruits, vegetables, tomatoes, potatoes	Helps to heal wounds, collagen maintenance, resistance to infection	Bleeding gums, slow healing of wounds, bruising, aching joints, nosebleeds, poor digestion
D 400 U	Fish-liver oils, egg yolks, organ meats, fish, fortified milk	Calcium and phosphorus metabolism (bone formation), heart action, nervous system maintenance	Rickets, poor bone growth, nervous system irritability
E 12-15 IU	Vegetable oils, green vegetables, wheat germ, organ meats, eggs	Protects red blood cells, inhibits coagulation of blood, cellular respiration	Muscular wasting, abnormal fat deposits in muscles, gastrointestinal disease, heart disease, impotency
F (No RDA)	Vegetable oils, wheat germ, seeds	Respiration of body organs, resilience and lubrication of cells, blood coagulation, glandular activity	Brittle nails and hair, dandruff, diarrhea, varicose veins, underweight, gallstones, acne
K No RDA	Green leafy vegetables, milk, kelp, safflower oil	Important in formation of blood clotting agents	Tendency to hemorrhage
P Bioflavonoids No RDA	Fruits	Strengthens capillaries, keeps connective tissue cells healthy, helps body utilize vitamin C	Similar to those of vitamin C, easy bruising and bleeding
Calcium 800-1.400 mg	Milk and milk products, bone meal	Strong bones, teeth, muscle tissue, regulates heart beat, muscle action and nerve function, blood clotting	Soft brittle bones, back and leg pains, heart palpitations, tetany

*RDA = recommended dietary allowances; IU = international unit; mg = milligram; mcg = microgram.

Continued on page 292

VITAMIN AND MINERAL INFORMATION CHART* *Continued from page 291*

Vitamin; RDA*	Best Sources	Functions	Deficiency Symptoms
Chromium No RDA	Corn oil, yeast, clams, whole grain cereals	Glucose metabolism (energy), increases effectiveness of insulin	Atherosclerosis, glucose intolerance in diabetics
Copper 2 mg	Seafood, whole grains, leafy green vegetables, liver, almonds	Formation of red blood cells, bone growth and health, works with vitamin C to form elastin	General weakness, impaired respiration, skin sores
Iodine	Seafood, iodized salt	Component of hormone thyroxine which controls metabolism	Goiter, dry skin and hair, nervousness, obesity
Iron 10-18 mg	Meats and organ meats, fish, leafy green vegetables	Hemoglobin formation, improves blood quality, increases resistance to stress and disease	Anemia (pale skin, fatigue) constipation, breathing difficulties
Magnesium 300-350 mg	Nuts, green vegetables, whole grains	Acid/alkaline balance, metabolism	Nervousness, tremors, easily aroused anger, disorientation, blood clots
Manganese No RDA	Green vegetables, egg yolks, legumes, whole grains	Enzyme activation, carbohydrate and fat production, sex hormone production, skeletal development	Dizziness, poor muscle coordination
Phosphorus 800 mg	Fish, meat, poultry, eggs, grains	Bone development, important in protein, fat and carbohydrate utilization	Poor bones and teeth, arthritis, rickets, appetite loss, irregular breathing
Potassium No RDA	Vegetables, grains, fruits, legumes	Fluid balance, controls activity of heart muscle, nervous system, kidneys	Poor reflexes, irregular heartbeat, dry skin, general weakness
Sodium No RDA	Table salt, seafood, meat, poultry	Regulates body fluid and acid base balance, maintains nervous, muscular, blood and lymph systems	Muscle weakness and shrinkage, nausea
Sulphur No RDA	Fish, eggs, nuts, cabbage, meat	Necessary for collagen formation, formation of body tissues	None known
Zinc 15 mg	Yeast, whole grains, wheat bran	Involved in digestion and metabolism, important in development of reproductive system, aids in healing	Retarded growth, prolonged wound healing, delayed sexual maturity